Review Manual *for*
Neurology in Clinical Practice
Third Edition

Review Manual *for* Neurology in Clinical Practice Third Edition

Karl E. Misulis, M.D., Ph.D.
Clinical Professor of Neurology, Vanderbilt University School of Medicine, Nashville, Tennessee; Neurologist, Semmes-Murphey Neurologic and Spine Institute, Jackson, Tennessee

Edited by
Walter G. Bradley, D.M., F.R.C.P.
Professor and Chairman, Department of Neurology, University of Miami School of Medicine; Chief, Neurology Service, University of Miami–Jackson Memorial Medical Center

Robert B. Daroff, M.D.
Chief of Staff and Senior Vice President for Academic Affairs, University Hospitals of Cleveland; Professor of Neurology and Associate Dean, Case Western Reserve University School of Medicine, Cleveland

Gerald M. Fenichel, M.D.
Professor of Neurology and Pediatrics, and Chairman, Department of Neurology, Vanderbilt University School of Medicine, Nashville, Tennessee; Neurologist-in-Chief, Vanderbilt University Hospital and Vanderbilt Children's Hospital, Nashville

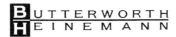

Boston   Oxford   Auckland   Johannesburg   Melbourne   New Delhi

Copyright © 2000 by Butterworth–Heinemann

 A member of the Reed Elsevier group

All rights reserved.

No part of this publication may be reproduced, stored in a retrieval system, or transmitted in any form or by any means, electronic, mechanical, photocopying, recording, or otherwise, without the prior written permission of the publisher.

Every effort has been made to ensure that the drug dosage schedules within this text are accurate and conform to standards accepted at time of publication. However, as treatment recommendations vary in the light of continuing research and clinical experience, the reader is advised to verify drug dosage schedules herein with information found on product information sheets. This is especially true in cases of new or infrequently used drugs.

 Recognizing the importance of preserving what has been written, Butterworth–Heinemann prints its books on acid-free paper whenever possible.

 Butterworth–Heinemann supports the efforts of American Forests and the Global ReLeaf program in its campaign for the betterment of trees, forests, and our environment.

Library of Congress Cataloging-in-Publication Data

Misulis, Karl E.
 Review manual for neurology in clinical practice third edition / Karl E. Misulis; edited
 by Walter G. Bradley, Robert B. Daroff, Gerald M. Fenichel.
  p. ; cm.
 Companion v. to: Neurology in clinical practice. 3rd ed. c2000.
 Includes index.
 ISBN 0-7506-7192-0 (alk. paper)
  1. Neurology—Examinations, questions, etc. 2. Nervous
 system—Diseases—Examinations, questions, etc. I. Bradley, W. G. (Walter George)
 II. Daroff, Robert B. III. Fenichel, Gerald M. IV. Neurology in clinical practice. V. Title.
  [DNLM: 1. Nervous System Diseases—Examination Questions. 2. Diagnostic
 Techniques, Neurological—Examination Questions. WL 18.2 M678r 2000]
 RC346. N4535 2000 Suppl.
 616.8'0076—dc21
                                                                    00-035808

British Library Cataloguing-in-Publication Data
A catalogue record for this book is available from the British Library.

The publisher offers special discounts on bulk orders of this book.
For information, please contact:
Manager of Special Sales
Butterworth–Heinemann
225 Wildwood Avenue
Woburn, MA 01801-2041
Tel: 781-904-2500
Fax: 781-904-2620

For information on all Butterworth–Heinemann publications available, contact our World Wide Web home page at: http://www.bh.com

10 9 8 7 6 5 4 3 2 1

Printed in the United States of America

Contents

Preface ix

Part I. Approach to Common Neurological Problems

1. Diagnosis of Neurological Disease 1
2. Episodic Impairment of Consciousness 3
3. Falls and Drop Attacks 7
4. Delirium 9
5. Clinical Approach to Stupor and Coma 11
6. Excessive Daytime Somnolence 13
7. Approaches to Intellectual and Memory Impairments 15
8. Developmental Delay and Regression in Infants 17
9. Behavior and Personality Disturbances 19
10. Depression and Psychosis in Neurological Practice 21
11. Cognitive-Motor Disorders, Apraxias, and Agnosias
    A. Cognitive-Motor Disorders and Apraxias 23
    B. Agnosias 25
12. Language Disorders
    A. Aphasia 27
    B. Developmental Speech and Language Disorders 29
13. Difficulties with Speech and Swallowing 31
14. Vision Loss 33
15. Abnormalties of the Optic Nerve and Retina 35
16. Eye Movement Disorders: Diplopia, Nystagmus, and Other Ocular Oscillations 37
17. Pupillary and Eyelid Abnormalities 41
18. Dizziness and Vertigo 43
19. Hearing Loss and Tinnitus without Dizziness and Vertigo 45
20. Disturbances of Taste and Smell 47
21. Disturbances of Lower Cranial Nerves 49
22. Cranial and Facial Pain 51
23. Brainstem Syndromes 53

24. Ataxic Disorders 57
25. Movement Disorders: Symptoms 59
26. Walking Disorders 61
27. Hemiplegia and Monoplegia 63
28. Paraplegia and Spinal Cord Syndromes 65
29. Proximal, Distal, and Generalized Weakness 67
30. Muscle Pain and Cramps 71
31. The Floppy Infant 73
32. Sensory Abnormalities of the Limbs, Trunk, and Face 75
33. Neurological Causes of Bladder, Bowel, and Sexual Dysfunction 77
34. Arm and Neck Pain 79
35. Low Back and Lower Limb Pain 81

Part II. Neurological Investigations and Related Clinical Neurosciences

36. Laboratory Investigations in Diagnosis and Management of Neurological Disease 83
37. Clinical Neurophysiology
    A. Electroencephalography and Evoked Potentials 85
    B. Electrodiagnosis of Neuromuscular Disorders 89
38. Neuroimaging
    A. Structural Neuroimaging 93
    B. Computed Tomographic and Magnetic Resonance Vascular Imaging 97
    C. Radiological Angiography 99
    D. Ultrasound Imaging of the Cerebral Vasculature 101
    E. Functional Neuroimaging 103
39. Neuropsychology 105
40. Neuro-Ophthalmology: Ocular Motor System 107
41. Neuro-Ophthalmology: Afferent Visual System 109
42. Neuro-Otology 111
43. Neurourology 113
44. Neuroepidemiology 115
45. Clinical Neurogenetics 119
46. Neuroimmunology 121
47. Neurovirology 125
48. Neuroendocrinology 127
49. Management of Neurological Disease 129
50. Principles of Neuropharmacology and Therapeutics 131
51. Principles of Pain Management 135
52. Principles of Neurointensive Care 137
53. Principles of Neurosurgery 139
54. Principles of Neurological Rehabilitation 143

Part III. Neurological Diseases

55. Neurological Complications of Systemic Disease
    A. In Adults   147
    B. In Children   151
56. Trauma of the Nervous System
    A. Basic Neuroscience of Neurotrauma   153
    B. Craniocerebral Trauma   155
    C. Spinal Cord Trauma   159
    D. Peripheral Nerve Trauma   161
57. Vascular Diseases of the Nervous System
    A. Ischemic Cerebrovascular Disease   163
    B. Intracerebral Hemorrhage   171
    C. Intracranial Aneurysms and Subarachnoid Hemorrhage   175
    D. Arteriovenous Malformations   179
    E. Stroke in Childhood   181
    F. Spinal Cord Vascular Disease   183
    G. Central Nervous System Vasculitis   185
58. Primary and Secondary Tumors of the Central Nervous System   187
    A. Pathology of Nervous System Tumors   189
    B. Molecular Biology of Nervous System Tumors   193
    C. Clinical Presentation and Therapy of Nervous System Tumors   195
    D. Clinical Presentation and Therapy for Spinal Tumors   199
    E. Clinical Presentation and Therapy of Peripheral Nerve Tumors   201
    F. Paraneoplastic Syndromes   203
    G. Quality of Life and Late Effects of Treatment   205
59. Infections of the Nervous System
    A. Bacterial Infections   207
    B. Viral Infections   215
    C. Fungal Infections   219
    D. Parasitic Infections   221
    E. Neurological Manifestations of Human Immunodeficiency Virus Infection   225
    F. Transmissible Spongiform Encephalopathies   229
60. Multiple Sclerosis and Other Inflammatory Demyelinating Disorders of the Central Nervous System   231
61. Anoxic and Ischemic Encephalopathies   235
62. Toxic and Metabolic Encephalopathies   239
63. Deficiency Diseases of the Nervous System   241
64. Effects of Toxins and Physical Agents on the Nervous System
    A. Effects of Occupational Toxins on the Nervous System   243
    B. Effects of Drug Abuse on the Nervous System   245
    C. Neurotoxins of Animals and Plants   247

      D. Marine Toxins 249

      E. Effect of Physical Agents on the Nervous System 251

65. Brain Edema and Disorders of Cerebrospinal Fluid Circulation 253
66. Developmental Disorders of the Nervous System 255
67. Developmental Disabilities 257
68. Inborn Errors of Metabolism of the Nervous System 259
69. Neurocutaneous Syndromes 265
70. The Dementias 267

    A. Primary Degenerative Dementia 269

    B. Dementia as Part of Other Degenerative Diseases 273

    C. Vascular Dementia 275

    D. Progressive Focal Cortical Syndromes 279

    E. Other Causes of Dementias 281

71. The Epilepsies 285
72. Sleep Disorders 293
73. Headache and Other Craniofacial Pain 297
74. Cranial Neuropathies 305
75. Movement Disorders 307
76. Cerebellar and Spinocerebellar Disorders 311
77. Disorders of Bones, Joints, Ligaments, and Meninges 313
78. Disorders of Upper and Lower Motor Neurons 317
79. Disorders of Nerve Roots and Plexuses 321
80. Disorders of Peripheral Nerves 325
81. Disorders of the Autonomic Nervous System 333
82. Disorders of Neuromuscular Transmission 335
83. Disorders of Skeletal Muscle 339
84. Neurological Problems of the Newborn 345
85. Neurological Problems of Pregnancy 349
86. Geriatric Neurology 351

Preface

Neurology in Clinical Practice has become a standard text for students and practitioners of neurology. Now, the third edition is even more up to date and complete, with new and completely rewritten chapters. This *Review Manual* is meant to be a companion to the master text. The guide can be used with reference to the text when needed or used for review after reading all or portions of the text.

The questions are organized by chapter and follow standard examination format. A brief explanation of the answer and page reference is given for each question.

I would like express my thanks to all of the authors of the individual chapters, to the editors of *Neurology in Clinical Practice*, and to the production and editorial staff of Butterworth–Heinemann for their fantastic work.

Karl E. Misulis

Review Manual *for*
Neurology in Clinical Practice
Third Edition

Chapter 1: Diagnosis of Neurological Disease

Question 1-1:
Which of the following can be initial manifestations of sarcoidosis?

A. Bell's palsy
B. Diabetes insipidis
C. Ophthalmoplegia
D. Peripheral neuropathy
E. Any of the above

Question 1-2:
Occam's razor presumes that a single explanation for a constellation of findings is more likely than multiple explanations. Which neurologic phenomenon appears to contradict this principle?

A. Multiple sclerosis
B. Sarcoidosis
C. Vasculitis
D. Small-cell lung cancer
E. All of the above

Question 1-3:
Which is the least important aspect of the screening neurologic examination?

A. Visual fields
B. Tendon reflexes
C. Olfaction
D. Muscle strength
E. Sensation to pin prick

Question 1-4:
Which of the following features can differentiate hard signs and soft signs?

A. Hard signs are subjective whereas soft signs are objective.
B. Hard signs include sensory testing; soft signs include reflexes.
C. Hard signs are clearly pathologic whereas soft signs may be within the normal variability of response.
D. Diagnosis depends on hard signs, whereas soft signs are of little to no diagnostic value.

Patient is a child with weakness progressive over months. EMG shows features of denervation.

Question 1-8:
Patient complains of diplopia and has ptosis.

Question 1-9:
Patient has a rash on the extensor surface of the fingers, elbows, and eyelids.

Answer 1-1: E.
Any of the above. All of the neurologic conditions described can be the presenting complaints of sarcoidosis. Of interest is that sarcoidosis is not the most common cause of any of these, but should be considered when more than one is present or when there are systemic features to suggest sarcoidosis, e.g., pulmonary lesions. Sarcoidosis is one of a few conditions that can affect the CNS or PNS focally or diffusely. (p5)

Answer 1-2: E.
Occam's razor as applied in neurology means that clinical findings should be attributed to one disease and one lesion, if possible. Therefore, a condition that cannot be explained by a single lesion appears to contradict Occam's razor. However, since many neurologic conditions can produce multifocal lesions, in the second sense, the theorem applies; a single condition produces multifocal lesions. Therefore, all of the entities listed could be thought of as exceptions to Occam's razor, when in reality the only answer that would be an actual exception would be the independent development of two unrelated lesions. For example, small-cell lung cancer has a tendency to produce multiple brain metastases, neoplastic meningitis, and neurologic paraneoplastic syndromes, all of which can be difficult to ascribe to a single lesion. (p7)

Answer 1-3: C.
Olfaction is rarely tested for during the screening neurologic examination, because most common neurologic conditions do not alter this cranial nerve function and there are non-neurologic causes of deficit. Also, most patients with absent or defective olfaction have the defect on the basis of nasal disease rather than an olfactory groove meningioma or other lesion in this location. Olfaction should be tested as part of the comprehensive neurologic examination and especially when examining patients with dementia associated with affective disturbance and patients who have had recent head injury. In reality, almost all of these patients will have brain CT or MRI, so the diagnostic utility of this examination finding is limited. The other listed examination components are integral to the screening examination. (p6)

Answer 1-4: C.
Objective and subjective distinction is important, and in general objective findings tend to be hard signs, but the classifications are not equivalent. (p6)

Answer 1-5: F.
ALS is associated with degeneration of upper lower motoneurons and lower motoneurons. (p6-7)

Answer 1-6: C.
Lambert-Eaton myasthenic syndrome is often a paraneoplastic syndrome associated with small-cell lung cancer. Patients present with weakness, often with a dry mouth. There are no sensory findings. (p5)

Answer 1-7: G.
Spinal muscular atrophy produces progressive weakness without sensory loss or corticospinal tract signs. SMA is the only one of the diseases that typically occurs in childhood. Myasthenia gravis and polymyositis can also occur in childhood, although these conditions should not show prominent neuropathic features on EMG. (p7)

Answer 1-8: A.
Myasthenia gravis is the only one of the listed conditions which typically produces diplopia. Guillain-Barré syndrome can produce ocular motor involvement, but this usually occurs with severe weakness and is unlikely to be a presenting complaint. (p7)

Answer 1-9: H.
Inflammatory myopathy may occur in association with other connective tissue disease or cancer. Dermatomyositis is characterized by inflammatory myopathy associated with the rash as described. The appearance is typical, such that the rash plus the proximal muscle weakness can often make the presumptive diagnosis prior to laboratory studies. (p7)

Chapter 2: Episodic Impairment of Consciousness

Question 2-1:
A 23-year-old female presents with recurrent blackouts. Which of the following features would be least indicative of seizure as a specific diagnosis?

A. Post-ictal confusion
B. Urinary incontinence
C. Post-ictal headache
D. Clonic activity
E. Focal neurologic signs

Question 2-2:
Which is the most common congenital cardiac malformation that causes loss of consciousness in children?

A. Mitral valve prolapse
B. Tetralogy of Fallot
C. Atrial-septal defect
D. Ventricular-septal defect

Question 2-3:
Absence and complex partial seizures can look similar. Differentiating features which support the diagnosis of absence seizures rather than complex partial seizures include all of the following except?

A. Duration of a few seconds
B. Generalized spike and wave complexes
C. Post-ictal confusion
D. Onset in youth
E. Simple automatisms

Question 2-4:
Which of the following arrhythmias causes syncope?

A. SA block
B. AV block
C. Paroxysmal supraventricular tachycardia
D. Paroxysmal ventricular tachycardia
E. All of the above

Question 2-5:
Which of the following statements regarding cardiac syncope is true?

A. Mitral valve prolapse is a common cause of syncope.
B. Carotid sinus massage is used to terminate supraventricular tachyarrhythmias.
C. Exercise is a common precipitant of tachyarrhythmias.
D. Syncope from Long-QT syndrome is most prominent in the middle-aged patients.
E. All are true.

Question 2-6:
Vertebrobasilar insufficiency causes syncope typically with other signs of brainstem dysfunction. Among causes of vertebrobasilar ischemia is which of the following?

A. Subclavian steal syndrome
B. Cervical spine disease
C. Takayasu's disease
D. All of the above

Answer 2-1: D.
All of the listed features can be seen in patients with seizures, however, clonic activity is the least specific for seizures. Any cause of anoxia can result in clonic activity, especially when prolonged. The other features are strongly supportive of the diagnosis of seizures. Prolonged anoxia from any cause can result in delayed recovery of cognitive function, although most causes of recurrent cardiac syncope do not cause sustained cerebral anoxia. Headache is commonly associated with seizures, although basilar migraine is also associated with headache. (p10)

Answer 2-2: B.
Tetralogy of Fallot is the most common congenital malformation implicated in syncope. The mechanism is right-to-left shunt producing hypoxia. Other congenital defects producing cyanosis can cause syncope, also. Mitral valve prolapse is over-rated as a cause for syncope. As a group, congenital defects are rare as causes of syncope in adolescents and adults. Diagnosis of congenital defects is supported by echocardiography. (p12)

Answer 2-3: C.
Post-ictal confusion is not expected in absence seizures whereas it is common with complex partial seizures. After an absence seizure, the patient often resumes the previous activity, starting from where they had just left off. In contrast, with complex partial seizures, the patient is often briefly confused, and has lost track of the task performed prior to the seizure. (p16)

Answer 2-4: E.
These are the four most common cardiac arrhythmias that can cause syncope. Not all patients are aware of cardiac irregularity. Cardiac syncope is suggested by acute onset, short duration, and absence of post-ictal confusion unless the duration of anoxia is prolonged. (p11)

Answer 2-5: C.
Exercise commonly precipitates supraventricular tachycardia. This is a helpful differentiating feature, since most neurologic causes of syncope are not precipitated by exercise. MVP is common, and fainting spells are frequently attributed to this condition, but this is over-diagnosed. Occasional patients with MVP will have ventricular arrhythmias. Carotid sinus massage is not recommended for SVT because of the possibility of cerebral embolism from dislodging atheroma. Long-QT syndrome can occur in older patients but is most common in children, in the first decade. (p11-12)

Answer 2-6: D.
These are all causes of vertebrobasilar ischemia. Subclavian steal can cause dizziness and occasionally syncope and classically is precipitated by ipsilateral arm exercise, although this is by no means a universal clinical finding. Cervical spine disease can produce compression of the vertebral arteries, which may be induced by neck movement, especially with extremes of rotation and flexion/extension. Takayasu's disease is one type of arteritis which can cause basilar ischemia. (p13)

Questions 2-7 through 2-10:
Following are a list of possible diagnoses for patients with syncope. Each question gives some additional clinical information. For each of the questions, select the most likely diagnosis on the basis of the additional information.

A. Micturition syncope
B. Tussive syncope
C. Vasovagal syncope
D. Hyperventilation-induced syncope
E. Paroxysmal SVT

Question 2-7:
A 54-year-old man with COPD has episodes of syncope precipitated by coughing fits.

Question 2-8:
A 23-year-old woman has episodes of syncope preceded by dizziness and dyspnea.

Question 2-9:
A 80-year-old man has several episodes of syncope when he gets up at night and uses the bathroom.

Question 2-10:
A 36-year-old man has episodes of unconsciousness precipitated by exercise.

Question 2-11:
Which of the following statements are true regarding complex partial seizures?

1. Interictal EEG shows focal discharges in most patients with complex partial seizures.
2. Prolactin level is not elevated in patients with complex partial seizures.
3. Complex partial seizures generally have a shorter duration than absence seizures.
4. There is usually an episode of post-ictal confusion following complex partial seizures.

Select: A = 1, 2, 3. B = 1, 3. C = 2, 4. D = 4 only. E = All

Question 2-12:
Pseudoseizures can be difficult to differentiate from epileptic seizures. Which of the following are supportive of the diagnosis of pseudoseizures?

1. Occurrence always while awake
2. Normal prolactin level after a clinical generalized tonic-clonic seizure
3. EEG during a seizure shows muscle activity but no electrocerebral discharge
4. Focal findings after a seizure which are not detected prior to the seizure

Select: A = 1, 2, 3. B = 1, 3. C = 2, 4. D = 4 only. E = All

Question 2-13:
Positional syncope could suggest which of the following?

1. Colloid cyst of the third ventricle
2. Cervical syrinx
3. Aqueductal stenosis
4. Atrial myxoma

Select: A = 1, 2, 3. B = 1, 3. C = 2, 4. D = 4 only. E = All

Answer 2-7: B.
Patients with tussive syncope often offer the history of presyncopal sensation and syncope in association with coughing. Sustained coughing fits are most common precipitants, but single coughs may precipitate syncope in susceptible individuals. Decreased cerebral perfusion is due to decreased venous return to the heart because of increased intrathoracic pressure during the coughing episode. (p14)

Answer 2-8: D.
Hyperventilation-induced syncope can be difficult to diagnose. Patients often do not offer the history of hyperventilation. Indirect hints to the diagnosis from reports of dyspnea or description by an observer are often key. (p14)

Answer 2-9: A.
Micturition syncope often presents with nocturnal syncope, which may even result in head injury. (p14)

Answer 2-10: E.
Paroxysmal SVT is associated with abrupt syncope that can be triggered by exercise. This clinical feature is unusual in most other causes of syncope. (p12)

Answer 2-11: D.
EEG is most sensitive for diagnosis of absence seizures, in which a 3-per-second spike-wave pattern is seen. The interictal EEG is almost always abnormal, especially with hyperventilation. In contrast, many patients with complex partial seizures have normal interictal EEGs. Prolactin level is most likely to be increased in patients with tonic-clonic seizures but is also increased in many patients with complex partial seizures. The increase in prolactin level is relative; a baseline level should be available for comparison. Absence seizures have a shorter duration than complex partial seizures, less than one minute in comparison to 1-3 minutes. Post-ictal confusion is common after complex partial seizures. (p16)

Answer 2-12: A.
Patients with epileptic seizures may have focal findings after an event that are not present between events. This may be because of depression of neuronal function in the focus of the seizure. Occurrence always while awake suggests pseudoseizures, since most seizure types are activated during sleep. Normal EEG patterns during a clinical seizure almost always indicate a pseudoseizure, although there are rare patients with partial seizures, who have a focus in the inferior frontal or medial temporal regions, that is not detected with scalp EEG electrodes. Fortunately, most pseudoseizures have a generalized tonic-clonic character, and the EEG is a good indicator. (p17)

Answer 2-13: E.
All can cause syncope, which is triggered by change in head and/or body position. Colloid cyst of the third ventricle and aqueductal stenosis are classic examples of causes of positional syncope, but cervical syrinx can do this as well, especially in children. (p18)

Chapter 3: Falls and Drop Attacks

Questions 3-1 through 3-4:
A 70-year-old right-handed man with stroke resulting in left hemiparesis has two episodes of falls which have incomplete history, and neither of which were observed by health-care workers. The list below includes possible reasons for the fall.

A. Recurrent TIA
B. Another CVA
C. Seizure secondary to the first CVA
D. Simple fall associated with poor coordination
E. Cardiac arrhythmia with decreased cerebral perfusion

The following additional pieces of clinical information would suggest which of the above diagnoses for the patient's falls?

Question 3-1:
Prolonged period of somnolence and confusion following the fall.

Question 3-2:
Presyncopal sensation and diaphoresis preceding the fall, with no sequelae.

Question 3-3:
Patient is noted to have a transient worsening of his left hemiparesis after one of the falls and to be unable to speak after another of the falls.

Question 3-4:
Patient falls twice at night on the way to the bathroom. There is no neurologic change, and the patient is able to walk when assisted to his feet.

Answer 3-1: C.
Seizure is the most likely if the patient has prolonged somnolence and confusion. While tonic-clonic activity is most suggestive of seizures, not all have motor activity. Also, the motor activity may not always be observed. (p20)

Answer 3-2: E.
Cardiac arrhythmia is most likely to produce presyncopal sensations. The diaphoresis also suggests a hyperadrenergic state which is most likely with cardiac causes and systemic hypotension. The lack of sequelae after the fall would argue against TIA or recurrent CVA. (p20)

Answer 3-3: A.
TIA is most likely to produce fall in association with new neurologic deficits. Seizures can also produce focal deficits, but some clonic activity would usually be expected. Also, after a seizure, there would usually be somnolence in addition to any focal deficit. (p20)

Answer 3-4: D.
A simple fall is most likely to occur at night. The most common scenario is an elderly patient on their way to the bathroom at night. The presence of a neurologic deficit from the stroke will make the fall even more likely. This is the situation during which patients are most likely to develop hip fractures. (p22)

Chapter 4: Delirium

Question 4-1:
Important risk factors for the development of delirium in elderly hospitalized patients include which of the following?

1. Age
2. Visual loss
3. Pre-morbid dementia
4. Dehydration

Select: A = 1, 2, 3. B = 1, 3. C = 2, 4. D = 4 only. E = All

Question 4-2:
Many prescription and over-the-counter medications have anticholinergic side effects. These can produce problems in elderly patients, especially when used in combination. Signs of anticholinergic excess include all of the following except?

A. Hypothermia
B. Dry mouth
C. Confusion
D. Flushing
E. Mydriasis

Question 4-3:
Which of the following statements regarding perioperative confusion are true?

1. Delirium develops in 30-40% of patients after CABG.
2. Delirium develops in 18% of patients after orthopedic surgery.
3. Delirium develops in about 7% of patients after cataract extraction.
4. Development of delirium depends on the route of administration of anesthetic.

Select: A = 1, 2, 3. B = 1, 3. C = 2, 4. D = 4 only. E = All

Questions 4-4 through 4-6:
A patient is admitted to the hospital for chest pain and is noted to be confused. The following list of diagnoses are among those which should be considered. Each question presents a small piece of additional clinical information. Select the diagnosis which is most likely for each question.

A. Hospitalization-related confusion
B. Dementia
C. Aphasia
D. Depression
E. Schizophrenia

Question 4-4:
Patient presents with complaints of memory loss for the past two months. Examination is normal except mental slowness and diffuse decrease in memory, affecting recent more than remote memory.

Question 4-5:
Patient presents with the inability to follow purely verbal commands yet can follow visual cues well.

Question 4-6:
Patient develops confusion and agitation at night while in the hospital, which resolves during the day. Patient tends to be awake much of night and sleeps part of the day. Patient sees bugs on the wall and has visions of children outside the window.

Answer 4-1: E.
Age is a risk factor for hospital-associated delirium even within the elderly population. Patients over 80 years of age are much more likely to become confused. Visual loss also predisposes to delirium, since adaptation to the environment depends on evaluation of the environment. Approximately half of hospitalized patients who develop delirium have an underlying dementia, and many of the rest have at least some cognitive difficulty. Dehydration is common in hospitalized patients because of reduced oral intake and is frequently correlated with azotemia and sodium disturbances. (p29)

Answer 4-2: A.
Patients with anticholinergic excess present with fever rather than hypothermia because of the inhibition of sweating. All of the other findings are typical of anticholinergic excess. The range of medications with anticholinergic effects is broad, ranging from tricyclic antidepressants to antihistamines, from medications used for parkinsonian tremor (trihexyphenidyl) to neuroleptics used in patients with dementia and delirium. (p32)

Answer 4-3: A.
The percentages of patients with delirium after surgeries is approximately correct. The frequency of delirium does not differ significantly on the route of anesthesia, probably because pre-operative medication and post-operative factors are in common, including sleep deprivation, pain, and analgesics, among others. (p33)

Answer 4-4: B.
Mild dementia predisposes to hospital-acquired confusion. Patients have difficulty with attention and concentration. Decompensation during hospitalization is typical. (p29)

Answer 4-5: C.
Wernike's aphasia is associated with the inability of the patient to respond to purely verbal commands with preserved ability to follow visual cues. This presentation may be misinterpreted as confusion. (p34)

Answer 4-6: A.
Hospital-acquired confusion is common in elderly patients. Patterned wallpaper can be misperceived as bugs, and occasionally spontaneous visual hallucinations can occur. Disturbance of the day/night cycle is expected. While mental status usually improves during the day, the improvement is not usually back to baseline. (p27)

Chapter 5: Clinical Approach to Stupor and Coma

Question 5-1:
A vegetative state is often the sequel of coma when patients have not improved to normal consciousness. Which of the following features are expected in this state?

1. Preserved sleep-wake cycles
2. Eyes open in response to stimulation
3. Intact regulation of cardiac and respiratory function
4. Ability to respond to commands only with eye blinks and vertical eye movements

Select: A = 1, 2, 3. B = 1, 3. C = 2, 4. D = 4 only. E = All

Question 5-2:
Oculocephalic testing in an unresponsive patient reveals conjugate movements to the right when the head is turned to the left yet no movement past the midline when the head is rotated to right. Which is the most likely site of lesion.

A. Right medulla
B. Right pons
C. Left pons
D. Right midbrain

Questions 5-3 and 5-4:
The Glasgow Coma Scale is an important tool for assessment of patients with decreased responsiveness. For the following vignettes, indicate what is the correct score.

Question 5-3:
Patient appears awake but is confused. Obeys commands briskly although the patient has to be re-directed to the task. Eyes are open immediately on examination.

A. 11
B. 12
C. 13
D. 14
E. 15

Question 5-4:
Patient is unresponsive to stimulation, does not open eyes or orient to the examiner. No speech. All limbs have extensor posturing in response to noxious stimulation.

A. 3
B. 4
C. 5
D. 6
E. 7

Question 5-5:
All of the following are features of the locked-in syndrome except which one?

A. Inability to accept input from the environment
B. Ability to communicate using eye blinks and vertical eye movements
C. Lesion in the ventral pons, bilaterally
D. Quadriplegia with lower cranial nerve palsies

Question 5-6:
Increased intracranial pressure with herniation affecting the brainstem is associated with which of the following features?

1. Decreased level of consciousness to the point of unresponsiveness
2. Asymmetric third and/or sixth cranial nerve palsies
3. Increased blood pressure
4. Decreased heart rate

Select: A = 1, 2, 3. B = 1, 3. C = 2, 4. D = 4 only. E = All

Answer 5-1: A.
Patients in the vegetative state have absence of cognitive function but retain sleep-wake cycles, regulation of cardiac and respiratory function, and will open eyes to stimulation. However, careful examination will reveal that the eye opening is an unpatterned response rather than a cognitive response. The ability to respond cognitively with only eye-blinks and vertical eye movements is characteristic of the locked-in syndrome rather than persistent vegetative state. (p38)

Answer 5-2: C.
Damage to the left paramedian pontine reticular formation results in inability to have conjugate movements of the eyes to that side when stimulated by passive rotation of the head to the right. The other lesions would not result in this deficit. (p49)

Answer 5-3: D.
The patient loses one point on verbal response for the confused conversation (V4); however, the patient receives full points for spontaneous eye opening (E4) and obeying motor commands (M6). (p45)

Answer 5-4: B.
The patient receives minimum points for verbal response (V1) and eye opening (E1) since there is complete failure of these responses. However, the patient does receive an additional point for the extensor response to stimulation (M2). (p45)

Answer 5-5: A.
Patients with the locked-in syndrome have the ability to accept input from the environment but marked deficit in ability to respond, hence the term, de-efferented state. All of the other features are typical of the locked-in syndrome. The most common cause is infarction of the pons bilaterally, often due to basilar artery thrombosis. This is seldom a stable state, patients showing improvement or deterioration, although long-term survival is possible. (p38)

Answer 5-6: E.
All of these are typical findings with herniation affecting the brainstem. Third and sixth cranial nerve palsies can develop, initially asymmetrically and ultimately bilaterally. Incipient herniation should be identified early because when the herniation extends lower than the midbrain the damage is usually irreversible. (p52)

Chapter 6: Excessive Daytime Somnolence

Question 6-1:
REM and NREM sleep have varied patterns, but there are some generalizations that can be made. Which of the following are true?

1. REM sleep is more prominent later in the sleep period.
2. NREM sleep is more prominent earlier in the sleep period.
3. NREM sleep accounts for up to 80% of total sleep time.
4. Hypotonia is more characteristic of REM sleep than NREM sleep

Select: A = 1, 2, 3. B = 1, 3. C = 2, 4. D = 4 only. E = All

Question 6-2:
Sleep patterns differ greatly between individuals, partly through training, partly through inheritance. Which of the following facts regarding sleep patterns are true?

1. The average amount of sleep in adults can be entrained by practice.
2. The total amount of sleep decreases throughout childhood.
3. Decreased sleep time is associated with health problems, but excessive sleep is not.
4. Longer sleepers spend relatively more time in Stage II sleep than slow-wave (Stage III-IV) sleep.

Select: A = 1, 2, 3. B = 1, 3. C = 2, 4. D = 4 only. E = All

Question 6-3:
Sleep spindles are a characteristic EEG finding during sleep. Which of the following is true for sleep spindles?

A. Sleep spindles are most prominent in early infancy and become less prominent with age.
B. Sleep spindles have a peak frequency of approximately 14 hertz.
C. Sleep spindles are most prominent from the parieto-occipital region.
D. Sleep spindles are most prominent in slow-wave sleep (Stage III-IV).

Question 6-4:
Partial sleep deprivation to less than 5 hours per night is expected to produce which of the following?

1. Impaired performance on cognitive tasks
2. Psychosis
3. Impaired attention and concentration
4. Persistent cognitive deficit if the period of deprivation exceeds two months

Select: A = 1, 2, 3. B = 1, 3. C = 2, 4. D = 4 only. E = All

Question 6-5:
Excessive daytime sleepiness (EDS) impairs the performance of many patients. Which of the following conditions predispose to impaired performance due to EDS?

1. Narcolepsy
2. Restless leg syndrome
3. Obstructive sleep apnea
4. Myotonic dystrophy

Select: A = 1, 2, 3. B = 1, 3. C = 2, 4. D = 4 only. E = All

Question 6-6:
Obstructive sleep apnea (OSA) is one common cause for EDS. All of the following are true except which?

A. Most patients with OSA are severely overweight.
B. Middle-aged men comprise the most commonly affected group.
C. Hypertension and cardiac arrhythmias are of increased likelihood in patients with OSA.
D. Hypoventilation results in frequent arousals.
E. OSA is the most common cause for EDS.

Question 6-7:
The Kleine-Levin syndrome is characterized by which of the following features?

1. Periodic hypersomnolence
2. Exacerbation of the disorder with age
3. Bulimia
4. Lesion of the ascending reticular activating system

Select: A = 1, 2, 3. B = 1, 3. C = 2, 4. D = 4 only. E = All

Answer 6-1: E.
All of these are true for the normal adult sleep cycle. Decreased tone can occur in NREM sleep, but profound hypotonia is most characteristic of REM sleep. (p60)

Answer 6-2: C.
The amount of sleep declines with age through childhood, beginning with at least 16 hours in infancy and approximately 7.5 hours for adults. Longer sleepers do spend relatively less proportionate time in slow-wave sleep than short sleepers. The amount of sleep differs between patients due to endogenous factors, and most individuals are not able to change their sleep requirements without affecting performance. Also, both excessive and deficient sleep quantities have been associated with increased frequency of MI, stroke, and cancer. (p60)

Answer 6-3: B.
Sleep spindles may have frequencies ranging from 12 to 18 hertz, and in early childhood may be a low as 10 hertz; 14 hertz is a good median frequency. Infants do not have sleep spindles, but they develop by the third month. Sleep spindles are most prominent in the fronto-central region. Spindles are seen in Stage II and are less prominent with progression into slow-wave sleep. (p60)

Answer 6-4: B.
Sustained partial sleep deprivation commonly results in mild deficits in cognitive performance, attention, and concentration. Psychosis is not expected with partial deprivation. Recovery from prolonged partial sleep deprivation results in normal cognition; permanent neurologic sequelae from sleep deprivation does not occur. (p62-63)

Answer 6-5: E.
All of these are associated with EDS and the potential for impaired cognitive performance. Some patients with myotonic dystrophy have two reasons for EDS: nocturnal hypoventilation and primary dysfunction of the ascending reticular activating system as part of the neurological defect. (p65)

Answer 6-6: E.
The most common cause for EDS is voluntary sleep deprivation, usually associated with occupation or life style; OSA is the second most common cause. All of the other facts are true for OSA. In addition to hypertension and cardiac arrhythmias, patients with OSA have an increased risk of stroke and congestive heart failure. (p65-66)

Answer 6-7: B.
The Kleine-Levin syndrome is characterized by episodes of hypersomnolence lasting 16-18 hours followed by enhanced appetite. The condition abates with age. While the exact locus of the deficit is not known, dysfunction is suspected in the limbic-hypothalamic system. (p67)

Chapter 7: Approaches to Intellectual and Memory Impairments

Questions 7-1 and 7-2:
Folstein's Mini-Mental State examination is probably the most commonly used bedside mental status assessment. A patient scores perfectly on all of the components except as noted for the following two questions. Select the answer for the mini-vignettes.

Question 7-1:
Misses two of the serial-7 calculations and does not know the city. What is the MMSE score?

A. 25
B. 26
C. 27
D. 28

Question 7-2:
Misses one element on registration but then is able to recall all three objects at five minutes. On the three-stage command, fails to place paper on the table but rather hands it back to the examiner. What is the MMSE score?

A. 26
B. 27
C. 28
D. 29

Question 7-3:
Which of the following features is characteristic of the split-brain patients?

A. Alien hand syndrome
B. Akinetic mutism
C. Conduction aphasia
D. Left-right confusion

Question 7-4:
Gerstmann's syndrome consists of which of the following elements?

1. Left-right disorientation
2. Finger agnosia
3. Acalculia
4. Agraphia

Select: A = 1, 2, 3. B = 1, 3. C = 2, 4. D = 4 only. E = All

Question 7-5:
A 26-year-old man with a history of severe head injury presents with an awake appearance, but he does not respond to the environment. There is little movement of the extremities. He recovers some alertness and motor functions but continues to exhibit apathy and decreased overall movement and becomes inappropriate in interpersonal relations. Disinhibition is of grave concern to the family. Which of the following are likely to be true?

1. The predominant lesion is in the temporal lobes bilaterally.
2. He exhibited akinetic mutism early in the course.
3. Intelligence is invariably reduced in this condition.
4. Neuropsychological testing likely shows concrete interpretation of proverbs.

Select: A = 1, 2, 3. B = 1, 3. C = 2, 4. D = 4 only. E = All

Answer 7-1: C.
Missing two of the calculations and one aspect of orientation results in a maximum score of 27. (p77)

Answer 7-2: C.
The patient loses one point for initial registration even though he remembers all three subsequently. The patient also loses the point for failing to place the paper on the table; this is the most common error in this task. (p77)

Answer 7-3: A.
Alien hand syndrome refers to the seeming independent movement of the left hand, which may oppose the volitional movements of the right hand, and is typically seen in split-brain patients. Other important causes include strokes involving projections through the corpus callosum and cortical-basal ganglionic degeneration. (p73)

Answer 7-4: E.
All of these are cardinal features of Gerstmann's syndrome, which is due to a lesion in the left parietal region. This is a clinical syndrome rather than a specific diagnosis and is usually due to stroke. (p73)

Answer 7-5: C.
The most likely area of maximum damage is in the orbitofrontal cortex. Intelligence is often at or near normal although some neuropsychological tests have a tendency to be abnormal. The inability to respond to the environment while appearing awake is termed akinetic mutism. (p73)

Chapter 8: Developmental Delay and Regression in Infants

Question 8-1:
Which of the following statements are true regarding developmental delay?

1. Fragile X syndrome is the most common chromosomal cause of mental retardation.
2. Chromosomal disorders account for about one third of cases of severe mental retardation.
3. All children with global developmental delay should have an MRI unless the diagnosis is clearly known.
4. Most cases of cerebral palsy are due to perinatal asphyxia.

Select: A = 1, 2, 3. B = 1, 3. C = 2, 4. D = 4 only. E = All

Question 8-2:
Clinical evaluation of the patient with progressive intellectual impairment includes determining whether the disorder affects gray matter, white matter, or both. Which of the following features suggest a disorder of the gray matter?

1. Seizures
2. Blindness
3. Personality change
4. Focal deficits

Select: A = 1, 2, 3. B = 1, 3. C = 2, 4. D = 4 only. E = All

Question 8-3:
Which is the most common cause of isolated speech delay?

A. Brainstem immaturity
B. Infarction of the dominant hemisphere
C. Hearing loss
D. Infantile autism

Question 8-4:
A 7-year-old child presents for evaluation of toe walking. The neurological examination is normal, except for the toe walking. Which is the most likely diagnosis?

A. Normal child
B. Muscular dystrophy
C. Tethered cord
D. Idiopathic shortening of the ankle tendon

Question 8-5:
Which is the most common cause of traumatic brain injury in infants?

A. Falls out of cribs and beds
B. Motor vehicle accidents
C. Child abuse
D. None of these

Answer 8-1: A.
Most cases of CP are caused by prenatal injury rather than perinatal asphyxia. The presumption that most CP is caused by perinatal injury is a common misconception. (p83)

Answer 8-2: B.
Seizures and personality change, along with intellectual decline, suggest a disorder predominantly of the gray matter. In contrast, blindness, focal deficits, and corticospinal tract signs suggest a disorder of the white matter. Determining the type of lesion narrows the differential diagnosis greatly. (p86)

Answer 8-3: C.
Hearing loss is the most common cause of isolated speech delay. Autism produces an impairment in reception and attention but not isolated speech delay. Brainstem immaturity is more of a problem in premature infants with respiratory and feeding disturbance than a problem for children later in life with isolated speech delay. (p81)

Answer 8-4: D.
Idiopathic shortening of the ankle tendon is the most likely diagnosis with this presentation, but there is the possibility of muscular dystrophy or tethered cord. Family history should be obtained, not only in reference to muscular dystrophy but also regarding ankle tendon shortening, which may be familial. (p83)

Answer 8-5: C.
Child abuse remains the most common cause of traumatic brain injury in infants, and remains an important cause through childhood. The medical and psychological effects of abuse may persist into adult life, even if there is no outward sign of neurologic dysfunction. (p85)

Chapter 9: Behavior and Personality Disturbances

Question 9-1:
Pseudoseizures are most typically seen in which of the following psychological settings?

1. Borderline personality
2. Histrionic personality
3. Depression
4. Obsessive-compulsive disorder

Select: A = 1, 2, 3. B = 1, 3. C = 2, 4. D = 4 only. E = All

Question 9-2:
Paranoid personality is characterized by which of the following features?

1. Heightened suspiciousness
2. Propensity for litigation
3. Avoidance of intimacy and failure of relationships
4. Ideas of reference

Select: A = 1, 2, 3. B = 1, 3. C = 2, 4. D = 4 only. E = All

Question 9-3:
Frontal lobe dysfunction can result from many types of lesions, and the pattern of deficits differs between entities. Which of the following symptoms are commonly seen with frontal lobe disorders?

1. Apathy
2. Emotional lability
3. Short attention span
4. Wernicke's aphasia

Select: A = 1, 2, 3. B = 1, 3. C = 2, 4. D = 4 only. E = All

Questions 9-4 through 9-6:
The following are some specific anatomic localizations that are seen commonly in practice. For the vignettes listed in the following questions, pick the most likely anatomic localization for the clinical findings.

A. Orbitofrontal
B. Medial frontal
C. Frontal convexity
D. Temporal

Question 9-4:
Akinetic with urinary incontinence.

Question 9-5:
Disinhibited, impulsive behavior. Poor judgment.

Question 9-6:
Hypersexuality, poor impulse control, hyperreligiosity, propensity to have complex partial seizures.

Answer 9-1: A.
Personality disorders are common in patients diagnosed with pseudoseizures, especially borderline and histrionic. Depression may also be associated with pseudoseizures, which probably fill a need in the individual for attentional focus and situational escape. OCD is often characterized by a preoccupation with health that may result in doctor visits, but the manifestations are rarely pseudoseizures. (p101)

Answer 9-2: E.
All of these are features that characterize patients with paranoid personality type. These patients often have difficulty with relationships because of their tendency to distrust others. Transient ideas of reference can develop, although they are not invariable. (p90)

Answer 9-3: A.
Apathy can occur with both frontal convexity or medial frontal damage. Emotional lability is especially common with orbitofrontal lesions. Short attention span can develop with almost any frontal lesion. Wernicke's aphasia develops from damage to the temporal lobe. (p92)

Answer 9-4: B.
Medial frontal lesions result in akinesia and often leg weakness and urinary incontinence; the later symptoms suggest myelopathy. (p91-92)

Answer 9-5: A.
Orbitofrontal lesions can produce disinhibited behavior, characterized by impulsiveness, poor judgment, and emotional lability. Poor attention with easy distractibility is common. (p92)

Answer 9-6: D.
Temporal lobe lesions can produce hypersexuality and hyperreligiosity, as well as a tendency to have complex partial seizures. An interictal personality disorder is common, as well. (p92-93)

Chapter 10: Depression and Psychosis in Neurological Practice

Question 10-1:
Features of mania include which of the following?

1. Easy distractibility
2. Pressure of speech
3. Euphoria
4. Increased daytime and nocturnal sleep

Select: A = 1, 2, 3. B = 1, 3. C = 2, 4. D = 4 only. E = All

Question 10-2:
Features of depression include which of the following?

1. Loss of interest in outside activities
2. Loss of sleep
3. Excessive sleep
4. Loquaciousness

Select: A = 1, 2, 3. B = 1, 3. C = 2, 4. D = 4 only. E = All

Question 10-3:
Which of the following pathological conditions can correlate with depression?

1. Meningioma
2. Alzheimer's disease
3. Stroke
4. Parkinson's disease

Select: A = 1, 2, 3. B = 1, 3. C = 2, 4. D = 4 only. E = All

Question 10-4:
Mania is usually primary, but some medical conditions can produce secondary mania. Which of the following is the most likely to produce secondary mania?

A. Left hemisphere infarct
B. Right hemisphere infarct
C. Hydrocephalus
D. Bilateral occipital infarcts

Question 10-5:
Which of the following statements regarding hallucinations are true?

1. Hypnopompic hallucinations are present on awakening and indicate physiologic or psychologic pathology.
2. Hypnagogic hallucinations are present on falling asleep and are typical of narcolepsy.
3. Delusions may be recognized to be false thoughts by some patients with degenerative conditions.
4. Olfactory hallucinations can be seen in schizophrenia as well as complex partial seizures.

Select: A = 1, 2, 3. B = 1, 3. C = 2, 4. D = 4 only. E = All

Question 10-6:
Carbamazepine and valproate are used in patients with behavioral disturbances. Which of the following are likely to respond to these agents?

1. Complex partial seizures
2. Bipolar disorder
3. Unipolar depression
4. Schizophrenia

Select: A = 1, 2, 3. B = 1, 3. C = 2, 4. D = 4 only. E = All

Question 10-7:
Psychotic features would be expected to develop earliest in patients with which neurologic disorder?

A. Alzheimer's disease
B. Parkinson's disease
C. Lewy body dementia
D. Multiple sclerosis

Answer 10-1: A.
Easy distractibility and pressured speech are typical findings in mania. Euphoria is typical although not invariable. In general, there is decreased sleep. Other typical findings include grandiosity, flight of ideas, and, in severe cases, psychomotor agitation. (p107)

Answer 10-2: A.
These features are characteristic of patients with depression. Decreased sleep is most common, although increase in sleep can occur. Decreased spontaneous speech and tendency to not engage in interpersonal relationships are common rather than an increase in conversation. (p106)

Answer 10-3: E.
All of these conditions are associated with an increased frequency of depression. Meningioma of the olfactory groove with frontal lobe dysfunction is a prototypic structural lesion that may produce depression without any hard physical findings. Alzheimer's disease and Parkinson's disease are both associated with an increased frequency of depression. In AD patients, the depression is present even in patients who are unaware of their dementia, indicating that the depression can be a fundamental part of the neurochemical defects rather than being merely reactive. Stroke is commonly associated with depression, especially with lesions of the right hemisphere. (p107-108)

Answer 10-4: B.
Secondary mania is most common with lesions of the right hemisphere, especially in the orbitofrontal and temporal regions, and involves the deep gray matter. (p108)

Answer 10-5: C.
Hypnagogic and hypnopompic hallucinations are not always pathologic; they can occur in some normal patients. Delusions are errant beliefs which are strongly held, and by definition, the patient has no insight into their unreality. However, some patients with degenerative diseases such as Parkinson's disease may have visual hallucinations that the patient realizes are not real. (p110-111)

Answer 10-6: A.
These AEDs have been used in complex partial seizures, which often have behavioral correlates, bipolar disorder, and relapsing unipolar depression. Some schizophrenics are given these agents, but this is not primary treatment for this disorder. Note that most use of AEDs for behavioral purposes is off label but well within accepted medical practice. (p109)

Answer 10-7: C.
Early appearance of psychosis is a clue to the diagnosis of Lewy body dementia. The other disorders can develop psychosis, but usually late in the course. Multiple sclerosis only rarely is associated with psychosis even at advanced stages. Patients with Parkinson's disease typically have psychotic features with advanced disease. (p112)

Chapter 11A: Cognitive-Motor Disorders, Apraxias, and Agnosias: Cognitive-Motor Disorders and Apraxias

Question 11A-1 through 11A-4:
The following are some cognitive-motor disorders that are encountered in common practice. For the vignettes that follow, select the disorder which correlates with the clinical features.

A. Akinesia
B. Ideomotor apraxia
C. Ideational apraxia
D. Motor impersistence
E. Motor extinction

Question 11A-1:
Patient occasionally moves, showing intact strength, but fails to respond to stimuli which should evoke the movement.

Question 11A-2:
The patient is able to perform tasks with each side independently but unable to make simultaneous tasks.

Question 11A-3:
The patient is able to extend his arm for only a few seconds.

Question 11A-4:
The patient has no weakness but is unable to successfully light a cigarette, being unable to perform the components of the task in the correct order.

Question 11A-5:
Ideomotor apraxia is often tested by asking the patient how to use tools. Which of the following statements regarding ideomotor apraxia are correct?

1. Patients with ideomotor apraxia usually do better using the actual tools than when doing pantomime to a verbal command.
2. Patients with ideomotor apraxia often have difficulty judging correct distance and direction when using tools.
3. Deficit in timing of movements for appropriate execution is a form of ideomotor apraxia.
4. Limb-kinetic apraxia is a form of ideomotor apraxia.

Select: A = 1, 2, 3. B = 1, 3. C = 2, 4. D = 4 only. E = All

Answer 11A-1: A.
Akinesia is the failure to initiate movement, which is not due to the upper or lower motor neurons. Damage to the motor neurons would cause weakness rather than akinesia, and the patient would never be able to make the movement, regardless of the stimulus and impetus. (p117)

Answer 11A-2: E.
Motor extinction is the motor correlate of sensory extinction. The patient is unable to make simultaneous movements of the two sides. (p119)

Answer 11A-3: D.
In the absence of weakness or easy fatigability, this patient has motor impersistence. This is the inability to maintain a motor command and is usually tested by asking the patient to protrude the tongue or extend a limb for 20 seconds. (p120)

Answer 11A-4: C.
Ideational apraxia is the inability to correctly order a series of movements. This is distinct from the similarly-named ideomotor apraxia in which there is the inability to performed a learned movement. (p123)

Answer 11A-5: A.
These three statements are true for ideomotor apraxia, probably the most common variety of apraxia, although seldom tested for in routine neurology practice. Limb-kinetic apraxia is not really an apraxia, per se, but rather a primary motor disorder where the patient loses the ability to make small coordinated graded movements, such as a pincher grasp. (p123-124)

Chapter 11B: Cognitive-Motor Disorders, Apraxias, and Agnosias: Agnosias

Question 11B-1:
Inability of the patient to recognize familiar faces is termed:

A. Associative visual agnosia
B. Prosopagnosia
C. Simultanagnosia
D. Aperceptive visual agnosia

Question 11B-2:
Associative visual agnosia is defective object recognition which is not due to a primary visual perceptive problem. Which of the following statements are true for this defect?

1. Patients have impaired copying abilities.
2. Prosopagnosia is a manifestation of associative visual agnosia.
3. Impaired face recognition is usually due to lesions in the posterior temporal or occipital regions of the left hemisphere.
4. Alexia may be present in patients with associative visual agnosia.

Select: A = 1, 2, 3. B = 1, 3. C = 2, 4. D = 4 only. E = All

Question 11B-3 through 11-B-6:
Following are some statements referring to auditory agnosia. Indicate whether each is true or false.

Question 11B-3:
Patients with pure word deafness have impaired ability to recognize complex sounds but preserved elemental auditory perception.

Question 11B-4:
Nonverbal auditory agnosia is characterized by impaired deficit in decoding elemental sounds.

Question 11B-5:
Most patients with nonverbal auditory agnosia also have deficits in decoding speech sounds.

Question 11B-6:
Auditory amusia is the auditory correlate to prosopagnosia.

Answer 11B-1: B.
Prosopagnosia is the inability to recognize faces. Other forms of object recognition are relatively preserved, although not perfectly. Associative agnosia is where patients have preserved perception but difficulty associating the perception with the relevant concept. Simultanagnosia is a defect in perception of a multi-element display, such as a complex picture. Patients with aperceptive visual agnosia have no problem recognizing faces. (p134)

Answer 11B-2: C.
Patients typically have preserved copying, even of objects with which they are not familiar; this is in distinction to aperceptive visual agnosias, where copying even simple objects is impaired. Impaired face recognition is usually a sign of right hemisphere or bilateral damage; left hemisphere damage produces more reading difficulty and impaired object recognition. (p133)

Answer 11B-3: False.
Pure word deafness is specific for words, which represent sound elements that have only an indirect association with the object. Patients can identify even complex sounds such as the phone ringing. (p136)

Answer 11B-4: False.
Nonverbal auditory agnosia is characterized by impaired comprehension of one or more classes of sounds, such as birds, telephones, etc. Some spheres of sound identification may be more affected than others. (p136)

Answer 11B-5: True.
While cases of pure nonverbal auditory agnosia have been reported, most have deficits in speech recognition as well. When the deficit is mainly nonverbal, the lesion is most likely in the right hemisphere. (p136)

Answer 11B-6: False.
Auditory amusia is the inability to recognize music, such as identification of specific melodies or a particular singing voice. This is most commonly due to bilateral lesions of the auditory association areas. The auditory correlate of prosopagnosia is phonagnosia, where the patient cannot recognize familiar voices, and has been localized to a lesion in the right parietal area. (p137)

Chapter 12A: Language Disorders: Aphasia

Question 12A-1:
Aphemia is a rare condition affecting language function. Which of the following are features of aphemia?

1. Causative lesion is in the dominant inferior frontal gyrus
2. Writing is preserved.
3. Auditory comprehension is normal.
4. Patient speaks with phoneme substitutions.

Select: A = 1, 2, 3. B = 1, 3. C = 2, 4. D = 4 only. E = All

Question 12A-2:
Wernicke's aphasia is characterized by all of the following except:

A. Lesion of the dominant superior temporal gyrus
B. Anomia
C. Deficit of auditory language comprehension with preservation of reading comprehension
D. Writing is impaired with poor spelling and impaired content of the prose

Question 12A-3:
Conduction aphasia can be recognized only if specifically tested for. Typical features include all of the following except:

A. Impaired repetition.
B. Coexistence of anomia
C. Lesion in the region of the arcuate fasciculus in the dominant hemisphere
D. Deficit in comprehension of purely verbal commands

Question 12A-4 through 12A-6:
For each of the following vignettes, select the language disorder from the list below which most closely fits the clinical description.

A. Transcortical motor aphasia
B. Thalamic aphasia
C. Transcortical sensory aphasia
D. Wernicke's aphasia

Question 12A-4:
Speech is impaired, with telegraphic output. Comprehension is good. Repetition is good.

Question 12A-5:
Speech is fluent, although with paraphrasic errors and echolalia. Comprehension is impaired. Repetition is normal.

Question 12A-6:
Fluent speech although poor information content. Poor comprehension. Poor repetition

Question 12A-7:
Which of the following lesion locations in the dominant hemisphere can result in fluent aphasia?

1. Superior temporal gyrus
2. Thalamus
3. Angular gyrus
4. Prefrontal cortex

Select: A = 1, 2, 3. B = 1, 3. C = 2, 4. D = 4 only. E = All

Question 12A-8:
Degenerative dementia can be characterized by which of the following language deficits?

1. Anomia
2. Progressive aphasia without dementia
3. Global aphasia
4. Alexia without agraphia

Select: A = 1, 2, 3. B = 1, 3. C = 2, 4. D = 4 only. E = All

Answer 12A-1: E.
These features are all typical of aphemia. More patients might be identified if writing was tested more commonly in patients with marked expressive deficit. (p145)

Answer 12A-2: C.
Reading comprehension is impaired in patients with Wernicke's aphasia, along with deficit of auditory language comprehension. All of the other features are true. The lesion is classically in the superior temporal gyrus, although extension into adjacent parietal lobule is common. Anomia is common in patients with dominant hemisphere lesions including the temporal lesions causing Wernicke's aphasia. Writing is impaired with poor content, just as spontaneous speech typically has poor content. Because of the requirement for spelling while writing, this deficit is obvious. (p145)

Answer 12A-3: D.
Comprehension is preserved. Conduction aphasia is demonstrated by asking the patient to repeat a phrase. Deficit in repetition is distinguished from a global expressive difficulty. The lesion typically involves the arcuate fasciculus and adjacent supramarginal gyrus. (p149)

Answer 12A-4: A.
Transcortical motor aphasia is characterized by disordered output but relative preservation of repetition. The lesion is typically in the frontal lobe, anterior to Broca's area. (p149-150)

Answer 12A-5: C.
Transcortical sensory aphasia is characterized by impaired comprehension with normal repetition. The speech is fluent. (p149-150)

Answer 12A-6: D.
Wernicke's aphasia is characterized by impaired comprehension and repetition. Although speech seems clear, paraphrasic errors are common and the information value of the speech is low. Thalamic aphasia could have been selected, although comprehension is usually better than with classic Wernicke's aphasia. (p145)

Answer 12A-7: B.
Lesion in the superior temporal gyrus gives Wernicke's aphasia, whereas lesion in the angular gyrus may give conduction aphasia, both fluent aphasias. (p145, 149)

Answer 12A-8: A.
Patients with degenerative dementias develop anomia early in the course of the disease. Progressive aphasia without dementia can be an initial presentation of some patients who ultimately have a degenerative dementia. Global aphasia develops with progression of degenerative dementias, although the stage at which the patient loses language differs between patients. Alexia without aphasia would not be expected, since writing difficulty develops early in the course of most degenerative dementias. (p153-154)

Chapter 12B: Language Disorders: Developmental Speech and Language Disorders

Question 12B-1:
Which of the following statements is true regarding stuttering?

A. Stuttering is more common in individuals without other language and developmental disorders.
B. Patients develop stuttering usually in adolescence.
C. Stuttering is a manifestation of a psychological disturbance rather than a true language or linguistic disorder.
D. Stuttering is often inherited.

Question 12B-2:
Which of the following features is not expected with the Landau-Kleffner syndrome?

A. Inability to understand language
B. Normal intellect
C. Hearing loss
D. Seizures

Question 12B-3:
Which of the following statements about acquired aphasia of childhood is true?

A. Most children with left hemisphere lesions do not recover language function.
B. Difficulties with school performance are common in children who recover from acquired aphasia.
C. When the dominant hemisphere is damaged at a very young age, language dominance can be transferred to the contralateral hemisphere in the majority of patients with normal language.
D. Language lateralization is not developed until adolescence.

Question 12B-4:
Which of the following is a risk factor for developmental language disorder in childhood?

A. Low birth weight
B. Prematurity
C. Parental mental retardation
D. Family history of developmental language disorders
E. All of the above

Answer 12B-1: D.
Stuttering is often inherited. The frequency is increased in patients with other language and developmental disorders. The dysfluency is evident early in development as language develops. Stuttering is a linguistic disorder rather than psychological. (p162)

Answer 12B-2: C.
Patients with LKS have impaired language comprehension with normal hearing. Their response to the auditory environment is usually normal in spheres other than language. (p163)

Answer 12B-3: B.
Many children with acquired aphasia have recovery of language function, but the children continue to have difficulty with school despite the improvement. Despite these limitations, most children with left hemisphere lesions have at least some return of language function. Transfer of dominance is associated with abnormal language function. Language lateralization begins before adolescence, but there are certainly maturational changes in lateralization with age. (p168)

Answer 12B-4: E.
All of these are risk factors for developmental language disorder according to the National Collaborative Perinatal Project. (p161)

Chapter 13: Difficulties with Speech and Swallowing

Question 13-1:
Which of the following clinical findings in speech difficulty indicates functional speech disorder?

A. Ability to sing clearly while speech is dysarthric
B. Speech improvement following ethanol intake
C. Episodes of normal speech while dysarthric at other times
D. Exacerbation of speech by anxiety
E. None

Question 13-2:
Diplophonia is the production of two tones of voice simultaneously. Which of the following statements about this disorder are true?

1. Unilateral vocal cord weakness is suspected.
2. The cause is usually a conscious effort, such that functional disorders are suspected.
3. Bilateral lesions of the recurrent laryngeal nerves may cause this.
4. Unilateral Horner's syndrome is common.

Select: A = 1, 2, 3. B = 1, 3. C = 2, 4. D = 4 only. E = All

Question 13-3 through 13-6:
The following are some important neurologic disorders. For the vignettes which follow, pick the disorder which would most likely be expected to produce the clinical description.

A. Alzheimer's disease
B. Parkinson's disease
C. Tenth cranial nerve lesion
D. Cerebellar degeneration
E. Myasthenia gravis
F. Essential tremor

Question 13-3:
Hoarse voice and low volume. Much worse with prolonged speech, better in the morning.

Question 13-4:
Weak voice with hoarseness and tendency to monotonic speech.

Question 13-5:
Tremulous voice with inappropriate fluctuations in volume.

Question 13-6:
Hoarse voice with diplophonia.

Question 13-7:
Oral apraxia, difficulty in performing certain oral movements on command, is associated with which of the following disorders?

1. Infarction in the left temporal lobe
2. Cortical-basal ganglionic degeneration (CBGD)
3. ALS
4. Infarction of frontal cortex in the region of Broca's area

Select: A = 1, 2, 3. B = 1, 3. C = 2, 4. D = 4 only. E = All

Answer 13-1: E.
None of these make the diagnosis of functional speech disorder. Singing usually is performed in a different frequency range than speech, so pathology affecting clarity and frequency content of speech may not affect patients when singing. Likewise, ethanol may improve vocal manifestations of essential tremor. Myasthenia gravis can have sufficient fluctuation that speech may be normal at times and markedly dysarthric at other times. Many causes of dysarthria, psychogenic and neurologic, are exacerbated by anxiety and stress. (p172)

Answer 13-2: B.
Diplophonia is produced by differences in set tension on the vocal cords, which indicates an imbalance in the neural control. The lesion is most commonly unilateral, although bilateral asymmetric lesions can produce the finding. Psychogenic speech disturbance can produce many findings, but diplophonia is not one of them; patients do not have such conscious or subconscious independent control over laryngeal muscles. Unilateral Horner's syndrome can develop with brainstem lesions, but not with isolated involvement of the recurrent laryngeal nerve. (p175)

Answer 13-3: E.
Myasthenia gravis typically gives a hoarse, low-volume voice which may be indistinguishable from a tenth cranial nerve lesion. However, the fluctuation with deterioration with sustained effort and improvement in the morning suggest myasthenia gravis. (p175)

Answer 13-4: B.
Parkinsonism commonly produces weakness of the voice more prominently than hoarseness. The loss of prosody is a clue to the diagnosis, which seems to be a component of the impaired motor function. The weak and hoarse features otherwise would not narrow the diagnosis greatly. (p175)

Answer 13-5: D.
Cerebellar degeneration is most likely to give a tremulous voice, with fluctuations in volume. Essential tremor is a common cause of tremulous voice, but without volume fluctuation. (p175)

Answer 13-6: C.
Tenth cranial nerve lesion presents with hoarse voice. The poor coordination between the vocal cords makes for a breathy, low-volume voice. The diplophonia develops from differences in tone of the two cords. Diagnosis is suspected clinically and is established by direct visualization of the cords. (p175)

Answer 13-7: C.
Oral apraxia is characteristic of some lesions in the inferior frontal region, in or near Broca's area. CBGD can also present with this, as well, and in these patients may predate most other clinical manifestations of the disease. Temporal lobe infarction affects comprehension and may affect the content of speech expression but does not cause oral apraxia. ALS typically produces a hoarse voice which sounds strained, and may have a gurgling sound because of silent aspiration and pooling of fluid on the cords. (p177)

Chapter 14: Vision Loss

Question 14-1:
Which of the following conditions would be considered in the differential diagnosis of patients with transient visual loss?

1. Amaurosis fugax (transient monocular blindness, TMB)
2. Retinal migraine
3. Uhthoff's phenomenon
4. Angle-closure glaucoma

Select: A = 1, 2, 3. B = 1, 3. C = 2, 4. D = 4 only. E = All

Question 14-2:
A patient has sudden central visual loss with relative sparing of peripheral vision and retinal hemorrhage. Which is the most likely diagnosis?

A. Anterior ischemic optic neuropathy
B. Central retinal vein occlusion
C. Retrobulbar optic neuritis
D. Posterior ischemic optic neuropathy
E. Retinal infarction due to migraine

Question 14-3:
Causes of acute bilateral visual loss include all of the following except which?

A. Occipital infarction
B. Pituitary apoplexy
C. Demyelinating disease
D. Ischemic optic neuropathy

Question 14-4:
Causes of gradually progressive visual loss include which of the following?

1. Optic nerve drusen
2. Pseudotumor cerebri
3. Paraneoplastic visual loss
4. Glaucoma

Select: A = 1, 2, 3. B = 1, 3. C = 2, 4. D = 4 only. E = All

Answer 14-1: E.
These are all potential causes of transient visual loss. TMB is usually due to carotid disease. Retinal migraine produces visual obscuration and is more likely to produce positive visual phenomena than carotid disease. Uhthoff's phenomenon is a decrease in visual acuity with increased body temperature and is characteristic of demyelinating disease. The tempo, duration, and pattern of visual loss would, of course, differ in comparison to that of ischemia. Angle closure glaucoma may produce attacks of monocular visual loss. (p188)

Answer 14-2: B.
This is a classic history for central retinal vein occlusion. Patients present with central visual field loss. Retinal hemorrhages are typical. Arterial occlusion producing anterior ischemic optic neuropathy may produce disk hemorrhages, but the pattern of visual loss is usually altitudinal rather than central. Retrobulbar optic neuritis commonly produces visual loss, but hemorrhages do not occur. (p190)

Answer 14-3: D.
Ischemic optic neuropathy is rarely bilateral. Bilateral occipital infarction produces cortical blindness often associated with memory deficit and confabulation (Anton's syndrome). Pituitary apoplexy can cause sudden visual loss, commonly associated with headache and encephalopathy, and diplopia. Demyelinating disease causes visual loss which is usually unilateral but may be bilateral, especially in Devic's disease. (p190)

Answer 14-4: E.
These are all potential causes of bilateral visual loss. Optic nerve drusen are due to extracellulary deposition of plasma proteins, which eventually results in visual loss in approximately 75% of patients. Pseudotumor cerebri produces insidious visual loss if untreated, and in a few unfortunate patients may progress despite normalization of the intracranial pressure. Paraneoplastic visual loss is due to antibodies against the retinal cells and optic neurons. Small-cell lung cancer is the most common associated malignancy. As with other paraneoplastic disorders, the visual manifestations may predate the diagnosis of the cancer by many months. Glaucoma is a common cause of progressive visual loss even with normal intraocular pressures. (p191)

Chapter 15: Abnormalities of the Optic Nerve and Retina

Questions 15-1 through15-4:
Following is a list of disorders that can affect optic nerve function. For the mini-vignettes that follow, select the disorder that is most likely.

A. Optic neuritis
B. Hyperviscosity syndrome
C. Diabetic papillopathy
D. Malignant hypertension
E. Peri-chiasmatic tumor

Question 15-1:
Monocular visual loss with optic disc swelling.

Question 15-2:
Bilateral visual loss with papilledema and encephalopathy.

Question 15-3:
Unilateral visual loss with segment defect in contralateral eye. Fundus is normal.

Question 15-4:
Bilateral disc edema with enlarged blind spot, in a young patient. No visual loss.

Answer 15-1: A.
Intrabulbar optic neuritis (papillitis) classically produces visual loss with optic nerve swelling, as distinct from the retrobulbar form, in which the disc appears normal. (p194)

Answer 15-2: D.
Malignant hypertension produces papilledema and can produce visual loss. Encephalopathy and focal signs are common but not requisite. (p196)

Answer 15-3: E.
Peri-chiasmatic tumor classically produces ipsilateral visual loss from optic nerve compression plus a segment defect in the opposite visual field, a junctional scotoma. (p197)

Answer 15-4: C.
Diabetic papillopathy presents with disc edema which is usually bilateral, although unilateral involvement can occur. These patients present with little visual loss, although there is enlargement of the blind spot. Diagnosis will be easy in diabetics, although other causes need to be eliminated. Optic neuritis, Devic's disease, and mass lesion are the main differential diagnoses. (p197)

Chapter 16: Eye Movement Disorders: Diplopia, Nystagmus, and Other Ocular Oscillations

Question 16-1:
Which of the following features is characteristic of patients with strabismus?

1. Consistent misalignment of the visual axes is most likely due to ophthalmological disorders.
2. Most people have a tendency to at least some misalignment, which can be manifest with illness and sedation.
3. Misalignment of the visual axes which changes with direction of gaze indicates a neurologic disorder.
4. The most common cause of vertical diplopia is inferior oblique palsy.

Select: A = 1, 2, 3. B = 1, 3. C = 2, 4. D = 4 only. E = All

Question 16-2:
A patient presents with diplopia and head tilt to the left and slightly forward. Which is the most likely location for the lesion?

A. Right inferior rectus
B. Left inferior rectus
C. Right trochlear nerve
D. Left trochlear nerve
E. Superior rectus

Question 16-3:
Which of the following conditions can produce acute bilateral ophthalmoplegia?

1. Multiple sclerosis
2. Pituitary apoplexy
3. Tricyclic overdose
4. Tick paralysis

Select: A = 1, 2, 3. B = 1, 3. C = 2, 4. D = 4 only. E = All

Question 16-4:
Which of the following statements regarding optokinetic nystagmus (OKN) are true?

1. Presence of OKN when reported visual acuity is only sufficient to count fingers indicates a psychogenic cause for the visual loss.
2. Testing for OKN with the pocket tape does not cover sufficient visual field to rule out psychogenic blindness.
3. In congenital nystagmus, OKN is expected to show a normal response.
4. Patients with parieto-occipital lesions causing hemianopia have defective OKN when the tape is moved toward the side of the lesion.

Select: A = 1, 2, 3. B = 1, 3. C = 2, 4. D = 4 only. E = All

Question 16-5:
A patient presents with unilateral Horner's syndrome, ophthalmoplegia, and sensory loss in a V1 distribution on the same side. What is the most likely location of the lesion?

A. Pituitary region
B. Medial pons
C. Posterior cavernous sinus
D. Superior orbital fissure
E. Cerebellopontine angle

Question 16-6:
Which of the following features are characteristic of patients with congenital nystagmus?

1. Congenital nystagmus usually develops in adolescence and is maximal in young adulthood.
2. Congenital nystagmus may be associated with myopia in infants.
3. Congenital nystagmus is enhanced by convergence.
4. Congenital nystagmus is usually horizontal.

Select: A = 1, 2, 3. B = 1, 3. C = 2, 4. D = 4 only. E = All

Answer 16-1: A.
The most common cause of vertical diplopia is superior oblique palsy. Misalignment which is consistent throughout directions of gaze is termed comitant strabismus, while misalignment which is gaze dependent is termed noncomitant strabismus and indicates a neurological disorder. (p204)

Answer 16-2: C.
The right trochlear nerve supplies the superior oblique muscle, which normally would intort the eye. Therefore, loss of this effect results in mild extortion of the eye by the unopposed inferior oblique. To make the vision conjugate, the patient tilts the head to the left to make the left eye intort. The forward tilt is also to compensate for the loss of the depressor action of the weak superior oblique, moving the other eye up to the same level as the abnormal eye. (p209)

Answer 16-3: E.
These conditions can all produce acute bilateral ophthalmoplegia. MS can produce acute ophthalmoplegia as well as visual loss. Pituitary apoplexy may also result in visual loss along with ophthalmoplegia. Tricyclic overdose commonly produces ophthalmoplegia, which triggers search for subarachnoid hemorrhage or other intracranial catastrophe when the patient presents to the ER. Tick paralysis can produce ophthalmoplegia as well as weakness of appendicular and axial muscles. (p215)

Answer 16-4: C.
Patients with poor vision to the point of counting fingers may still have preserved OKN in some circumstances. In congenital nystagmus, the direction of the fast phase may be paradoxical, i.e., in the direction of the tape movement. The pocket OKN tape is commonly used for possible psychogenic ophthalmoplegia or blindness, but this technique is helpful only if positive. If negative, whole-field stimulation should be performed. OKN is defective in patients with parieto-occipital lesions, when the movement is toward the side of the lesion. (p215)

Answer 16-5: D.
The findings could be caused by a lesion at the superior orbital fissure or in the anterior aspect of the cavernous sinus. Posterior cavernous sinus lesions would be expected to produce dysfunction of V2 with or without V3 in addition to V1. (p214)

Answer 16-6: C.
Congenital nystagmus is usually horizontal but may be vertical or circumductory in rare patients. This disorder is associated with a number of other ocular disorders including infantile myopia. However, the nystagmus is thought to be an associated problem, and not caused by the visual disorder. Congenital nystagmus can occasionally develop in adolescence but more commonly is present at birth, although it may not be noticed during the first months. Congenital nystagmus is usually damped by convergence, and this feature is used to help patients overcome the nystagmus. (p218)

Questions 16-7 through 16-9:
A list of potential diagnoses is presented below for patients with abnormal ocular movements. For each of the mini-vignettes, select the most likely diagnosis.

 A. Vestibular nystagmus
 B. Spasmus nutans
 C. Latent nystagmus
 D. Congenital nystagmus
 E. Physiological nystagmus

Question 16-7:
A patient presents with dizziness which sounds presyncopal. Examination shows nystagmus with extreme lateral gaze to each side. No other ocular motor abnormality is noted.

Question 16-8:
An 18-month-old has horizontal pendular nystagmus and obvious lateral head nodding.

Question 16-9:
An infant is noted to have horizontal pendular nystagmus without other neurologic or ophthalmologic deficit.

Answer 16-7: E.
Physiological nystagmus is characterized by end-point nystagmus, which is classically with lateral gaze, but can also be present with vertical gaze. The nystagmus is typically in the same plane as the gaze, but a torsional component can be present. (p220)

Answer 16-8: B.
Spasmus nutans is a high-frequency, low-amplitude pendular nystagmus that develops in children between the ages of 6 and 12 months and usually abates within 2 years. When it appears as the fully developed triad, the nystagmus is associated with torticollis and titubation. Spasmus nutans is a benign disorder, but investigation is usually required to rule out structural causes. (p219)

Answer 16-9: D.
Congenital nystagmus is usually present at birth and is usually horizontal. The condition can be sporadic or inherited. (p218)

Chapter 17: Pupillary and Eyelid Abnormalities

Questions 17-1 through 17-4:
Some important causes of anisocoria are listed below. For the mini-vignettes which follow, select the diagnosis which is most likely.

A. Pharmacologic mydriasis
B. Cerebral herniation
C. Horner's syndrome
D. Holmes-Adie syndrome
E. Benign episodic unilateral mydriasis

Question 17-1:
A patient presents with episodic dilation of one pupil associated with migraine-like headache. No other neurologic deficit is identified.

Question 17-2:
A patient presents with one widely dilated pupil without other deficit or pain. No precipitating factors, but the patient had been fishing.

Question 17-3:
Patient presents with pupil larger on the right with the eye appearing more open than on the left. No other neurologic abnormalities.

Question 17-4:
A patient presents with dilation of the left pupil and left hemiparesis with somnolence.

Questions 17-5 through 17-8:
Following is a list of some important causes of ptosis. For each of the mini-vignettes, select the disorder which is the most likely cause.

A. Dehiscence of the levator palpabrae aponeurosis
B. Myasthenia gravis
C. Guillain-Barré syndrome
D. Oculomotor nerve palsy
E. Horner's syndrome

Question 17-5:
A patient presents with bilateral although asymmetric ptosis and complains of diplopia when both eyes are open.

Question 17-6:
A patient presents with unilateral ptosis following a motor vehicle accident. Examination shows extensive bruising plus the unilateral ptosis but no other ocular motor abnormality.

Question 17-7:
A patient with unilateral ptosis also has mydriasis and complains of diplopia.

Question 17-8:
A 28-year-old female presents with ptosis and facial weakness and is found to be areflexic.

Answer 17-1: E.
Benign episodic unilateral mydriasis presents with brief episodes of unilateral dilation, which is often associated with visual blurring and can be associated with headache. The absence of other signs of CN-3 palsy is reassuring, but aneurysmal compression of the nerve is often considered. (p230)

Answer 17-2: A.
Pharmacologic mydriasis is the most likely cause. The patient may have used transdermal scopolamine patches while fishing. Transfer of drug to the eye can produce hours of mydriasis. The pupil does not constrict with pilocarpine eye drops. (p230)

Answer 17-3: C.
Horner's syndrome is present on the left, which is characterized by miosis and ptosis, and there may be ipsilateral anhydrosis. (p232)

Answer 17-4: B.
Right hemisphere mass lesion with incipient uncal herniation results in left hemiparesis because of a direct effect of the mass lesion and compression of CN-3 against the tentorium. Sometimes, the oculomotor nerve affected is ipsilateral to the lesion, but in this case displacement of the midbrain results in compression of the contralateral oculomotor nerve, a false localizing sign. (p229)

Answer 17-5: B.
Myasthenia gravis produces ptosis which may be bilateral or unilateral, usually with other ocular motor deficits that do not fall into the anatomic distribution of one cranial nerve lesion. (p234)

Answer 17-6: A.
Dehiscence of the aponeurosis can occur as a result of trauma but can also develop with advanced age. The absence of other findings makes this diagnosis. If the pupil ipsilateral to the ptosis was smaller, Horner's syndrome would have been present, and post-traumatic causes of Horner's syndrome would have to be considered including lower cervical and plexus lesions and carotid dissection. (p234)

Answer 17-7: D.
Oculomotor (third) nerve palsy produces unilateral ptosis, mydriasis, and loss of appropriate oculomotor function. (p229)

Answer 17-8: C.
Guillain-Barré syndrome should always be considered in a patient with weakness and areflexia. Myasthenia can also produce decreased reflexes, but unless the weakness is profound, the reflexes should be elicitable. (p234)

Chapter 18: Dizziness and Vertigo

Question 18-1:
Benign positional vertigo is one of the most common causes of dizziness. Which of the following are true for this disorder?

1. Position change exacerbates the vertigo.
2. Symptoms are worse later in the day.
3. Duration of evoked nystagmus is usually less than 30 seconds.
4. The vertigo becomes progressively worse with successive movements.

Select: A = 1, 2, 3. B = 1, 3. C = 2, 4. D = 4 only. E = All

Question 18-2:
Post-traumatic vestibulopathy is associated with all of the following features except which?

A. Symptoms are alleviated by successive movements.
B. Development is usually immediately after the injury; occurrence beginning weeks after the injury indicates a functional component.
C. Prognosis is good, with improvement expected in weeks to months.
D. Patients often respond to exercise therapy.
E. Temporal bone fracture may be associated.

Question 18-3:
Which of the following features are characteristic of Ménière's disease?

1. Causative pathology is thought to be movement of canaliths
2. Pressure sensation in the ear
3. Episodes of vertigo with occasional loss of consciousness
4. Fluctuating hearing loss

Select: A = 1, 2, 3. B = 1, 3. C = 2, 4. D = 4 only. E = All

Question 18-4:
Brainstem ischemia is an uncommon cause of vertigo, but recognition has tremendous therapeutic and prognostic implications. Which of the following features suggest a brainstem lesion?

1. Diplopia
2. Perioral numbness
3. Transient hemianopia
4. Horizontal or vertical nystagmus without a torsional component

Select: A = 1, 2, 3. B = 1, 3. C = 2, 4. D = 4 only. E = All

Question 18-5:
Which of the following features are typical of acute peripheral vestibulopathy?

1. Tendency to fall to the side of the involved ear during Romberg testing
2. Nystagmus with a fast phase away from the side of the involved ear
3. Past-pointing to the side of the involved ear when pointing to an object with the eyes closed
4. Facial weakness ipsilateral to the involved ear

Select: A = 1, 2, 3. B = 1, 3. C = 2, 4. D = 4 only. E = All

Answer 18-1: B.
Position change exacerbates the vertigo, and, essentially, without movement the symptoms are minimal. The duration of the nystagmus after change in head position is between 3 and 30 seconds. Symptoms are worse in the morning and become better later in the day. The vertigo becomes better with successive provocative movements, and this feature is employed as a part of treatment. (p242)

Answer 18-2: B.
Post-traumatic vestibulopathy is usually noticed immediately after a significant head injury but can develop weeks later without implicating a functional component to the symptoms. Symptoms can be very similar to that of benign positional vertigo including improvement with successive movement and response to exercise therapy. In general, the prognosis is good. (p244)

Answer 18-3: C.
Ménière's disease is characterized by attacks of vertigo with tinnitus and fluctuating hearing loss and is often preceded by a feeling of pressure in an ear. Pathology is thought to be endolymphatic hydrops rather than canalith movement. Patients may fall, but loss of consciousness does not occur. (p245)

Answer 18-4: E.
Diplopia is always a red flag for brainstem dysfunction, but an exact description should be elicited. Some patients offer to admit to diplopia when they mean blurred vision. Perioral numbness signifies parenchymal brainstem damage from damage to the trigeminal projections. Transient hemianopia indicates occipital ischemia, since the PCAs are the terminal branches of the basilar artery. The character of the nystagmus can aid differentiation of central from peripheral causes. Peripheral vestibulopathy always has a torsional component; brainstem nystagmus may not. (p246)

Answer 18-5: A.
Facial weakness or any other cranial neuropathy would suggest a cause for the symptoms other than inner ear (labyrinthine) dysfunction. (p239)

Chapter 19: Hearing Loss and Tinnitus without Dizziness or Vertigo

Question 19-1:
Which of the following statements are true regarding the bedside examination of hearing?

1. For the Rinne test, the tuning fork is held on the midline of the skull.
2. Bedside testing can usually localize the lesion to sensorineural or conductive hearing loss.
3. For the Weber test, the tuning fork is held on the mastoid then in the air lateral to the tragus.
4. Hearing should be tested only with a tuning fork at 512 Hz.

Select: A = 1, 2, 3. B = 1, 3. C = 2, 4. D = 4 only. E = All

Questions 19-2 through 19-4:
Following are mini-vignettes that present features of conductive and sensorineural hearing loss. For the features listed select the best answer from the following list.

A. Sensorineural hearing loss
B. Conductive hearing loss
C. Both
D. Neither

Question 19-2:
Loudness recruitment is enhanced, such that patients may have difficulty especially in loud environments with conflicting audio inputs.

Question 19-3:
Patients frequently have tinnitus.

Question 19-4:
Hearing aid may help audio perception.

Question 19-5:
Tinnitus is one of the more frustrating neurologic complaints, for the physician as well at the patient. Which of the following statements concerning tinnitus are true?

1. Tinnitus is a benign condition for most patients.
2. More than 90% of patients with tinnitus have some degree of hearing loss.
3. Non-audiologic tinnitus can be due to turbulence of blood flow.
4. There is not treatment for tinnitus.

Select: A = 1, 2, 3. B = 1, 3. C = 2, 4. D = 4 only. E = All

Answer 19-1: C.
Bedside testing can usually distinguish sensorineural from conductive hearing loss. The only tuning fork which should be used for routine bedside hearing testing has a frequency of 512 Hz; lower frequencies can produce vibration which can be mistaken for sound. Regarding the Rinne and Weber tests, the statements are reversed. (p253-254)

Answer 19-2: A.
Sensorineural hearing loss produces loudness recruitment, where relatively modest changes in input magnitude produce relatively large differences in perceived volume. The enhanced volume may result in confusion of the normal gating mechanisms such that perception of these loud sounds is relatively impaired compared to perception of softer sounds. Loudness recruitment usually indicates dysfunction at the level of the cochlea. (p257-258)

Answer 19-3: C.
Both conductive and sensorineural hearing loss may have associated tinnitus. In general, the frequency of the tinnitus is higher in patients with sensorineural hearing loss than in conductive hearing loss, in which case the frequency may be low enough to be perceived as buzzing or hissing rather than ringing. (p257-258)

Answer 19-4: C.
Hearing aid is used predominantly for patients with conductive hearing loss, but patients with sensorineural hearing loss may also benefit. (p257-258)

Answer 19-5: A.
Tinnitus is benign for most patients. Tinnitus is not always of ear or nerve origin, and vascular causes have to be considered, including AVM, fistula, and transmitted bruit from the carotid or vertebral arteries. More than 90% of patients with tinnitus have some hearing deficit. Tinnitus is difficult to treat, hence the frustration for patient and physician, but there are treatment modalities. (p260)

Chapter 20: Disturbances of Taste and Smell

Question 20-1:
Impaired olfactory testing can be a clinical finding of which of the following neurologic disorders?

1. Alzheimer's disease
2. Multiple sclerosis
3. Parkinson's disease
4. Olfactory groove meningioma

Select: A = 1, 2, 3. B = 1, 3. C = 2, 4. D = 4 only. E = All

Question 20-2:
Taste afferents from the posterior third of the tongue are carried in which of the following nerves?

A. Vagus
B. Lingual nerve
C. Trigeminal nerve
D. Glossopharyngeal nerve
E. Nervus intermedius

Question 20-3:
Which of the following statements regarding taste and smell after trauma are true?

1. Most patients with anosmia after head injury recover their olfactory function.
2. A common mechanism of anosmia after head injury is shearing of the olfactory nerves at the cribriform plate.
3. Taste loss is common after head injury.
4. Traumatic loss of taste may be associated with numbness of the tongue as well.

Select: A = 1, 2, 3. B = 1, 3. C = 2, 4. D = 4 only. E = All

Answer 20-1: E.

These disorders are all associated with olfactory findings, although not in all patients. The obvious answer is olfactory groove meningioma, but the anosmia may not be perceived by the patient if the damage is unilateral; specific testing is required. MS is associated with olfactory abnormalities in 40% of patients and correlates with the number of plaques in the inferior frontal and temporal regions. Alzheimer's disease and Parkinson's disease are two neurodegenerative conditions that frequently have olfactory deficits. (p265-266)

Answer 20-2: D.

The glossopharyngeal nerve (CN-9) carries the taste afferents from the posterior third of the tongue, pharynx, and soft palate. (p267)

Answer 20-3: C.

Shearing of the olfactory nerves is a common mechanism of olfactory loss after head injury, with inferior frontal fractures and direct contusion being other mechanisms. Traumatic loss of taste can be associated with numbness of the tongue if the lingual nerve is directly damaged, which can rarely occur with jaw fractures. Unfortunately, most patients with post-traumatic anosmia do not recover, and the chance of recovery declines with increasing time without recovery. Traumatic loss of taste is much less common than loss of smell. Patients may complain of loss of taste, but loss of smell is the usual cause of this perception. (p265, 268)

Chapter 21: Disturbances of Lower Cranial Nerves

Question 21-1:
Axons in the facial nerve supply all of the following functions except which?

A. Submandibular gland
B. Palatine gland
C. Lacrimal gland
D. Parotid gland

Question 21-2:
The facial nerve supplies all of the following functions except which?

A. Efferent to the levator palpabra superioris
B. Efferent to the depressor angularis oris
C. Afferents to the nucleus solitarius
D. Efferents from the superior salivatory nuclei

Question 21-3:
Which of the following are true regarding facial palsy?

1. Hyperacusis is due to dysfunction of the tensor tympani.
2. Ramsay-Hunt syndrome is due to zoster of the geniculate ganglion.
3. Bell's palsy with complete paresis at onset has a poor prognosis with less than 50% recovery.
4. Bell's palsy is increased in incidence during pregnancy.

Select: A = 1, 2, 3. B = 1, 3. C = 2, 4. D = 4 only. E = All

Question 21-4:
Which of the following statements are true for the glossopharyngeal nerve?

1. It exits the brainstem in the medulla.
2. The stylopharyngeus is not testable on routine examination.
3. The tympanic nerve is the first branch of the glossopharyngeal.
4. The glossopharyngeal nerve carries afferents for the gag reflex.

Select: A = 1, 2, 3. B = 1, 3. C = 2, 4. D = 4 only. E = All

Question 21-5:
Which of the following are recognized causes of spinal accessory nerve palsy?

1. Radiation therapy
2. Carotid dissection
3. Neck lymph node dissections
4. Shoulder injuries

Select: A = 1, 2, 3. B = 1, 3. C = 2, 4. D = 4 only. E = All

Question 21-6:
Which of the following structures pass through the jugular foramen?

1. CN-9
2. CN-10
3. CN-11
4. CN-12

Select: A = 1, 2, 3. B = 1, 3. C = 2, 4. D = 4 only. E = All

Answer 21-1: D.
All of these glands are supplied by axons of the facial nerve except the parotid gland, which is supplied by branches of the glossopharyngeal nerve which travel with branches of the trigeminal nerve. Visceral efferent fibers of the facial nerve depart from the superior salivatory nucleus. Some of these join the greater superficial petrosal nerve to the sphenopalatine ganglion to supply the lacrimal and palatine glands. Other efferents travel in the chorda tympani to supply the submandibular gland. (p271)

Answer 21-2: A.
The levator palpabra superioris is supplied by branches of the oculomotor nerve and is the only facial muscle not supplied by the facial nerve. All of the other listed functions are supplied by the facial nerve including innervation of the depressor angularis oris. Afferents to the nucleus solitarius carry taste from the anterior 2/3 of the tongue. Efferents from the superior salivatory nucleus supply the salivary glands. (p271-272)

Answer 21-3: C.
Ramsay-Hunt syndrome is varicella zoster involvement of the geniculate ganglion. The prognosis is poorer than with garden-variety Bell's palsy. Hyperacusis is due to dysfunction of the stapedius muscle. About 70% of patients with complete paresis at onset have full recovery; the prognosis is even better for patients with incomplete paresis at onset. Bell's palsy is four times more likely during pregnancy and the postpartum period than in controls. (p274)

Answer 21-4: E.
All of these statements are true. The glossopharyngeal nerve exits the brainstem between the inferior olive and the inferior cerebellar peduncle in the medulla. The stylopharyngeus is not routinely testable. The tympanic nerve is the first branch of the glossopharyngeal after it exits the jugular foramen. The afferents of the gag reflex are carried in the glossopharyngeal nerve and the efferents are carried in the vagus. (p276-277)

Answer 21-5: E.
All of these can produce injury to the spinal accessory nerve, producing a droopy shoulder and impaired abduction of the arm. Patients will have pain in the shoulder and neck area and difficulty with stabilization of the scapula. Radiation therapy to the neck and shoulder typically has a greater effect on nerves in the upper part of the neck, including the upper plexus and spinal accessory nerve. Carotid dissection can produce spinal accessory nerve palsy, although this is not a consistent finding. Lymph node dissections in the posterior triangle and shoulder injuries with downward displacement of the shoulder are the most common causes of spinal accessory nerve damage. (p279)

Answer 21-6: A.
The glossopharyngeal (CN-9), vagus (CN-10), and spinal accessory (CN-11) nerves pass through the jugular foramen on the way to the retropharyngeal space. The hypoglossal nerve (CN-12) passes through the hypoglossal canal medial and posterior to the jugular foramen. After exiting the skull, the hypoglossal nerve is in proximity to these other nerves. (p283)

Chapter 22: Cranial and Facial Pain

Questions 22-1 through 22-5:
Below are some important headache diagnoses. For the mini-vignettes, select the one diagnosis which is most likely. Note that the vignettes may not represent the most typical presentations of these disorders.

  A. Classic migraine (migraine with aura)
  B. Common migraine (migraine without aura)
  C. Complicated migraine
  D. Cluster headache
  E. Hemicrania continua
  F. Temporal arteritis
  G. Pseudotumor cerebri
  H. Venous sinus thrombosis
  I. Subarachnoid hemorrhage
  J. Brain tumor

Question 22-1:
A 23-year-old female presents with severe headache with prominence in the retroauricular area. Headache began 2 days ago; today has mild right hemiparesis.

Question 22-2:
A 48-year-old man has a headache in the left peri-orbital region. He has had similar headaches for years. The headaches last 30-45 minutes, can occur multiple times per day, and may awaken him from sleep. He has never gone for more than a few days without the headaches.

Question 22-3:
A 30-year-old man presents with acute onset of headache during intercourse. It is a throbbing pain, associated with nausea, vomiting, and photophobia. Examination is normal except for elevated blood pressure and marked tenderness and stiffness of the neck. Headache is relieved by an injection of sumatriptan.

Question 22-4:
A 34-year-old female presents with a third episode of headache which is preceded by expressive difficulty. The language disturbance abates while the headache phase is developing. Examination during the headache is normal except for distress and obvious photophobia.

Question 22-5:
A 25-year-old female has a long history of common migraines and would occasionally wake with a headache. She now complains of headaches most commonly in the morning and has difficulty with weakness of her left arm. Examination is normal.

Question 22-6:
Which one of the following statements is true regarding imaging in headache?

  A. MRI is the imaging modality of choice for most patients with acute onset of headache.
  B. CT may show areas of decreased attenuation in prolonged migraine.
  C. Magnetic resonance angiography on modern machines can show virtually all aneurysms.
  D. MRI is superior to CT in delineation of clinically significant sinus disease.
  E. Skull films can eliminate many important causes of subacute and chronic headache.

Answer 22-1: H.
Venous sinus thrombosis is the most likely diagnosis. This condition typically presents with progressive headache, out of proportion to any previous headaches. Focal signs and/or seizures may develop and strongly suggest the diagnosis when present. Brain tumor would also have to be considered, although the progression would typically not be so fast. (p286)

Answer 22-2: D.
Cluster headache is suspected by the brief unilateral periorbital headaches. While they are referred to as cluster, not all patients have headache remissions, as with this patient with chronic cluster. The awakening from sleep is atypical for most headache types but is typical for cluster headache. (p286)

Answer 22-3: I.
Subarachnoid hemorrhage is most likely because of the abrupt onset, severity, neck stiffness, and onset during intercourse. Coital headache can present similarly but is usually not associated with prominent neck symptoms. The response to sumatriptan is not diagnostic of migraine, since patients with subarachnoid hemorrhage and other serious causes of headache may respond to the triptans. Therefore, a therapeutic trial with triptans is not warranted. (p286)

Answer 22-4: A.
Classic migraine presents with focal neurologic signs or symptoms before the headache, and the most common are visual. However, somatosensory, motor, and even language symptoms may occur. (p287)

Answer 22-5: J.
Brain tumor would be most likely in the scenario of a patient with morning headache, especially if she complains of focal neurologic deficits. The previous migraines are not reassuring, since migraines would not be expected to produce daily morning headaches. Pseudotumor would be the most likely alternative diagnosis from this list, but papilledema would be expected, and the examination was described as normal. While visual deficits are common with pseudotumor cerebri, focal weakness does not occur. (p289)

Answer 22-6: B.
CT may occasionally show regions of decreased attenuation with prolonged migraine, lasting several days, which resolves following resolution of the headache. This is an unusual finding. In general, brain imaging is not needed for most patients with headache, but when atypical features are present, imaging with CT may be indicated. (p289-290)

Chapter 23: Brainstem Syndromes

Question 23-1:
Which of the following are components of the dorsal midbrain (Parinaud's) syndrome?

1. Loss of upgaze
2. Lid retraction
3. Light-near dissociation of pupil response
4. Convergence-retraction nystagmus

Select: A = 1, 2, 3. B = 1, 3. C = 2, 4. D = 4 only. E = All

Question 23-2:
Internuclear ophthalmoplegia is characterized by all of the following features except which?

A. Medial rectus palsy may produce similar clinical findings.
B. Skew deviation can develop in patients with INO.
C. The lesion is of the MLF ipsilateral to the side of the adduction weakness.
D. Most patients with INO complain of horizontal diplopia.
E. Vertical pursuit is impaired in most patients with INO.

Question 23-3:
Potential causes of internuclear ophthalmoplegia include which of the following?

1. Multiple sclerosis
2. Cerebral hemorrhage with herniation
3. Lacunar infarction
4. Myasthenia gravis

Select: A = 1, 2, 3. B = 1, 3. C = 2, 4. D = 4 only. E = All

Question 23-4:
A patient presents with left-body hemisensory loss associated with pain in the same distribution. The pain is always present but is exacerbated by sensory stimulation. There is no weakness or reflex abnormality. Which is the correct diagnosis?

A. Diencephalic syndrome
B. Thalamic syndrome
C. Parinaud's syndrome
D. One-and-a-half syndrome

Question 23-5:
Lesions at the foramen magnum can produce a variety of motor and sensory findings, which may be subtle initially. Which of the following are true for foramen magnum syndrome?

1. Neck stiffness is common.
2. Relapsing-remitting symptoms indicate MS as the cause.
3. Development of symptoms during pregnancy suggests meningioma.
4. Cranial nerve palsies are common.

Select: A = 1, 2, 3. B = 1, 3. C = 2, 4. D = 4 only. E = All

Answer 23-1: E.
All are true. Dorsal midbrain syndrome has a wide differential diagnosis, but some of the most important causes are pineal tumors, aqueductal stenosis, vascular malformation, stroke, trauma, and MS. The full composite of clinical findings is not always present but may include the four signs listed above. (p294)

Answer 23-2: D.
Most patients with INO do not complain of diplopia, but if they do, horizontal diplopia is the most common variety. All of the other statements are true. Vertical pursuit is commonly affected because the MLF carries information regarding vertical gaze in addition to its relay for lateral gaze. Skew deviation can develop in some patients, and the diplopia may be vertical. (p295)

Answer 23-3: A.
MS and small-vessel disease producing lacunar infarction are typical causes of INO. Brainstem compression from cerebral herniation can also cause INO, a false localizing sign. The physician would expect an intrinsic lesion of the brainstem. Myasthenia gravis can cause ocular motor deficit which might look like INO but is not INO, per se. (p295)

Answer 23-4: B.
Thalamic syndrome may have some transient weakness associated with the sensory loss and pain. The sensory loss may be dissociated, with pain and temperature differentially affected from light touch and vibration. (p297)

Answer 23-5: B.
Neck stiffness and craniocervical junction pain are common in patients with foramen magnum lesions. Meningiomas may grow to the point of becoming symptomatic during pregnancy. While MS typically has a relapsing-remitting presentation, this is not the only disorder, and tumors at the craniocervical junction may have relapsing-remitting symptomatology. This is because the mechanical effects of the mass lesion are altered by posture and movement. (p298)

Questions 23-6 through 23-10:
Following are some important ischemic stroke syndromes. For the mini-vignettes which follow, select the best anatomic localization from the list.

A. Median midbrain
B. Lateral midbrain
C. Medial pons
D. Lateral pons
E. Medial medulla
F. Lateral medulla

Question 23-6:
Ipsilateral paralysis of the tongue. Contralateral hemiparesis sparing face. Contralateral sensory loss sparing face.

Question 23-7:
Ipsilateral appendicular ataxia and internuclear ophthalmoplegia. Contralateral hemiparesis.

Question 23-8:
Ipsilateral appendicular ataxia, Horner's syndrome, facial numbness. Contralateral hemisensory loss, symmetric gag reflex.

Question 23-9:
Ipsilateral facial numbness, Horner's syndrome, appendicular ataxia, dysphagia, and palatal weakness. Contralateral hemisensory loss sparing face.

Question 23-10:
Ipsilateral ptosis. Diplopia. Contralateral hemiparesis and appendicular ataxia.

Answer 23-6: E.
Medial medullary syndrome is due to occlusion of the vertebral artery or one of its branches. Other findings include upbeat nystagmus when the eyes are in the primary position. The sensory loss involves tactile, vibratory, and proprioceptive modalities. (p306)

Answer 23-7: C.
Medial pontine infarct produces the listed findings plus additional symptoms which may reveal the rostro-caudal extent of the lesion. Lower pontine lesions may produce ipsilateral gaze palsy which together with the INO gives the one-and-a-half syndrome. The cause is usually occlusion of a small penetrating branch of the basilar artery. (p304)

Answer 23-8: D.
Lateral pons infarction is usually due to occlusion of branches of the basilar artery which wrap laterally around the brainstem. Other symptoms may include paralysis of ipsilateral muscles of mastication giving chewing difficulty. The normal gag reflex rules out lateral medullary syndrome. Inferior pontine infarction from anterior inferior cerebellar artery occlusion may additionally produce vertigo, nausea, vomiting, and ipsilateral deafness. (p304)

Answer 23-9: F.
The lateral medullary (Wallenberg's) syndrome is usually from occlusion of the posterior inferior cerebellar artery or vertebral artery. Classic findings are listed in the question and may also include loss of ipsilateral taste and possible numbness on the contralateral face, as well. Vertigo, nausea, and vomiting are common. (p306)

Answer 23-10: A.
Medial midbrain infarction is usually due to occlusion of small penetrating branches of the basilar artery or mesencephalic arteries. Other signs may include supranuclear gaze paresis. Third nerve palsy is the critical clue to localization. (p302)

Chapter 24: Ataxic Disorders

Question 24-1:
A patient presents with chronic cerebellar ataxia affecting gait and limb movements. Further examination also reveals ptosis and incomplete external ophthalmoplegia. Which of the following diagnoses is most likely?

A. Wernicke's encephalopathy
B. Mitochondrial encephalomyopathy
C. Ataxia-telangiectasia
D. Niemann-Pick disease type C
E. Multiple sclerosis

Question 24-2:
Nystagmus is expected with dysfunction of which component of the cerebellum?

A. Cerebrocerebellum
B. Spinocerebellum
C. Vestibulocerebellum
D. Vermis
E. All of the above

Question 24-3:
Cardiomyopathy associated with cerebellar ataxia suggests which of the following conditions?

A. Leigh disease
B. Mitochondrial encephalomyopathy
C. Adrenoleukomyeloneuropathy
D. Friedreich's ataxia

Question 24-4:
Which of the following conditions could be reasonably suspected in a patient with episodic ataxia?

1. Vertebrobasilar TIAs
2. Drug ingestion
3. Multiple sclerosis
4. Colloid cyst

Select: A = 1, 2, 3. B = 1, 3. C = 2, 4. D = 4 only. E = All

Answer 24-1: B.
External ophthalmoplegia plus cerebellar ataxia suggests mitochondrial encephalomyopathy. The lack of acute presentation would argue against Wernicke's encephalopathy. Ataxia-telangiectasia produces ataxia plus ocular motor apraxia and inability to suppress the vestibulo-ocular reflex, giving a particular head-thrusting movement. Niemann-Pick disease type C can produce supranuclear gaze palsies. Ptosis would be unexpected in multiple sclerosis. (p314)

Answer 24-2: C.
Damage to the vestibulocerebellum is associated with nystagmus, whereas damage to other newer portions of the cerebellum typically produce ataxia without nystagmus. In addition, damage to the vestibulocerebellum can produce inability to suppress the vestibulo-ocular reflex. (p313)

Answer 24-3: D.
Friedreich's ataxia is associated with cardiomyopathy. Mitochondrial encephalomyopathies may have cardiac involvement, but the problem is typically conduction defect rather than cardiomyopathy. (p315)

Answer 24-4: E.
All of these are potential causes of episodic ataxia. Colloid cyst can produce intermittent ventricular obstruction. Other causes could include dominantly inherited periodic ataxia, urea cycle abnormalities, aminoaciduria, Leigh disease, and mitochondrial encephalomyopathies. (p316)

Chapter 25: Movement Disorders: Symptoms

Questions 25-1 through 25-3:
The following are some important types of tremor. For each of the mini-vignettes that follow, select the most likely diagnosis.

A. Parkinson's tremor
B. Physiologic tremor
C. Essential tremor
D. Dystonic tremor
E. Orthostatic tremor

Question 25-1:
A 74-year-old man presents with tremor which is prominent in the legs upon prolonged standing. It is relieved by walking or sitting.

Question 25-2:
A 36-year-old woman complains of tremor of the hands when she eats or does fine manipulative activities. The tremor may interfere with her fine manipulative skills.

Question 25-3:
A 72-year-old man complains of tremor of the hands which is almost always present. It is most prominent when he is walking or at rest, and less prominent when using his hands.

Question 25-4:
Tardive dyskinesia is characterized by all of the following features except:

A. Movements are repetitive and stereotyped.
B. Oro-buccal-lingual dyskinesias are a common manifestation.
C. Most patients manifest impersistence of tongue protrusion.
D. Gait is not markedly impaired as part of the disease process.
E. Movements can be voluntarily suppressed.

Question 25-5:
A 42-year-old man has episodes of brief single muscle jerks without disturbance of consciousness. The episodes have been present for years, although gradually worsening. He has found that alcohol has some beneficial effect on the symptoms. There is no family history. Examination is normal except for some very mild dystonia affecting the right arm, evident when he is walking. Which is the most likely diagnosis?

A. Hepatic failure
B. Essential myoclonus
C. Ramsay Hunt syndrome
D. Huntington's disease
E. Cortical-basal-ganglionic degeneration

Questions 25-6 through 25-8:
Below are some common conditions which affect leg movement. For each of the following questions, select the best answer.

A. Restless legs syndrome
B. Akathisia
C. Painful legs and moving toes
D. Periodic movements of sleep

Question 25-6:
Repetitive, slow movements of the legs in sleep plus occasional myoclonic movements of the feet when awake.

Question 25-7:
Motor restless, with a need to move the legs or walk.

Question 25-8:
Dysesthesias are common, along with burning pain. Patient has a subjective need to move the legs.

Answer 25-1: E.
Orthostatic tremor typically manifests in the legs with prolonged standing. Most patients have relief with walking or sitting. This is an unusual tremor in clinical practice partly because patients seldom complain of it to their physician, and when the tremor is not observed in the primary care physician's office, referral to a neurologist is unlikely to be made. (p325)

Answer 25-2: C.
Essential tremor produces tremor which is noticed predominantly in the hands and is prominent with activity. While essential tremor is a minor annoyance for many patients, for others it can interfere with occupational skills or activities of daily living. (p325)

Answer 25-3: A.
Parkinson's tremor is the most likely diagnosis. He has the typical resting tremor of the hands which is damped by activity involving the hands. Walking and standing do not dampen the tremor in the way that limb activity does. (p324)

Answer 25-4: C.
Most patients with TD do not have impersistence of tongue protrusion despite even marked oral dyskinesias. Impersistence is more commonly seen in Huntington's disease. Movements commonly affect oral, buccal, and lingual muscles and are typically repetitive and stereotyped. Gait is surprisingly unaffected, despite the movements. The movements can be voluntarily suppressed for brief periods, but they return when the patient attends to other tasks. (p329-330)

Answer 25-5: B.
Essential myoclonus is characterized by brief muscle jerks which are present over years. Many patients have a positive family history. Dystonia can be an associated finding. Ethanol may help not only the myoclonus but also the dystonia. (p336)

Answer 25-6: D.
Periodic movements of sleep are slow movements which may arouse the patient. Patients may also have some myoclonic movements of the feet in the waking state. (p337)

Answer 25-7: B.
Akathisia is characterized by a need to move without specific sensory symptoms. This is commonly related to neuroleptic therapy, but can also occur with SSRIs and in Parkinson's disease. (p337)

Answer 25-8: A.
Restless legs syndrome is typically associated with a pins-and-needles sensation and burning pain. The other conditions usually do not have sensory involvement. (p337)

Chapter 26: Walking Disorders

Question 26-1:
Difficulty in initiating gait is seen in which of the following conditions?

1. Sensory ataxia
2. Frontal lobe dysfunction
3. Spastic gait
4. Parkinson's disease

Select: A = 1, 2, 3. B = 1, 3. C = 2, 4. D = 4 only. E = All

Question 26-2:
Which of the following features suggest secondary (symptomatic) parkinsonism rather than idiopathic Parkinson's disease?

1. Lack of festination
2. Lack of hesitation on gait initiation
3. Broad-based gait
4. Lack of freezing episodes

Select: A = 1, 2, 3. B = 1, 3. C = 2, 4. D = 4 only. E = All

Question 26-3:
Dopa-responsive dystonia is characterized by all of the following except which?

A. Brisk tendon reflexes
B. Dystonia is prominent in the legs
C. Onset in childhood
D. Diurnal fluctuation, worse later in the day
E. Develop after arising from a chair and initiating gait

Question 26-4:
Frontal ataxia has a broad differential diagnosis. Which of the following statements are true for ataxia due to frontal lobe dysfunction?

1. Bradykinesia is common.
2. Rigidity is common.
3. Gait is narrow based with short steps.
4. Brisk reflexes are commonly present.

Select: A = 1, 2, 3. B = 1, 3. C = 2, 4. D = 4 only. E = All

Question 26-5:
Which of the following are true for cerebellar ataxia?

1. Hemisphere lesions produce predominantly appendicular ataxia
2. Paraneoplastic cerebellar degeneration may cause predominantly gait and leg ataxia, relatively sparing arm coordination.
3. Ataxia due to lesion of the vermis may have relatively preserved appendicular coordination.
4. The phylogenetically oldest portion of the cerebellum serves appendicular coordination.

Select: A = 1, 2, 3. B = 1, 3. C = 2, 4. D = 4 only. E = All

Answer 26-1: C.
Both frontal lobe dysfunction and Parkinson's disease may produce difficulty in initiating gait. Other parkinsonism syndromes may have this as well, such as progressive supranuclear palsy, but it is not as prominent as in Parkinson's disease. (p344)

Answer 26-2: B.
Lack of festination and wider-based gait suggest that a patient with an otherwise parkinsonian gait has secondary parkinsonism rather than idiopathic Parkinson's disease. Difficulty with gait initiation and freezing are commonly seen in secondary parkinsonism, so they cannot be used as distinguishing features. (p348)

Answer 26-3: E.
Dystonia which develops mainly after arising from a chair and initiating gait is kinesigenic rather than dopa-responsive. All of the other features are characteristic of patients with dopa-responsive dystonia. However, predicting who will respond is so imprecise that therapeutic trial in any child with leg dystonia is warranted. (p349)

Answer 26-4: E.
All of these are true for frontal lobe ataxia. The gait may superficially resemble parkinsonism. The rigidity is often termed gegenhalten, and has a different character than the cogwheel rigidity of parkinsonism. (p345)

Answer 26-5: A.
Lesions of the cerebellar hemisphere produce predominantly limb incoordination rather than gait ataxia. Vermis lesions produce predominantly gait ataxia with relative preservation of appendicular coordination. Paraneoplastic cerebellar degeneration commonly produces gait and leg ataxia. (p347)

Chapter 27: Hemiplegia and Monoplegia

Question 27-1:
Which clinical findings suggest L5 radiculopathy?

1. Weakness of extensor hallucis longus
2. Weakness of flexion of the big toe
3. Loss of sensation on the dorsum of the foot
4. Decreased ankle reflex

Select: A = 1, 2, 3. B = 1, 3. C = 2, 4. D = 4 only. E = All

Question 27-2:
What is the most likely diagnostic consideration in a patient with arm pain plus weakness of the finger and wrist flexors and interossei?

A. C8 radiculopathy from cervical spondylosis
B. Radiation plexitis
C. Mononeuropathy multiple
D. Tumor infiltration of the brachial plexus

Question 27-3:
Subcortical cause for hemiparesis is suggested by which of the following clinical findings?

A. Pure motor deficit, i.e., no sensory loss
B. Approximately equal weakness of arm and leg
C. Aphasia
D. Neglect
E. Answers A and B

Question 27-4:
All of the following features suggest a central rather than peripheral etiology for arm weakness except which?

A. Finger coordination affected more than strength
B. Increased arm tendon reflexes
C. Pronator drift
D. Absence of sensory deficit

Question 27-5:
EMG is performed on a patient with right arm weakness. Findings are as tabulated below. Where is the lesion?

	Fibs	Polys	Recruit
Extensor digitorum communis	2+	2+	Reduced
Biceps	0	0	Normal
Triceps	0	0	Normal
Brachioradialis	2+	2+	Reduced
Extensor carpi radialis	2+	2+	Reduced
Extensor carpi ulnaris	2+	2+	Reduced
Anconeus	1+	1+	Reduced
Abductor pollicis brevis	0	0	Normal

A. Radial nerve at the spiral groove of the forearm
B. Posterior interosseus nerve
C. Anterior interosseus nerve
D. Posterior cord of brachial plexus

Question 27-6:
Left hemiparesis from a cortical lesion, such as MCA CVA, would be expected to produce all of the following findings except:

A. Deltoid weakness more prominent than hand intrinsic muscle weakness
B. Deficits in visuospatial orientation
C. Depression
D. Left hemianopia
E. Neglect

Answer 27-1: B.

The L5 nerve root innervated the extensor hallucis longus. Weakness of this muscle is the most sensitive and specific finding of L5 radiculopathy. The dermatomal distributions of sensory loss are variable, but in general, sensory loss, when present, is on the dorsum of the foot. Toe flexion is served by intrinsic muscles of the foot which are supplied by the S1 nerve root. The ankle reflex is also predominantly mediated by S1. No reflex abnormalities are common from L5 radiculopathy. (p362)

Answer 27-2: D.

Weakness of the median-innervated finger and wrist flexors plus weakness of the ulnar-innervated intrinsic muscles suggests a single lesion at the brachial plexus. Tumor can infiltrate the brachial plexus, typically from a cancer at the superior pole of the lung, or from lymph node involvement by systemic tumor. This type of tumor is typically quite painful. C8 radiculopathy would be unlikely to produce a profound deficit. Radiation plexitis usually affects the upper plexus rather than the lower plexus, because of lesser attenuation in the superior plexus by surrounding tissues. This type of plexopathy is usually painless, in contrast to tumor infiltration. Mononeuropathy multiplex can produce ipsilateral median and ulnar neuropathies, but when median neuropathy is a component of mononeuropathy multiplex, the involvement is commonly distal to the innervation of the long flexors. (p362)

Answer 27-3: E.

Cortical lesions typically produce sensory as well as motor symptoms, since there is not defined separation of the motor and sensory regions, supplied by different arterial branches. Therefore, pure-motor deficit suggests a subcortical infarction, in the internal capsule, basal ganglia, or brainstem. Since the subcortical tracts lack the topographic organization of the cerebral cortex, the weakness spans the arm and leg approximately equally. Signs of cortical dysfunction are distinctly absent with subcortical infarction, so aphasia (expected with dominant hemisphere cortical lesions) and neglect (expected with non-dominant hemisphere cortical lesions) are absent. (p356)

Answer 27-4: D.

Sensory deficit is variable in both central and peripheral lesions. With some cortical and subcortical lesions, the involvement of sensory systems may be so mild that the motor findings eclipse any sensory findings. With some peripheral lesions, sensory findings may be minimal, especially radial neuropathies, anterior interosseus syndrome, and very distal ulnar neuropathy, after sensory supply to digits 4 and 5 has separated. The other findings are present in patients with central lesions rather than peripheral lesions. Two of the prime clinical features differentiating central from peripheral lesions are coordination and tendon reflexes. Central lesions produce coordination deficit out of proportion to weakness. Central lesions also produce increase in the tendon reflexes of affected muscles, opposite that expected in patients with peripheral lesions. (p365)

Answer 27-5: A.

Radial nerve at the spiral groove of the forearm. Wrist extensors can be impaired by several lesions, the most common of which is compression at the spiral groove, "Saturday night palsy." The posterior interosseus nerve innervates most of the wrist and finger extensors, but it does not supply the brachioradialis and extensor carpi radialis, which are innervated by the radial nerve proximal to the posterior interosseus nerve. The anterior interosseus nerve is a motor branch of the median nerve and does not supply wrist and finger extensors. The posterior cord of the brachial plexus gives rise to the axillary and radial nerves. Because of the proximal location of the lesion, the triceps and anconeus should be affected. In some patients with Saturday night palsy, the innervation to the triceps may be affected; in this instance, preservation of the deltoid signifies that the lesion is distal to the departure of the axillary nerve. (p364)

Answer 27-6: A.

With hemiparesis or monoparesis from cerebral cortical lesions, distal muscles are usually affected more prominently than proximal muscles, especially for the arm. With MCA lesions, proximal muscles of the leg may be more affected than distal muscles because the vascular supply to the proximal leg overlaps between MCA and ACA, whereas cortex serving the lower leg is clearly in the ACA distribution. (p355-357)

Chapter 28: Paraplegia and Spinal Cord Syndromes

Questions 28-1 through 28-4:
Below are listed some clinically important nerve root levels. For the following muscles, select the root which is most responsible for its innervation.

A. C3
B. C4
C. C5
D. C6
E. C7
F. L3
G. L4
H. L5
I. S1

Question 28-1:
Tibialis anterior.

Question 28-2:
Deltoid.

Question 28-3:
Gastrocnemius.

Question 28-4:
Brachioradialis.

Question 28-5:
Which of the following statements regarding dermatomal sensory innervation are true?

1. Digit 5 of the hand is supplied by C8.
2. In the upper chest, the C4 and T2 dermatomes are contiguous.
3. The nipple is at the T4 level.
4. The umbilicus is at the T10 level.

Select: A = 1, 2, 3. B = 1, 3. C = 2, 4. D = 4 only. E = All

Question 28-6:
A lesion of the L2 nerve root would be expected to produce which of the following findings?

1. Sensory loss in the upper thigh
2. Weakness of knee extension
3. Weakness of hip flexion
4. Loss or diminution of knee reflex

Select: A = 1, 2, 3. B = 1, 3. C = 2, 4. D = 4 only. E = All

Question 28-7:
Anterior spinal artery syndrome is associated with which of the following findings?

1. Dysfunction of autonomic pathways
2. Dysfunction of the spinothalamic tracts
3. Dysfunction of the corticospinal tracts
4. Dysfunction of the dorsal columns

Select: A = 1, 2, 3. B = 1, 3. C = 2, 4. D = 4 only. E = All

Answer 28-1: G.
The tibialis anterior is responsible for foot dorsiflexion, and is innervated predominantly by L4, although there is some contribution from L5. (p368)

Answer 28-2: C.
The deltoid is responsible for arm abduction, and receives its major innervation from C5. (p368)

Answer 28-3: I.
The gastrocnemius receives its major innervation from S1, although there are a few fibers from L5. (p368)

Answer 28-4: D.
Brachioradialis is responsible for flexion of the forearm. Major innervation is from C6. (p368)

Answer 28-5: E.
All of the statements are true. Digit 5 is innervated by C8, digit 3 is innervated by C7, and digit 1 (thumb) is innervated by C6. The nipple (T4) and umbilicus (T10) levels are good points to remember. (p369)

Answer 28-6: B.
L2 lesion often produces no sensory loss but, when present, results in sensory loss in the upper thigh. Hip flexion is also affected. However, knee extension is not affected, since little or no innervation to the quadriceps is supplied by L2; most of the innervation is by L3. Similarly, the knee reflex would not be affected by lesion of L2, but rather by lesion of L3 and a contribution of L4. (p370)

Answer 28-7: A.
These three pathways are among the most important pathways affected by the anterior spinal artery syndrome. The dorsal columns are spared. (p375)

Chapter 29: Proximal, Distal, and Generalized Weakness

Question 29-1:
A 36-year-old black male is evaluated for weakness and is found on routine evaluation to have a CK of 480 U/l. Which of the following clinical formulations is most likely?

A. The CK is elevated sufficiently that the differential diagnosis would have to include inflammatory myopathy, muscular dystrophy, and other myopathies.
B. The CK is abnormal, but the low level of increase would be consistent with non-myopathic conditions including denervation and even minor muscle trauma unrelated to the weakness.
C. The CK is normal for age and race, and therefore is not supportive of a primary muscle disorder.

Question 29-2:
Clinical assessment of patients being treated for inflammatory myopathy is key, but which of the following laboratory tests is best for following patients during the treatment regimen?

A. CK
B. EMG
C. Muscle biopsy
D. None of these are helpful

Questions 29-3 through 29-5:
The following questions concern a single patient. Select the best answer for each question on the basis of the information provided, not using information from subsequent questions.

A 27-year-old female presents for evaluation of weakness and is found on examination to have weakness most prominent in the deltoid, biceps, quadriceps, and iliopsoas. Distal muscles are judged to have normal strength. CK is mildly increased. EMG shows some short-duration polyphasic potentials in the right deltoid and biceps, with some longer-duration polyphasic potentials in the right quadriceps.

Question 29-3:
What is the best clinical formulation for the information provided?

A. The patient most likely has a myopathy.
B. The patient most likely has a neuropathy with the CK increase being due to partial denervation.
C. The patient has mixed myopathic and neuropathic findings, which indicates a multi-system disease with both neuronal and muscle involvement.

Question 29-4:
Muscle biopsy is performed to help with the diagnosis. Which muscle would be the best to sample?

A. Left quadriceps
B. Right quadriceps
C. Right deltoid
D. Left gastrocnemius

Question 29-5:
Muscle biopsy is performed and shows inflammatory reaction with scattered fiber necrosis. Perifascicular atrophy is not seen. Which is the most likely diagnosis?

A. Polymyositis
B. Dermatomyositis
C. Limb girdle dystrophy
D. Motoneuron disease

Answer 29-1: C.
There is a substantial difference between the normal values for males vs females and blacks vs non-blacks. Upper limit of normal for a black male is 520 U/l. (p387)

Answer 29-2: A.
CK is the most helpful of these for evaluation of patients during treatment of inflammatory myopathy. CK is expected to decrease as weakness improves. Subsequently, the CK may be helpful when a patient becomes weaker. A second phase of weakness associated with elevated CK suggests exacerbation of the polymyositis, such that increasing immunosuppressant treatment is indicated. On the other hand, if the increased weakness is accompanied by no increase in CK, alternative causes should be considered, such as corticosteroid myopathy or other metabolic causes of weakness. (p387)

Answer 29-3: A.
Myopathy is the most likely diagnosis even though the studies cannot be confirmatory. Biopsy would be the next step in diagnosis. (p388)

Answer 29-4: A.
The left quadriceps would be the best muscle of those listed. Alternatives would be the left deltoid and biceps. The right quadriceps and deltoid should not be biopsied because they were the subjects of recent EMG examination, and changes can accompany the needle sticks. The left gastrocnemius is not optimal for muscle biopsy because of the propensity of this muscle to exhibit some minor pathological changes even in the absence of true disease. (p388)

Answer 29-5: A.
This pathological description is typical for inflammatory myopathy, although the typical features of dermatomyositis are not seen. This biopsy evidence in conjunction with the clinical information already provided makes polymyositis the most likely diagnosis. (p388)

Question 29-6:
Which of the following neuromuscular disorders is least likely to give fluctuating weakness, as opposed to constant (static) weakness?

A. Myasthenia gravis
B. Lambert-Eaton myasthenic syndrome
C. Periodic paralysis
D. ALS

Question 29-7:
Which features are helpful in differentiating ALS from multifocal motor neuropathy?

1. Bulbar deficits suggest ALS rather than MMN.
2. NCV is very different between the conditions.
3. Hyperreflexia suggests ALS rather than MMN.
4. Sensory deficits suggest MMN.

Select: A = 1, 2, 3. B = 1, 3. C = 2, 4. D = 4 only. E = All

Answer 29-6: D.
All patients with neuromuscular disease will have some fluctuations; however, MG, LEMS, and periodic paralysis are the most likely to fluctuate widely in capacity. Patients with ALS are least likely to have variable improvements in function, although with exertion, the fatigue is often a prominent feature. (p390)

Answer 29-7: A.
Sensory deficits are not expected in either condition. The other statements are true and are helpful for differentiating the two disorders. Since the bulbar signs and reflex signs are not invariably present early in ALS, the NCV remains the most important differentiating tool. (p391)

Chapter 30: Muscle Pain and Cramps

Question 30-1:
Which of the following clinical features are typical of polymyalgia rheumatica?

1. Muscle pain
2. Low-grade fever
3. Elevated erythrocyte sedimentation rate
4. Onset in young adult life

Select: A = 1, 2, 3. B = 1, 3. C = 2, 4. D = 4 only. E = All

Question 30-2:
Which of the following agents have been associated with rhabdomyolysis?

1. Simvastatin
2. Propofol
3. Cocaine
4. Lithium

Select: A = 1, 2, 3. B = 1, 3. C = 2, 4. D = 4 only. E = All

Question 30-3:
Myotonia congenita often presents with complaints of muscle cramps. Which of the following best describes the EMG findings in myotonia congenita?

A. Increased insertional activity with myotonic discharges. Spontaneous fibrillation potentials and positive sharp waves with fasciculations. Large-amplitude polyphasic potentials. Reduced recruitment.
B. Normal insertional activity except for myotonic discharges. Polyphasic motor unit potentials. Normal or early recruitment.
C. Normal insertional activity except for myotonic discharges. Normal motor unit potentials. Normal recruitment.
D. Increased insertional activity with myotonic discharges. Low-amplitude polyphasic motor unit potentials. Early recruitment.

Question 30-4:
Which of the following disorders is most likely to produce muscle pain?

A. Becker's muscular dystrophy
B. Lovastatin myopathy
C. Mitochondrial myopathy
D. Duchenne's muscular dystrophy
E. Polymyositis

Question 30-5:
Which of the following disorders which cause muscle cramps are characterized by electrical silence on EMG?

1. Brody's syndrome
2. Hypothyroidism
3. Myophosphorylase deficiency
4. Stiff-man syndrome

Select: A = 1, 2, 3. B = 1, 3. C = 2, 4. D = 4 only. E = All

Answer 30-1: A.
PMR is characterized by pain and stiffness in muscles and joints, often with weight loss and mild fever. Sedimentation rate is often elevated. Onset is usually after age 50. (p400)

Answer 30-2: E.
All of these agents have been associated with producing rhabdomyolysis and may produce a myopathy with chronic use. Ethanol is the most common cause of chemical-induced rhabdomyolysis. While simvastatin was singled out in this question, other statin drugs also have been implicated. (p400)

Answer 30-3: C.
The EMG of patients with myotonia congenita is normal except for the myotonia. (p399)

Answer 30-4: B.
Myopathy secondary to some drugs and ethanol is more likely to produce a painful myopathy with rhabdomyolysis than the other chronic myopathies. While some patients with Becker's dystrophy will have muscle pain, this is usually not a common feature in the dystrophies. Inflammatory myopathies may have pain as a component of the symptoms, especially in patients with connective tissue diseases and in childhood dermatomyositis. (p399)

Answer 30-5: A.
The first three disorders can produce silent cramps on EMG, although thyroid disorders can produce myotonic changes as well. Stiff-man syndrome is characterized by excessive electrical discharges rather than silent cramps. (p399)

Chapter 31: The Floppy Infant

Question 31-1:
Which of the following disorders producing neonatal hypotonia have findings which may be seen in the parents?

1. Congenital myopathy
2. Myotonic dystrophy
3. Neonatal myasthenia gravis
4. Non-ketotic hyperglycinemia

Select: A = 1, 2, 3. B = 1, 3. C = 2, 4. D = 4 only. E = All

Question 31-2:
Which of the following statements are true regarding reflexes in the newborn period?

1. Upgoing plantar responses are normal at this age.
2. Tendon reflexes are usually elicitable shortly after birth.
3. Central hypotonia is associated with normal or exaggerated tendon reflexes.
4. The tonic neck reflex disappears at about 3 months of age.

Select: A = 1, 2, 3. B = 1, 3. C = 2, 4. D = 4 only. E = All

Questions 31-3 through 31-5:
For the following mini-vignettes, select the best answer from the list of potential diagnoses of neonatal hypotonia.

A. Stroke
B. Congenital hypomyelinating neuropathy
C. Congenital myasthenia
D. Cervical spine injury
E. Spinal muscular atrophy

Question 31-3:
Neonate with bilateral flaccid leg and arm weakness. Good suck.

Question 31-4:
Neonate with hypotonia, absent tendon reflexes, and poor suck and respirations. Poor response to sensory stimulation and weakness which is most prominent distally.

Question 31-5:
Diffuse weakness of all extremities, most prominent distally. Poor suck. No sensory involvement. Normal reflexes.

Answer 31-1: A.
The first three may all have physical findings identified in parents. Non-ketotic hyperglycinemia is not associated with findings in parents. Patients with neonatal myasthenia gravis from passive transfer of maternal antibodies have mothers with the stigmata of systemic myasthenia gravis. Parents of neonates with dominantly inherited congenital myopathies may have subtle weakness, a history of anomalies, or a history of delay in walking and achieving other motor milestones. (p410)

Answer 31-2: E.
All of these statements are true. While the hallux may move upward in response to plantar stimulation, this normal response has a different character than the Babinski response; the flaring of the toes is not expected. Tendon reflexes are usually present after birth, although the biceps and ankle reflexes develop after the knee reflex. Patients with substantial hypotonia in the presence of normal or brisk reflexes suggests central hypotonia, i.e., CNS dysfunction. The tonic neck reflex is present at birth and abates by about 3 months. (p407)

Answer 31-3: D.
High cervical spine injury can produce weakness of all extremities, sparing bulbar muscles. Cause is usually birth trauma. (p411)

Answer 31-4: B.
Congenital hypomyelinating neuropathy is the most likely cause of this presentation. Sensory examination is difficult in neonates, but documentation of impaired sensory function makes muscle disorders less likely. The loss of reflexes argues against central disorders. (p411)

Answer 31-5: E.
Spinal muscular atrophy is the most likely listed cause of diffuse weakness with normal reflexes. The normal sensory examination supports this, but the sensory examination is imprecise in neonates. Congenital myasthenia or congenital myopathy could produce similar findings, but hyporeflexia would be expected. Central hypotonia could give similar results but is not on the list; this would usually produce hypotonia which is out of proportion to weakness, whereas with SMA, the weakness is a prominent component to the hypotonia. Other findings suggesting a central cause would be seizures. (p412)

Chapter 32: Sensory Abnormalities of the Limbs, Trunk, and Face

Question 32-1:
Which of the following sensory nerve types carry nociceptive sensation?

1. A-alpha
2. A-delta
3. A-beta
4. C

Select: A = 1, 2, 3. B = 1, 3. C = 2, 4. D = 4 only. E = All

Questions 32-2 through 32-4:
Nerve damage is classified depending on severity. The three basic types are:

A. Neurotmesis
B. Axonotmesis
C. Neurapraxia

For each of the three questions below, select the type of neural injury which best correlates with the statement.

Question 32-2:
Poorest prognosis for good neurologic recovery.

Question 32-3:
Common mechanism of crush injury damage.

Question 32-4:
Mechanism of nerve dysfunction in most compressive injuries.

Question 32-5:
Which of the following nerves is not a branch of the sciatic nerve?

A. Superficial peroneal
B. Saphenous
C. Sural
D. Lateral cutaneous nerve of the calf
E. All are branches of the tibial

Answer 32-1: C.
A-delta and C fibers carry pain information, although they also carry some non-nociceptive information, especially tactile for the A-delta and thermal for the C fibers. A-alpha fibers carry large-fiber tactile information from the skin plus some muscle spindle afferent information. A-beta fibers carry some cutaneous mechanoreceptive information and, in addition, some muscle and joint afferents. (p419)

Answer 32-2: A.
Neurotmesis is the most severe of the mechanisms of neural injury. The nerve trunk is severed so that there is transection of not only the axons but also the myelin and connective tissue supporting structures which would otherwise provide a guide for axonal regeneration. (p421)

Answer 32-3: B.
Axonotmesis is usually due to crush or stretch of the nerve resulting in disruption of the axons without damage to the surrounding connective tissue. Recovery is aided by the connective tissue, although time for axonal regeneration is long. (p421)

Answer 32-4: C.
Neurapraxia is usually due to damage from non-structural causes, with reversible deficit in neuronal conduction. This form has the best prognosis for good neurologic recovery. (p421)

Answer 32-5: B.
The saphenous nerve is a branch of the femoral nerve. The others are all cutaneous branches of the sciatic nerve. (p422)

Chapter 33: Neurological Causes of Bladder, Bowel, and Sexual Dysfunction

Question 33-1:
Which of the following conditions commonly produces erectile dysfunction early in the disease process?

1. Amyloid polyneuropathy
2. Diabetes
3. Multiple sclerosis
4. Parkinson's disease

Select: A = 1, 2, 3. B = 1, 3. C = 2, 4. D = 4 only. E = All

Question 33-2:
A 34-year-old man with probable MS complains of inability to get and maintain an erection during attempted intercourse despite preserved nocturnal erections. Which of the following clinical assessments is most likely to be correct?

A. The patient has psychogenic erectile dysfunction as evidenced by preserved erectile abilities. Causes may include mental status effects of MS or situational depression from the disease.
B. The patient likely has extensive demyelination in the white matter of the frontal lobes which is responsible for conscious erectile function but not nocturnal erections.
C. The patient has an incomplete lesion of the spinal cord which affects descending parasympathetics. Variability in parasympathetic activity may result in the dissociated loss of erectile ability.

Question 33-3:
Sexual dysfunction is common in patients with epilepsy, especially in patients with complex partial seizures. Which of the following sexual dysfunctions are seen with increased frequency in patients with epilepsy?

1. Hypersexuality
2. Decreased sexual interest
3. Erectile dysfunction
4. Fetishism

Select: A = 1, 2, 3. B = 1, 3. C = 2, 4. D = 4 only. E = All

Question 33-4:
Bladder and bowel dysfunction is common in neurodegenerative diseases, including Parkinson's disease. Select the incorrect statement regarding parkinsonism.

A. Bladder dysfunction in PD usually is in the setting of moderate to advanced disease.
B. The most common urodynamic abnormality is detrusor hyperreflexia.
C. Bladder dysfunction in PD is more common than in MSA.
D. Urinary frequency is common.

Question 33-5:
Bladder dysfunction in the absence of other clinical findings is likely to be a finding in which of the following conditions?

A. MS
B. MSA
C. Diabetic neuropathy
D. All of the above

Answer 33-1: E.
All of these have been associated with a high frequency of erectile dysfunction. Approximately 60% of patients with MS and PD have erectile dysfunction. Diabetes mellitus is the most common cause of erectile dysfunction seen in andrology clinics. Amyloidosis produces prominent autonomic involvement with erectile dysfunction as one component. (p436)

Answer 33-2: C.
A dissociation between erections with conscious arousal and nocturnal erections has promoted the idea that the deficit is psychogenic, but with incomplete cord lesions, this discrepancy is possible, and in fact common, with early MS. Cord lesions are correlated more with erectile dysfunction than are hemisphere lesions. (p436)

Answer 33-3: E.
All of these are felt to be of increased prevalence in patients with epilepsy. (p432)

Answer 33-4: C.
Bladder dysfunction is more common in MSA than in PD. All of the other statements are true. In fact, if a patient with parkinsonism has bladder dysfunction out of proportion to the movement disorder, MSA should be considered. (p432)

Answer33-5: B.
In MSA, bladder dysfunction may precede other symptoms by years, whereas for all of the other conditions, bladder dysfunction is expected to be associated with other signs of neurologic dysfunction. In MS, spinal cord involvement correlates with bladder dysfunction, and other signs of myelopathy are expected. In diabetic neuropathy, distal neuropathic symptoms are expected. However, because of the frequency of distal neuropathic findings in diabetics, the onset of bladder dysfunction should not be assumed to be due to neuropathy without other investigation. (p432, 434, 436)

Chapter 34: Arm and Neck Pain

Question 34-1:
Which of the following diagnostic studies is least helpful for diagnosis of acute cervical radiculopathy?

A. EMG
B. MRI
C. CT
D. Myelography

Question 34-2:
A 54-year-old man presents with weakness in the left biceps and deltoid muscles. He initially had severe pain in the shoulder and upper arm radiating to the thumb. The pain has abated, but he is now developing progressive weakness and has loss of the biceps tendon reflex. Except for some dysesthesias and a vague altered sensory perception over the shoulder, there are no sensory findings. Which is the most likely diagnosis?

A. C5 disk herniation
B. C6 disk herniation
C. Neoplastic infiltration of the upper trunk of the brachial plexus
D. Acute brachial plexopathy affecting the C5 and C6 nerve roots

Questions 34-3 through 34-5:
The following three questions concern brachial plexus damage in patients with cancer. In many of these patients, the main differential diagnoses are neoplastic infiltration of the plexus versus radiation plexopathy. For the three questions, select which of the alternatives best applies.

A. Neoplastic infiltration of the plexus
B. Radiation plexopathy
C. Both
D. Neither

Question 34-3:
Myokymia is a common EMG finding.

Question 34-4:
Upper plexus involvement is more prominent.

Question 34-5:
Horner's syndrome is present.

Question 34-6:
Carpal tunnel syndrome would be expected to produce which of the following clinical findings?

1. Electric sensation in digits 1 and 2 with percussion of the wrist crease over the median nerve
2. Decreased sensation over the thenar eminence
3. Increased distal latency of motor fibers to the abductor pollicis brevis
4. Denervation of the median-innervated portion of the flexor digitorum profundus

Select: A = 1, 2, 3. B = 1, 3. C = 2, 4. D = 4 only. E = All

Answer 34-1: A.

The three imaging procedures are likely to support the diagnosis of acutely herniated disk. EMG is a helpful adjunct but may be normal in one third of patients with definite radiculopathy. This is because the changes of acute denervation (fibrillation potentials) take up to 4 weeks to appear, and those of chronic reinnervation (long duration, high amplitude polyphasic potentials) may take several months. Reduced recruitment can be due to pain and does not prove the presence of nerve root damage. (p441)

Answer 34-2: D.

Acute brachial plexopathy is the most likely diagnosis with a history of weakness which develops after a phase of pain. The resolution of the pain is the main clue. Cervical radiculopathy commonly presents with pain prior to the weakness, although the pain would not be expected to abate prior to the weakness. With neoplastic infiltration of the brachial plexus, the lower plexus (lower trunk, medial cord) is more commonly affected. Upper plexus involvement, if it occurs, would not be expected to produce weakness at a time of resolution of the pain; pain is often severe with neoplastic infiltration. (p444)

Answer 34-3: B.

Myokymic discharges have a characteristic appearance and are one of the differentiating features between neoplastic infiltration and radiation plexopathy. (p443)

Answer 34-4: B.

Radiation plexopathy is most likely to be associated with the upper plexus because of the lesser amount of surrounding tissue present to attenuate the radiation. (p443)

Answer 34-5: A.

Neoplastic infiltration is more likely to produce Horner's syndrome than radiation plexopathy because the former most commonly affects the lower plexus carrying the sympathetic efferents, whereas the latter most commonly affects the upper plexus. (p443)

Answer 34-6: B.

Tinel's sign is a dependable clinical sign of CTS. Increased distal latency of motor and sensory axons is a common electrophysiological finding in CTS. However, sensory loss is not present over the thenar eminence, since the palmar branch of the median nerve exits the main trunk of the nerve proximal to the transverse carpal ligament which is implicated in producing median nerve compression with CTS. Denervation of the median-innervated portion of the FDP is not expected since this, too, has its nerve supply proximal to the wrist, by the anterior interosseus nerve. (p446-447)

Chapter 35: Low Back and Lower Limb Pain

Question 35-1:
Which of the following statements regarding lumbar radiculopathy is not true?

A. L3 radiculopathy can produce a depressed knee reflex.
B. Patients with fibromyalgia usually have spine-area pain spanning multiple dermatomal distributions.
C. A knee reflex graded 3 is pathologic and indicates a corticospinal lesion.
D. Weakness of the extensor hallucis may be the only clinical sign of L5 radiculopathy.
E. Isolated back pain without extremity pain, numbness, or weakness is seldom due to focal lumbar radiculopathy.

Question 35-2:
Neurogenic claudication due to spinal stenosis and peripheral arterial claudication can usually be differentiated by history and examination. Which of the following statements are true concerning these entities?

1. Both produce pain which is prominent with walking but is alleviated by sitting.
2. Both can produce distal leg pain.
3. Standing is most likely to alleviate pain of peripheral vascular claudication.
4. Both are related to reduced blood flow and change in metabolic pathways for energy production.

Select: A = 1, 2, 3. B = 1, 3. C = 2, 4. D = 4 only. E = All

Question 35-3:
Which of the following statements is true regarding the straight-leg–raising test?

1. Pain with straight-leg raising of the contralateral leg is more sensitive for radiculopathy than ipsilateral straight-leg raising.
2. Forced dorsiflexion of the foot causes a positive straight-leg–raising test to become positive at a lower angle of inclination.
3. A positive reverse straight-leg–raising test suggests L5 or S1 radiculopathy.
4. Severe pain with straight-leg raising at 90 degrees is less sensitive for radiculopathy than positive response at a lower angle.

Select: A = 1, 2, 3. B = 1, 3. C = 2, 4. D = 4 only. E = All

Questions 35-4 through 35-6:
Most muscles are innervated by more than one nerve root, and some by three or more. For the following three questions, select the nerve root combination which provides the major innervation.

A. L1-L2
B. L2-L3
C. L3-L4
D. L4-L5
E. L5-S1
F. S1-S2

Question 35-4:
Tibialis anterior.

Question 35-5:
Gastrocnemius.

Question 35-6:
Adductor magnus.

Answer 35-1: C.
A knee reflex of 3 is hyperactive but not definitely pathologic. Factors to take into account in assessing the clinical relevance of a grade 3 reflex include state of the patient (e.g., anxious), symmetry of the findings, and comparison to the other reflexes on the same side. An anxious individual with diffuse hyperreflexia probably does not have a corticospinal lesion. The other statements are true. (p454, 456-458)

Answer 35-2: E.
All of these statements are true. Both produce pain which is alleviated by sitting, although patients with peripheral vascular disease will have improvement usually even with standing, as long as the patient is not walking. Both neurogenic claudication and vascular claudication can produce leg pain, although neurogenic claudication is more likely to produce back pain than vascular disease. Vascular claudication is due to changes in metabolism of the ischemic muscle. At least part of the pathophysiology of neurogenic claudication is related to neural ischemia and resultant metabolic changes. (p462)

Answer 35-3: C.
Exacerbation of the straight-leg–raising test by forced foot dorsiflexion is Bragard's test, and results in a positive response at a lower inclination. Straight-leg raising is most sensitive when positive at a level of inclination of 30-70 degrees. A positive straight-leg raising with lifting of the contralateral leg is more specific for lumbar radiculopathy but less sensitive. A positive reverse straight-leg–raising test suggests proximal femoral neuropathy or upper lumbar root damage rather than L5-S1 radiculopathy. (p456)

Answer 35-4: D.
L4 and L5 nerve roots provide motor innervation for the tibialis anterior as well as associated muscles including peroneii via the peroneal nerve. (p453)

Answer 35-5: F.
S1 and S2 provide major innervation for the gastrocnemius and soleus via the tibial nerve. (p453)

Answer 35-6: B.
L2 and L3 supply the adductor magnus and adductor longus through the obturator nerve. (p453)

Chapter 36: Laboratory Investigations in Diagnosis and Management of Neurological Disease

Question 36-1:
Which of the following statements are true regarding vascular imaging studies?

1. Diagnosis of suspected AVM is best performed by MRI with MRA.
2. Duplex ultrasound has diagnostic sensitivity for carotid plaque and ulceration which is comparable to that of conventional angiography.
3. Magnetic resonance angiography tends to overestimate the level of carotid stenosis.
4. Conventional angiography should be performed on all patients with transient cerebral ischemia in the carotid circulation.

Select: A = 1, 2, 3. B = 1, 3. C = 2, 4. D = 4 only. E = All

Question 36-2:
Which of the following statements are true regarding brain biopsy?

1. Biopsy is usually needed to differentiate suspected cerebral degenerative disease if the diagnosis is not obvious clinically.
2. Biopsy for suspected herpes encephalitis is usually not necessary prior to treatment trial with acyclovir.
3. Biopsy should be performed in AIDS patients if toxoplasmosis or CNS lymphoma is suspected.
4. Stereotactic brain biopsy is usually preferable to open biopsy for intraparenchymal lesions.

Select: A = 1, 2, 3. B = 1, 3. C = 2, 4. D = 4 only. E = All

Question 36-3:
Markedly elevated CSF protein content may suggest all of the following except which?

A. Guillain-Barré syndrome
B. Pseudotumor cerebri
C. Chronic inflammatory demyelinative polyradiculoneuropathy
D. Spinal cord compression

Answer 36-1: A.

AVM is best diagnosed by MRI with MRA, although conventional angiography is usually performed prior to surgical or radiosurgical or interventional radiological treatment. Duplex ultrasound can be very sensitive for diagnosis of extracranial carotid disease, although the accuracy depends greatly on the skills of the technician and interpreting physician. MRA is a good tool for evaluating vascular malformations but tends to overestimate the degree of carotid stenosis. Also, small aneurysms may be missed on MRA, which would be visualized on conventional angiography. Cerebral angiography is a useful test for evaluation of patients with suspected high-grade stenosis or ulcerated plaque but does not need to be performed on all patients with transient cerebral ischemia. (p468-469)

Answer 36-2: C.

Biopsy for suspected herpes encephalitis is mainly reserved for atypical cases or cases which do not appear to respond to acyclovir. Imaging with MRI or CT plus CSF findings can usually make the diagnosis, especially since HSV-PCR on the CSF is available with relatively short turnaround. Stereotactic biopsy is usually performed rather than open biopsy unless the suspected etiology, lesion location, and other factors suggest that the lesion might be completely removed. Cerebral degenerative diseases are usually not susceptible to definitive curative treatment, so biopsy is rarely warranted. In AIDS patients, the differentiation between toxoplasmosis and CNS lymphoma is not always easy, but biopsy can await response to empiric treatment for toxoplasmosis. (p469)

Answer 36-3: B.

Pseudotumor cerebri produces increased intracranial pressure but does not result in elevated protein. The other three disorders commonly result in marked increase in CSF protein. (p468)

Chapter 37A: Clinical Neurophysiology: Electroencephalography and Evoked Potentials

Question 37A-1:
Focal attenuation of EEG activity can be suggestive of which of the following disorders?

1. Overlying subdural hematoma
2. Meningioma
3. Old cerebral cortical injury
4. Anoxic encephalopathy

Select: A = 1, 2, 3. B = 1, 3. C = 2, 4. D = 4 only. E = All

Question 37A-2:
A 24-year-old woman has recurrent episodes of loss of consciousness, which clinically seem to be simple faints. The primary care physician orders a Holter monitor, MRI, and EEG. The studies are normal except for the EEG, which shows occasional central spikes without sustained repetitive discharges. Which would be the most appropriate diagnostic and therapeutic formulation?

A. Before deciding on AED treatment, inpatient video-EEG monitoring should be performed.
B. If the patient has a family history of epilepsy, the risk of seizures is sufficiently high that she should be placed on an AED.
C. The patient had a seizure causing the apparent faint and should be placed on an AED.
D. The patient should not be considered for AED treatment unless she develops clinical seizure activity.

Question 37A-3:
Which of the following statements regarding EEG abnormalities and epilepsy are true?

1. Interictal EEG may be consistently normal in patients with definite epilepsy.
2. Approximately 10% of patients without epilepsy have epileptiform discharges on the EEG.
3. EEG results are of prognostic value if a patient with epilepsy has not had seizures for 4 years.
4. Focal slowing suggests the diagnosis of epilepsy even in the absence of spikes.

Select: A = 1, 2, 3. B = 1, 3. C = 2, 4. D = 4 only. E = All

Question 37A-4:
All of the following suggest non-epileptic seizures except which?

A. Muscle artifact without epileptiform discharges during a seizure
B. A 10-Hz posterior rhythm during and immediately after a seizure
C. Seizures occurring multiple times per day until monitoring begins, then no seizures until the monitoring session has ended
D. Seizures only while sleeping and never when awake

Question 37A-5:
EEG is often performed to assess patients in coma. Which of the following statements are true regarding EEG in this setting?

1. A burst suppression pattern indicates a poor prognosis for recovery regardless of cause.
2. Rhythmic epileptiform discharges in the absence of clinical convulsive activity represent CNS destruction rather than actual seizures.
3. Diffuse alpha pattern during apparent coma suggests a psychogenic cause.
4. Periodic discharge patterns after hypoxia indicate a poor prognosis.

Select: A = 1, 2, 3. B = 1, 3. C = 2, 4. D = 4 only. E = All

Answer 37A-1: A.
Anoxic encephalopathy would be expected to produce generalized slowing rather than focal attenuation. The other three are typical differential diagnoses to be considered in patients with focal attenuation. (p475)

Answer 37A-2: D.
The EEG should probably not have been ordered. EEG is not indicated if the clinical history suggests simple faint. Unfortunately, patients may have asymptomatic spikes and sharp waves on their EEG which are detected when the patient has an EEG ordered for a marginal indication, such as a fall, behavioral disorder, or headache. Patients with a family history of seizures are especially likely to have these discharges. The patient should not be placed on AEDs unless she has clinical seizure activity. Inpatient video-EEG monitoring is done mainly for two reasons: 1) differentiating episodes as seizures or pseudoseizures and 2) precise localization of discharge focus prior to seizure surgery. (p475-476)

Answer 37A-3: B.
Interictal EEG is abnormal in the vast majority of patients with epilepsy, although repeat recordings and special techniques may have to be employed, including sleep-deprivation, inpatient video-EEG recording, ambulatory EEG monitoring, sphenoidal electrodes, or subdural electrodes. If a patient is being considered for discontinuation of AED therapy, EEG is of prognostic value, although if the EEG shows some spikes, the patient is not certain to have seizures upon withdrawal of the AED. The percentage of nonepileptic patients with epileptiform discharges on EEG is approximately 2%. Focal slowing suggests a focal structural lesion rather than epilepsy, although epilepsy can coexist. The reverse can also occur, where a focal structural lesion can produce sharp waves and spikes without the patient manifesting clinical seizure activity. (p476)

Answer 37A-4: D.
In general, epileptic seizures are more common during sleep than during the waking state, and nonepileptic seizures occur typically when awake, although there are exceptions to this rule. The other features are typically associated with nonepileptic seizures, with a couple of cautionary notes: Muscle and movement artifact may obscure epileptiform discharges. Seizures happen at unpredictable times, and some patients with real seizures may not have them during a time of monitoring. (p477)

Answer 37A-5: D.
After hypoxia, a periodic discharge pattern, burst-suppression, or alpha coma suggests poor prognosis for good neurologic recovery. However, a burst-suppression pattern can be seen with certain medications and in other conditions that do not have a dismal prognosis. Rhythmic epileptiform discharges on EEG may indicate nonconvulsive seizures, which are probably underdiagnosed in ICU patients. As mentioned already, alpha coma in patients with hypoxia has a poor prognosis for good recovery. The alpha rhythm in coma is central and does not react to passive eye opening, whereas in the awake patient, the alpha is posterior and will react to a variety of external stimuli. (p482-483)

Question 37A-6:
Which of the following statements are true regarding the EEG in aging?

1. The posterior dominant rhythm slows with advancing age.
2. Periodic sharp-wave complexes in a patient with dementia suggests Creutzfeldt-Jakob disease.
3. Normal elderly patients have increases in theta and delta activity.
4. A normal posterior dominant rhythm and absence of other slow activity in a patient with apparent dementia suggests pseudodementia.

Select: A = 1, 2, 3. B = 1, 3. C = 2, 4. D = 4 only. E = All

Question 37A-7:
Which evoked potential modality is least likely to be helpful in identifying a clinically silent lesion in a patient with MS?

A. Visual evoked potentials
B. Somatosensory evoked potentials
C. Brainstem auditory evoked potentials

Question 37A-8:
Which of the following findings would be expected to occur in a patient with acoustic neuroma?

1. Prolongation of the III-V interpeak interval
2. Loss of all waves beyond wave I
3. Loss of all waves including wave I
4. Prolongation of the I-III interpeak interval

Select: A = 1, 2, 3. B = 1, 3. C = 2, 4. D = 4 only. E = All

Answer 37A-6: A.
The posterior dominant rhythm slows slightly with advancing age, and there is an increase in the amount of theta and delta activity. Periodic sharp waves in a patient with dementia are strongly suggestive of CJD. Patients with early AD commonly have normal EEG patterns including a normal posterior dominant rhythm. For this reason, the EEG is only really helpful in differentiating pseudodementia from dementia if abnormal. (p484)

Answer 37A-7: C.
The BAEP is least likely of these three to show a clinically silent lesion in patients with MS. In fact, the VEP and SEP are so much better that performance of the BAEP is not necessary. The MRI can miss a demyelinating lesion in the optic nerve or spinal cord more often than in the brainstem, so these evoked potentials have greater clinical utility for diagnosis of MS. (p490-491)

Answer 37A-8: C.
The typical finding in patients with acoustic neuromas is disruption of conduction beyond wave I, such that the I-III interpeak interval may be prolonged or there may be loss of waves after I. However, wave I is present in these patients. Increased III-V interpeak interval would not be expected since the segment which serves this conduction is in the brainstem. (p489-490)

Chapter 37B: Clinical Neurophysiology: Electrodiagnosis of Neuromuscular Disorders

Question 37B-1:
Demyelinating neuropathy would be expected to produce which of the following neurophysiologic findings?

1. Increased F-wave latency
2. Slowed nerve conduction velocities
3. Increased distal motor latency
4. Dispersal of the compound motor action potential

Select: A = 1, 2, 3. B = 1, 3. C = 2, 4. D = 4 only. E = All

Question 37B-2:
The Martin-Gruber anastomosis is encountered in every busy clinical and EMG practice. While there are several described forms, which of the following are generally true of this anomaly?

1. Median motor fibers cross to the ulnar nerve in the forearm.
2. Median sensory fibers usually do not cross with the motor axons.
3. The CMAP elicited on the thenar eminence by proximal stimulation is of greater magnitude than that elicited by stimulation at the wrist.
4. The collision technique can block conduction of the crossed fibers, allowing for accurate NCV calculation.

Select: A = 1, 2, 3. B = 1, 3. C = 2, 4. D = 4 only. E = All

Question 37B-3:
Which of the following findings would be expected in patients with inflammatory myopathy?

1. Small-amplitude polyphasic motor unit potentials
2. Decreased insertional activity
3. Fibrillation potentials and positive sharp waves
4. Reduced recruitment pattern

Select: A = 1, 2, 3. B = 1, 3. C = 2, 4. D = 4 only. E = All

Question 37B-4:
Increased jitter on single-fiber EMG can occur in all of the following except which?

A. Myasthenia gravis
B. Lambert-Eaton myasthenic syndrome
C. Partial denervation
D. Muscular dystrophy
E. All of the above

Question 37B-5:
Fasciculation potentials have been described in which of the following conditions?

1. ALS
2. SMA
3. Acetylcholinesterase toxicity
4. In the legs in cervical myelopathy

Select: A = 1, 2, 3. B = 1, 3. C = 2, 4. D = 4 only. E = All

Question 37B-6:
Myokymic discharges are common in which of the following disorders?

1. Radiation plexopathy
2. Brainstem tumor
3. Multiple sclerosis
4. Neoplastic infiltration of a plexus

Select: A = 1, 2, 3. B = 1, 3. C = 2, 4. D = 4 only. E = All

Question 37B-7:
Which one of the following statements regarding complex repetitive discharges is true?

A. Pathophysiology is thought to involve synaptic transmission between membrane surfaces.
B. It has a sound suggestive of a dive bomber on an audio monitor.
C. It is specifically associated with axonal neuropathies.
D. Each potential is the discharge of a single muscle fiber.
E. All statements are false.

Answer 37B-1: E.

All of these are expected in patients with demyelinating neuropathy. F-wave latency prolongation indicates increased time for proximal conduction. Increased distal motor latency is another manifestation of the slowed nerve conduction velocities. Dispersal of the compound motor action potential waveform is because the change in conduction velocity is to a different extent in different axons. (p503)

Answer 37B-2: E.

All of the answers are correct. The Martin-Gruber anomaly is suspected when the appearance of the CMAPs with proximal and distal stimulation have a markedly different appearance and magnitude. The collision technique offers correction for the NCV calculation. Sensory fibers may join the motor fibers, but this is not common. (p504)

Answer 37B-3: B.

Inflammatory myopathy is typically characterized by small-amplitude polyphasic potentials with voluntary activation along with spontaneous fibrillation potentials and positive sharp waves at rest. Insertional activity is typically increased rather than decreased, as a manifestation of increased irritability of the membrane. Early recruitment is typical rather than reduced recruitment, the latter being more typical of neuropathic processes. (p518)

Answer 37B-4: E.

All of these conditions can produce increased jitter on single-fiber EMG. While neuromuscular transmission defects such as myasthenia gravis and Lambert-Eaton myasthenic syndrome are the classically described causes of increased jitter, denervation can be, as well. (p510)

Answer 37B-5: E.

Fasciculations can be seen with any of these conditions. The first two, forms of motoneuron disease, typically produce fasciculations. Acetylcholinesterase produces fasciculations due to hyperstimulation at the neuromuscular junction. Cervical myelopathy produces fasciculations by loss of descending control over segmental reflex systems. In this circumstance, the fasciculations are generated by discharge originating in the spinal cord rather than at the motor endplate. (p513)

Answer 37B-6: A.

Neoplastic infiltration typically does not produce myokymic discharges, a fact that helps to differentiate this condition from radiation plexopathy, in which myokymic discharges are common. Brainstem tumor and MS may produce facial myokymia. (p513)

Answer 37B-7: E.

All of the answers are false. The pathophysiology is thought to involve nonsynaptic (ephaptic) transmission between membrane surfaces, such that adjacent muscle fibers are activated; therefore, each potential is the sum of several muscle fiber action potentials. Complex repetitive discharges can occur in axonal neuropathies, but this is by no means a specific finding, and can occur in neuropathies as well as a variety of myopathies. (p513)

Questions 37B-8 through 37B-10:
The next 3 questions deal with motor unit potential characteristics. For the mini-vignettes, select the best answer from the following list:

A. Myopathy
B. Neuropathy
C. Both
D. Neither

Question 37B-8:
Brief, small-amplitude polyphasic potentials are typical.

Question 37B-9:
High-amplitude, long-duration polyphasic potentials are typical.

Question 37B-10:
Doublet potentials may be seen.

Answer 37B-8: A.
Brief, small-amplitude polyphasic potentials are typically seen in patients with myopathy, although some motor units with a myopathic appearance can occasionally be seen in patients with neuropathy. (p515)

Answer 37B-9: B.
Neuropathy typically produces high-amplitude, long-duration polyphasic potentials. Neuropathy can cause some motor unit potentials to appear myopathic, but myopathy does not cause neuropathic motor unit potentials. (p515)

Answer 37B-10: C.
Doublet motor unit potentials may occur in neuropathy and in some myopathies, especially myotonic dystrophy. (p514)

Chapter 38A: Neuroimaging: Structural Neuroimaging

Question 38A-1:
A 76-year-old man presents for evaluation of dementia. MRI shows atrophy which is somewhat more pronounced than would be expected for age with symmetric enlargement of the temporal horns and sylvian fissures. There are multiple small areas of increased signal intensity on T2-weighted images in the periventricular white matter. Which is the most likely diagnosis?

A. Vascular dementia
B. Alzheimer's disease
C. Multiple sclerosis
D. None of these

Question 38A-2:
A patient with profound hyponatremia is admitted and treated with 3% saline. He develops bulbar dysfunction followed by corticospinal tract signs. MRI is performed which shows extensive regions of increased signal intensity on T2-weighted images in the pons but also in the white matter of the hemispheres. Which is the most likely diagnosis?

A. Multiple sclerosis
B. Acute disseminated encephalomyelitis
C. Central pontine myelinolysis
D. Small-vessel infarcts from vasculitis

Question 38A-3:
A 32-year-old female is evaluated for suspected neurologic complications of Lyme disease. She has positive Lyme serology, but there is no history that can be elicited for a rash. MRI shows areas of increased signal intensity on T2-weighted images, some of which enhance. In addition, there is some enhancement of the basilar meninges. Which is the most likely diagnosis?

A. Multiple sclerosis
B. Lyme disease
C. Adrenoleukodystrophy
D. Cryptococcal meningitis
E. Acute disseminated encephalomyelitis

Question 38A-4:
Which of the following features are helpful for differentiation of PML from HIV-related demyelination on MRI?

1. HIV-related demyelination in the absence of PML is uncommon, present in less than 15% of patients with AIDS.
2. HIV-related demyelination is more subcortical, whereas PML is more periventricular.
3. HIV-related demyelination develops at a later stage of the disease whereas PML is usually an early complication.
4. HIV-related demyelination is more symmetric while PML is more multifocal and patchy.

Select: A = 1, 2, 3. B = 1, 3. C = 2, 4. D = 4 only. E = All

Question 38A-5:
A 34-year-old male with AIDS presents with headache and confusion and is found on MRI to have areas of low signal on T1-weighted images which are bright on T2-weighted images. These are found in the basal ganglia, midbrain, and dentate nuclei. Neither these lesions nor the meninges enhance. Which of the following is the most likely diagnosis?

A. HIV encephalopathy
B. Toxoplasmosis
C. Cryptococcal meningitis
D. PML

Question 38A-6:
Hydrocephalus in children due to aqueductal stenosis is usually due to what condition?

A. Chiari II malformation
B. Encephalocele
C. Intrauterine infection
D. Idiopathic occurrence

Answer 38A-1: B.
The imaging findings are typical of Alzheimer's disease. The atrophy and white matter changes are common with age, and do not, by themselves, indicate vascular dementia. (p544)

Answer 38A-2: C.
CPM often shows MRI findings not only in the pons but also in the other white matter regions of the brain. Therefore, the extent of the white matter changes should not dissuade the clinician from making the diagnosis of CPM on the basis of this finding. (p547)

Answer 38A-3: B.
Lyme disease is the most likely diagnosis despite the absence of a reported rash. First, not all patients will remember the rash, and second, neurologic complications can develop even in the absence of a rash. The meningeal enhancement would be characteristic of Lyme disease but not of most of the other entities listed here. (p554)

Answer 38A-4: D.
HIV-related demyelination is usually periventricular whereas PML is patchy and usually subcortical. Stage of disease is not helpful for differential diagnosis. HIV-related demyelination is common, with up to 70% of patients with AIDS showing some MRI findings, regardless of neurologic findings. (p557)

Answer 38A-5: C.
This is a typical description for cryptococcal meningitis. The finding of the lesions in the basal ganglia would suggest that the demyelinating lesions of HIV encephalopathy and PML were not present. Cryptococcal meningitis in AIDS patients rarely shows enhancement on MRI because of the failure to mount an inflammatory response. Toxoplasmosis would be expected to produce variable signal characteristics on T2-weighted images plus more prominent enhancement than was described here. (p556-558)

Answer 38A-6: A.
Chiari II malformation is the most common cause of aqueductal stenosis and subsequent hydrocephalus in young children. Tumors, infections, and idiopathic causes are less common. (p561)

Question 38A-7:
Fat suppression techniques on MRI are used for which of the following purposes?

A. Visualization of the extracranial vessels
B. Identification of MS plaques and zones of cerebral edema
C. Visualization of skull based and orbital lesions
D. Identification of aneurysms and vascular formations

Question 38A-8:
Which of the following statements correctly distinguishes the appearance of brain MRI on T2-weighted and Flair images?

A. MS plaques appears bright on T2-weighted images and dark on Flair images.
B. CSF appears bright on T2-weighted images and dark on Flair images.
C. Periventricular white matter vascular disease is more conspicuous on T2-weighted images than Flair images.
D. Flair images are used mainly for uncooperative patients because of the short scan time, whereas T2-weighted images require the patient to remain motionless.

Question 38A-9:
Which are the most common imaging characteristics of medulloblastomas?

A. High-density on CT. Isointense on T2-weighted MRI.
B. Low-density on CT. High-intensity on T2-weighted MRI.
C. Low-density on CT. Low-intensity on T2-weighted MRI.

Question 38A-10:
Which of the following findings on MRI can be seen in patients with Parkinson's disease?

1. Normal for age
2. Decreased width of the pars compacta
3. Altered signal characteristics of the putamen
4. Prominent frontal and temporal atrophy

Select: A = 1, 2, 3. B = 1, 3. C = 2, 4. D = 4 only. E = All

Questions 38A-11 through 38A-15:
The following questions are statements which are True or False. Select the best answer for each question.

Question 38A-11:
MRI is less sensitive to subarachnoid blood than CT.

Question 38A-12:
MRI in acute herpes encephalitis shows increased intensity on T2-weighted images in the anterior temporal and inferior frontal lobes.

Question 38A-13:
Brain MRI is normal in patients with AIDS who do not have neurologic symptoms.

Question 38A-14:
MRI with contrast is the best screening test for cerebral metastases of systemic neoplasm.

Question 38A-15:
Nerve root avulsions may be detected better on post-myelographic CT scanning than on MRI.

Answer 38A-7: C.
Fat suppression techniques are used to visualize structures in normally fat-rich areas. The main applications are in the orbits, skull base, neck, and spinal canal. (p523)

Answer 38A-8: B.
Fluid-attenuated inversion recovery (FLAIR) images produce attenuation of CSF signal, whereas white matter lesions remain bright. This accentuates the appearance of periventricular white matter lesions. CSF is bright on T2-weighted images. MS plaques typically appear bright on both sequences. Echo-planar images are used for uncooperative patients because of the brief scan time. (p524-525)

Answer 38A-9: A.
Medulloblastomas typically have a high-density appearance on uncontrasted CT but substantial enhancement. T2-weighted MRI shows a nearly isointense lesion with a homogenous or mixed appearance. (p532)

Answer 38A-10: A.
Frontal and temporal atrophy are characteristic of Pick's disease rather than Parkinson's disease. The combination of decreased width of the pars compacta and altered signal characteristics of the putamen is most commonly seen in Parkinson's-plus syndromes. (p545)

Answer 38A-11: True.
MRI does not show subarachnoid blood acutely because methemoglobin has not yet formed in sufficient quantities to be visualized. (p551)

Answer 38A-12: True.
MRI is much more sensitive than CT early in herpes encephalitis. Late in the disease, atrophy may be the predominant imaging finding. (p552)

Answer 38A-13: False.
MRI is abnormal in about 70% of patients with AIDS, regardless of the presence of neurologic symptoms. (p557)

Answer 38A-14: True.
MRI is more sensitive than CT for detection of metastases and is the preferred diagnostic procedure for this purpose. A normal contrast-enhanced CT may give a false sense of security. (p528)

Answer 38A-15: True.
CT with intrathecal contrast may show both nerve root avulsions and dural tears more clearly than MRI. (p525)

Chapter 38B: Neuroimaging: Computed Tomographic and Magnetic Resonance Vascular Imaging

Question 38B-1:
Which of the following statements regarding magnetic resonance angiography are true?

1. MRA tends to overestimate the degree of carotid artery stenosis.
2. MRA can detect virtually all intracranial aneurysms in a cooperative patient.
3. MRA and carotid doppler sonography (CDS) have comparable sensitivity and specificity.
4. Flow gap is usually due to technical issues rather than pathology.

Select: A = 1, 2, 3. B = 1, 3. C = 2, 4. D = 4 only. E = All

Question 38B-2:
Which of the following are true regarding comparisons between CT angiography and MRA?

1. CT angiography is less susceptible than MRA to errors introduced by tortuosity of the vessels.
2. CT angiography has better visualization of tandem lesions than MRA.
3. CT angiography has better localization of the level of the carotid bifurcation than MRA.
4. CT angiography is less sensitive for level of moderate- to high-grade stenosis than MRA.

Select: A = 1, 2, 3. B = 1, 3. C = 2, 4. D = 4 only. E = All

Questions 38B-3 through 38B-6:
The following statements are True or False. Select the best answer.

Question 38B-3:
MRA cannot visualize venous thrombosis well.

Question 38B-4:
Spinal vessels cannot usually be visualized well on MRA.

Question 38B-5:
CT angiography provides information on direction of flow which MRA cannot identify.

Question 38B-6:
CT angiography is relatively insensitive for ulcerated plaque.

Answer 38B-1: B.
MRA is frequently used as a screen for aneurysms, but angiography remains the gold standard for evaluation. Small aneurysms may be missed on MRA, although there is currently debate about the clinical importance of these small aneurysms. A flow gap is usually due to restriction of flow but does not necessarily indicate high-grade stenosis. Therefore, the flow gap is not a technical problem, but is not always of significance. (p601-602)

Answer 38B-2: B.
CT angiography is more sensitive for determining the level of moderate to severe carotid stenosis than MRA. Tandem lesions are not as easily seen on CT angiography as on MRA. (p610)

Answer 38B-3: False.
MRA venography with spin-echo imaging is able to establish the diagnosis of venous thrombosis in most cases. (p605)

Answer 38B-4: True.
Spinal vessels usually cannot be visualized because of their small size. (p607)

Answer 38B-5: False.
The statement is backward. MRA provides information on direction of flow which CT angiography cannot provide. (p611)

Answer 38B-6: True.
The limitation of CT angiography in identification of ulcerated plaque is an important limitation of this technique. (p610)

Chapter 38C: Neuroimaging: Radiological Angiography

Question 38C-1:
Which of the following are possible causes of carotid stenosis?

1. Neurofibromatosis
2. Takayasu's arteritis
3. Fibromuscular dysplasia
4. Neurofibromatosis

Select: A = 1, 2, 3. B = 1, 3. C = 2, 4. D = 4 only. E = All

Question 38C-2:
Which of the following statements regarding carotid cavernous fistula are true?

1. It may develop from trauma.
2. It may develop from rupture of a carotid artery aneurysm.
3. It can be treated by balloon embolization.
4. The patient often has no symptoms.

Select: A = 1, 2, 3. B = 1, 3. C = 2, 4. D = 4 only. E = All

Question 38C-3:
Which of the following are associated with increased risk of cerebral aneurysms?

1. Polycystic kidney disease
2. Fibromuscular dysplasia
3. Marfan's syndrome
4. Coarctation of the aorta

Select: A = 1, 2, 3. B = 1, 3. C = 2, 4. D = 4 only. E = All

Questions 38C-4 through 38C-6:
The following questions concern arterial anatomy. Select the best answer from the following list:

A. Aorta
B. Subclavian artery
C. Innominate artery
D. Common carotid artery
E. Internal carotid artery
F. External carotid artery
G. Vertebral artery

Question 38C-4:
The right common carotid artery usually arises from which vessel?

Question 38C-5:
The superior thyroidal artery arises from which vessel?

Question 38C-6:
Which vessel courses through the cavernous sinus?

Answer 38C-1: E.
All of these are potential causes of carotid stenosis, although atherosclerosis and hypertension are more common causes. (p633)

Answer 38C-2: A.
Carotid-cavernous fistula can develop from trauma, rupture of an intracavernous aneurysm, or weakness of the vessel wall. The patient usually hears a bruit and has other symptoms including ptosis and deficits in CN 3, 4, and 6. (p635-636)

Answer 38C-3: E.
All of these are associated with an increased risk of intracranial aneurysms. Other important predisposing factors include Ehlers-Danlos syndrome, collagen vascular disease, neurofibromatosis, and pseudoxanthoma elasticum. (p640)

Answer 38C-4: C.
The right CCA usually arises from bifurcation of the innominate artery. (p619)

Answer 38C-5: F.
The superior thyroidal artery is usually the first branch of the external carotid artery. (p619)

Answer 38C-6: E.
The internal carotid artery has a segment within the cavernous sinus. (p620)

Chapter 38D: Neuroimaging: Ultrasound Imaging of the Cerebral Vasculature

Question 38D-1:
What is the expected sensitivity of carotid duplex ultrasonography for detecting high-grade carotid stenosis?

A. 60%
B. 75%
C. 90%
D. 99%

Question 38D-2:
Which of the following is the best indication of the degree of stenosis?

A. Ultrasound imaging of the vessel walls
B. Flow velocity
C. Volume flow rate
D. None of these

Question 38D-3:
Which of the following are clinical uses for transcranial doppler ultrasonography?

1. Assessment of vasospasm in patients with subarachnoid hemorrhage
2. Search for tandem lesions in patients with CDS evidence of extracranial carotid disease
3. Intraoperative monitoring during carotid endarterectomy
4. Detection of subclavian steal

Select: A = 1, 2, 3. B = 1, 3. C = 2, 4. D = 4 only. E = All

Questions 38D-4 through 38D-6:
The following questions are True or False. Select the best answer.

Question 38D-4:
Ultrasound imaging of the vertebral vessels usually cannot demonstrate stenosis of these vessels.

Question 38D-5:
Increasing carotid artery stenosis produces progressive decrease in velocity of flow.

Question 38D-6:
Calcified plaque may prevent visualization of vascular structures and flow beneath the plaque.

Answer 38D-1: C.
Ideally, ultrasonography should have a 90% sensitivity for detecting tight carotid stenosis. This is a standard which should be met. All laboratories should have assessment procedures to determine that their data are in this general range, since this technique is highly dependent on the abilities of the technician, equipment, and reading physician. (p650)

Answer 38D-2: C.
Volume flow rate is a better correlate to the level of clinically significant stenosis than the other features. This is routinely determined in many labs, especially when initial screening suggests that the stenosis exceeds 50%. (p652)

Answer 38D-3: E.
All of these are clinical uses for TCD. Although not in widespread use, they are in routine clinical use in many institutions. (p657)

Answer 38D-4: True.
The vertebral arteries can usually be identified on ultrasound imaging, but detailed visualization is not possible. There are no current widely accepted criteria for classification of vertebral artery stenosis. (p653)

Answer 38D-5: False.
Increasing stenosis produces increasing velocity of flow, beginning with elevation of peak systolic velocity, and also increasing diastolic velocity with severe stenosis. (p650)

Answer 38D-6: True.
Calcified plaque may block the transmission of the sound waves through the soft tissues, thereby preventing adequate visualization. (p653)

Chapter 38E: Neuroimaging: Functional Neuroimaging

Questions 38E-1 through 38E-4:
The following questions compare functional imaging techniques. For each of the questions, select the best answer from the following list.

A. PET
B. SPECT
C. Functional MRI
D. None of these

Questions 38E-1:
Best spatial resolution.

Questions 38E-2:
A normal study in a patient being evaluated for dementia essentially rules out Alzheimer's disease.

Questions 38E-3:
Least sensitivity to patient cooperation and motion.

Questions 38E-4:
Best absolute quantification of neuronal function.

Question 38E-5:
Which of the following best described the patterns of change in PET in patients with complex partial seizures?

A. Focal zone of hypometabolism in the interictal state which becomes hypermetabolic during seizures
B. Focal zone of hypometabolism in the interictal and ictal state
C. Focal zone of hypermetabolism in the interictal state which becomes hypometabolic during seizures

Answer 38E-1: C.
Functional MRI has the best spatial resolution and SPECT the worst. PET is intermediate between these two extremes. (p666)

Answer 38E-2: D.
Both PET and SPECT commonly show abnormalities in patients with AD, and there are suggestions that pre-symptomatic patients may have abnormalities on functional imaging. However, clinically certain AD may occasionally be associated with a normal PET, so even this technique cannot rule out the diagnosis. (p667)

Answer 38E-3: B.
Functional MRI is the most sensitive to degradation of images by motion, and SPECT is the least sensitive. (p666)

Answer 38E-4: A.
PET is the only one of these techniques which allows for absolute quantification of the metabolism. The other techniques give relative assessments of metabolic data. (p666)

Answer 38E-5: A.
PET typically shows regions of hypometabolism which correlate with the seizure focus. This area develops increased local blood flow and glucose utilization during the seizure. (p671)

Chapter 39: Neuropsychology

Question 39-1:
Memory loss with otherwise relatively normal neurologic function can be caused by which of the following conditions?

1. Herpes encephalitis
2. Anoxia
3. Alcoholism
4. Brain tumor

Select: A = 1, 2, 3. B = 1, 3. C = 2, 4. D = 4 only. E = All

Question 39-2:
Where is the lesion that typically produces Gerstmann's syndrome?

A. Left frontal lobe
B. Left temporal lobe
C. Left parietal lobe
D. Bilateral anterior temporal lobes

Question 39-3:
Which of the following statements regarding visual perceptive deficits are correct?

1. True color perception deficit is due only to congenital retinal abnormality.
2. Ishihara plates are most sensitive for central (CNS) causes of color perceptive deficit.
3. Visual form agnosia prevents patients from navigating through complex environments.
4. Prosopagnosia is usually due to a right posterior cerebral lesion.

Select: A = 1, 2, 3. B = 1, 3. C = 2, 4. D = 4 only. E = All

Question 39-4:
Which of the following statements regarding cortical function are true?

1. Left hemisphere lesions may produce constructional apraxia.
2. Left hemisphere lesions often give more difficulty with writing to dictation than copying written material.
3. Ideomotor apraxia can be manifest on examination as difficulty mimicking the examiner's movements.
4. Left hemisphere neglect does not occur.

Select: A = 1, 2, 3. B = 1, 3. C = 2, 4. D = 4 only. E = All

Question 39-5:
What proportion of left-handed individuals have the left hemisphere dominant for language function?

A. 90%
B. 70%
C. 30%
D. 10%

Answer 39-1: E.
All of these conditions can produce a prominent amnestic syndrome. Herpes encephalitis and alcoholism are the most commonly described causes, although anoxic encephalopathy can produce amnesic syndrome, as well. Tumors can produce this with bilateral limbic-hippocampal or diencephalic involvement directly, as well as a remote effect of systemic neoplasia, i.e., limbic encephalitis. More common unilateral occurrence of tumors would not be expected to produce an amnestic syndrome. (p680)

Answer 39-2: C.
Gerstmann's syndrome is typically due to a lesion in the left parietal lobe. (p687)

Answer 39-3: D.
Only D is correct; prosopagnosia, inability to recognize familiar faces, is due to a right hemisphere lesion, in the posterior region. True color perceptive defect can be due to central lesions as well as retinal lesions. The Ishihara plates are designed to identify predominantly color perceptive deficits related to retinal lesions, but deficits with central processing can also result in abnormal interpretation of the Ishihara plates. Patients with visual-form agnosia are often able to navigate through novel environments despite their deficit in interpretation of forms. (p689-690)

Answer 39-4: A.
Patients with left hemisphere lesions which preserve writing may have writing to dictation impaired more than copying. Ideomotor apraxia is manifest as difficulty performing new tasks as demonstrated by the examiner; this is in contrast to ideational apraxia, which more involves the performance of a sequence of movements composing a previously learned task. Left hemisphere lesions are less likely to produce constructional apraxia than right hemisphere lesions, but this deficit can occur but has a different character than constructional apraxia due to a lesion of the right hemisphere. (p694)

Answer 39-5: B.
Approximately 70% of left-handed individuals have the left hemisphere dominant for language function, in comparison to 96% of right-handed individuals. (p682)

Chapter 40: Neuro-Ophthalmology: Ocular Motor System

Question 40-1:
Which of the following statements are true regarding vestibular control of eye movements?

1. The vestibular system stabilizes gaze during head movements.
2. The vestibular system initiates eye movements in response to a novel visual stimulus.
3. Rotation of the head to the side activates the ampulla of the horizontal semicircular canal on the same side as the rotation.
4. Activation of the horizontal vestibular canal results in excitation of ipsilateral abducens nucleus and inhibition of the contralateral abducens nucleus.

Select: A = 1, 2, 3. B = 1, 3. C = 2, 4. D = 4 only. E = All

Question 40-2:
Which of the following centers coordinates vertical eye movements?

A. Paramedian pontine reticular formation
B. Oculomotor nucleus
C. Edinger-Westphal nucleus
D. Midbrain reticular formation

Question 40-3:
A term newborn with otherwise normal neurologic function is noted to have disconjugate eye movements with episodes of esotropia and other times of exotropia. In the awake state, there is a tendency for the eyes to turn tonically downward, while in the sleeping state the eyes are in the primary position. What is the most likely diagnosis?

A. Anoxic encephalopathy with supranuclear eye movement dysfunction
B. Midbrain hemorrhage
C. Neuroblastoma
D. Normal neonate

Question 40-4:
A patient presents with the following ocular motor deficits: inability to look left with either eye, inability to look right with the left eye, otherwise intact vertical eye movements. Which of the following are true for this patient?

1. The patient most likely has a lesion in the dorsal pons.
2. The patient has one-and-a-half syndrome.
3. The patient has an internuclear ophthalmoplegia.
4. The patient may have ocular myasthenia.

Select: A = 1, 2, 3. B = 1, 3. C = 2, 4. D = 4 only. E = All

Question 40-5:
Which is the most common cause of oculogyric crisis?

A. Post-encephalitic parkinsonism
B. Head injury
C. Neuroleptic use
D. Lithium toxicity

Answer 40-1: B.

The vestibular system is responsible for stabilization of visual fixation during head movements, but not for initiation in response to stimuli, which is the province of the frontal eye fields and associated connections with other cortical areas. A horizontal semicircular canal is stimulated by warming of the ipsilateral ear or rotation of the head to that side. The last statement is exactly backward; stimulation of one horizontal semicircular canal results in activation of the contralateral abducens and inhibition of the ipsilateral abducens nucleus such that the eyes look toward the opposite side. (p700)

Answer 40-2: D.

The MRF provides the supranuclear control of vertical eye movements. The oculomotor nucleus supplies most of the individual muscles involved in vertical eye movements but does not coordinate the movements. The Edinger-Westphal nucleus innervates the sphincter muscle of the pupil and the ciliary muscle. (p706)

Answer 40-3: D.

These findings are normal. Divergent gaze with variation in the magnitude and direction of divergence is common. Tonic downward eye deviation in the awake state with correction in sleep with otherwise normal ocular motor function is present in about 2% of neonates, and probably represents delayed maturation of the ocular motor system. (p707-708)

Answer 40-4: E.

All of the statements are true. The one-and-a-half syndrome is a combination of an INO plus a gaze palsy such that the only intact horizontal eye movement is abduction of the contralateral eye. The most common cause is a lesion of the dorsal pontine tegmentum. Ocular myasthenia can produce similar results if both medial recti and one lateral rectus are affected predominantly. (p714)

Answer 40-5: C.

All of these are potential causes of oculogyric crisis, but neuroleptic use is the most common cause, especially with haloperidol. Other important causes include carbamazepine toxicity, neurosyphilis, and the autosomal dominant rapid-onset dystonia-parkinsonism. (p717)

Chapter 41: Neuro-Ophthalmology: Afferent Visual System

Question 41-1:
What proportion of retinal fibers cross at the chiasm?

A. 23%
B. 47%
C. 53%
D. 57%

Question 41-2:
The primary visual cortex is which Brodman area?

A. Area 16
B. Area 17
C. Area 18
D. Area 19

Question 41-3 through 41-5:
The following are some common locations for lesions which can produce visual field defects. For the mini-vignettes which follow, select the most likely anatomic location.

A. Optic nerve
B. Optic chiasm
C. Posterior optic tract
D. Posterior optic radiations
E. Temporal lobe
F. Occipital lobe
G. None of the above

Question 41-3:
Left eye has a temporal field defect, right eye has little vision in the temporal or nasal field.

Question 41-4:
Left and right eyes have visual field defects which are almost exactly superimposable. Preservation of central vision.

Question 41-5:
Bilateral nasal hemianopia.

Question 41-6:
What effect does hemianopia from an occipital lobe lesion have on visual acuity?

A. None
B. Reduced at the fovea but normal in the unaffected field
C. Reduced through the preserved visual field
D. Varies depending on whether cortex serving central vision is affected

Answer 41-1: C.
Approximately 53% of optic nerve axons cross in the optic chiasm. These subserve the temporal field for each eye. (p721)

Answer 41-2: B.
Area 17 is the primary visual cortex which receives the afferent axons from the optic radiations. From here, projections extend to the visual association areas. (p721)

Answer 41-3: B.
Lesions in or near the optic chiasm can produce markedly incongruous visual field defects. A lesion near the right side of the optic chiasm may affect the crossing fibers from the left eye as well as the entirety of the optic nerve fibers from the right eye. (p728)

Answer 41-4: D.
Lesion of the optic radiations produces congruous hemianopia, in contrast to lesion of the optic tract, which produces incongruous hemianopia. (p728)

Answer 41-5: G.
Binasal hemianopia is usually due to ocular disease such as ischemic optic neuropathy or glaucoma. Occasionally, this defect can be due to hydrocephalus, cranial-based tumors, or other perichiasmal structural lesions. (p728)

Answer 41-6: A.
Isolated hemianopia does not produce a change in visual acuity, although patients may complain of a vague change in vision. They often do not complain of a hemianopia, per se. (p726)

Chapter 42: Neuro-Otology

Question 42-1:
Which of the following is most effective in producing long-term improvement in positional vertigo?

A. Meclizine
B. Cyclizine
C. Scopolamine
D. Promethazine
E. Exercise therapy

Question 42-2:
Which one of the following statements concerning brainstem auditory evoked potentials is true?

A. Increased I-III interpeak latency is a sensitive screen for acoustic neuroma.
B. Absence of all waves is supportive of brain death.
C. Wave I is generated by charge movement in the cochlea.
D. Wave V is generated by thalamocortical projections.

Question 42-3:
A patient with complaint of hearing loss has audiologic evaluation which demonstrates normal speech discrimination at moderate volumes but decreased speech discrimination at high volumes. Which is the most likely clinical correlate to these findings?

A. Cochlear lesion
B. CN-8 lesion
C. Psychogenic hearing loss
D. Normal patient

Answer 42-1: E.

Exercise therapy is the most effective technique for producing long-term improvement in positional vertigo. Meclizine and cyclizine are antihistamines which are commonly used first line, but they have little or no effect on the long-term course of the condition. Scopolamine may be the most effective acute suppressant of positional vertigo. Promethazine is an antiemetic which is helpful for symptom relief but has no effect on long-term symptoms. (p740-741)

Answer 42-2: A.

Acoustic neuroma is strongly suspected in patients with increased I-III interpeak interval, although this finding is not specific, and there are other possible findings. Absence of all waves beyond wave I or distortion of following wave forms can occur, making measurement of this interval impossible. BAEP can be supportive of brain death, but not if there is no wave I, since one cannot rule out failure of transduction of the auditory stimulus to a neural signal. Wave I is generated by the distal portion of CN-8. Wave V is thought to be generated in or near the midbrain. (p739)

Answer 42-3: B.

A retro-cochlear lesion such as an eighth cranial nerve lesion is most likely with a breakdown in speech discrimination at high volumes; this is termed rollover. Cochlear lesion would elevate the threshold, but the rollover would not be expected. (p737)

Chapter 43: Neurourology

Question 43-1:
A 24-year-old female with complaints of urinary incontinence and hesitancy is referred to you by a urologist for neurologic evaluation. Examination shows normal strength, sensation, coordination, and reflexes. Which is the most likely diagnosis?

A. Multiple sclerosis
B. Transverse myelitis
C. Peripheral neuropathy
D. Functional disorder

Question 43-2:
Which of the following drugs are used for detrusor hyperreflexia?

1. Oxybutinin
2. Desmopressin
3. Propantheline
4. Imipramine

Select: A = 1, 2, 3. B = 1, 3. C = 2, 4. D = 4 only. E = All

Question 43-3:
A patient with MS presents with urinary incontinence which initially responds to oxybutinin 5 mg tid. After a few days, the incontinence returns despite the medication. Which is the most likely cause and remedy?

A. The dose of oxybutinin is low and needs to be increased.
B. The patient may now be developing urinary retention which needs intermittent catheterization.
C. The patient had a new MS attack and should be treated with solumedrol.
D. The cause of the exacerbation is psychogenic.

Question 43-4:
A 37-year-old man with spinal cord injury has detrusor hyperreflexia and incomplete emptying. Which of the following treatments would be best for long-term management?

A. Condom catheter
B. Urethral catheter
C. Suprapubic catheter
D. Intermittent catheterization

Question 43-5:
Which of the following statements are true regarding male erectile dysfunction (MED)?

1. Sildenafil (Viagra) is ineffective for patients with myelopathy.
2. Physical methods are generally used before trying vasoactive agents.
3. Normal nocturnal penile tumescence suggests a functional cause to the erectile dysfunction.
4. Patients with male erectile dysfunction often have ejaculatory failure.

Select: A = 1, 2, 3. B = 1, 3. C = 2, 4. D = 4 only. E = All

Answer 43-1: D.
The probability of an organic neurologic disorder when neurologic examination is normal is very low. The most likely diagnosis is functional disorder providing that primary urologic disorders have been ruled out. (p743)

Answer 43-2: E.
All of these agents are used for patients with detrusor hyperreflexia. Oxybutinin and propantheline are used most prominently; desmopressin is not in common use but is a good alternative. Imipramine is also used as second line for some patients. (p752)

Answer 43-3: B.
Patients with myelopathy from MS often have both detrusor hyperreflexia, which responds to oxybutinin, and incipient urinary retention, which may be exacerbated by the anticholinergic medication, resulting in overflow. (p754)

Answer 43-4: D.
Intermittent catheterization is the best choice for most patients in this situation, often in conjunction with an anticholinergic medication. Selected patients may require chronic indwelling catheters, but intermittent catheterization is preferable, especially if the patient has the upper extremity strength and coordination to perform the procedure himself. (p754)

Answer 43-5: D.
MED patients often have associated ejaculatory failure. Sildenafil is the drug of choice for most patients with MED secondary to myelopathy from trauma or MS. Vasoactive agents are usually tried prior to trying physical methods. Normal nocturnal penile tumescence is consistent with a psychogenic diagnosis, but is not diagnostic since patients with incomplete myelopathy may exhibit this finding. (p756)

Chapter 44: Neuroepidemiology

Question 44-1:
Which population group has the highest death rate from stroke?

A. White males
B. White females
C. Black males
D. Black females

Question 44-2:
Which of the following statements are true regarding stroke epidemiology?

1. Rates of stroke death have declined in the United States for all races and both sexes.
2. Incidence of cerebral hemorrhage in Asia is twice that in the West.
3. Death rates from stroke in eastern Europe have increased.
4. Japan has a lower death rate from stroke than the United States.

Select: A = 1, 2, 3. B = 1, 3. C = 2, 4. D = 4 only. E = All

Question 44-3:
Which of the following statements are true for brain tumors in the United States?

1. Incidence peaks at the second to third decade.
2. Approximately 80% of primary brain tumors are gliomas.
3. Five-year survival for childhood primary brain tumors is unchanged.
4. The reported incidence of brain tumors is increasing in the US.

Select: A = 1, 2, 3. B = 1, 3. C = 2, 4. D = 4 only. E = All

Question 44-4:
Which of the following statements are true regarding epidemiology of seizures?

1. Age-specific incidence of epilepsy peaks at the third and fourth decades.
2. Death rate for seizures has declined in recent years.
3. New AEDs have decreased seizure mortality in recent years.
4. There is a greater death rate in patients with epilepsy independent of motor vehicle accidents.

Select: A = 1, 2, 3. B = 1, 3. C = 2, 4. D = 4 only. E = All

Question 44-5:
Which of the following statements regarding febrile seizures is not true?

A. Risk of febrile seizures in the US is approximately 2%.
B. Recurrent seizures occur in about one third of patients with a single febrile seizure.
C. Risk of later epilepsy is approximately 35%.
D. Febrile seizures are more common in males than females.

Question 44-6:
Which of the following statements regarding epidemiology of MS is not true?

A. Risk of a primary relative of a patient with MS developing the same disease is less than 5%.
B. Concordance among monozygotic twins is approximately 60%.
C. Females are more commonly affected than males.
D. Whites are more commonly affected than blacks.

Answer 44-1: C.
Black males have the highest death rate from stroke of these groups, followed by black females, white males, and while females. (p761)

Answer 44-2: A.
Japan has a higher death rate from stroke than the US, although the rate has dropped substantially. The other statements are true. (p761)

Answer 44-3: D.
The increasing incidence of brain tumors in the US is not completely explained. Improved diagnostics accounts for only part of the increase. Age-related incidence peaks at about 60 years. Approximately 50% of primary brain tumors are gliomas. The 5-year survival of childhood brain tumors has improved dramatically from 35% twenty years ago to approximately 61% now. (p763-764)

Answer 44-4: C.
Patients with epilepsy have an increased frequency of death independent of traffic fatalities, but this is declining. The decline is felt to be independent of the new anti-epileptic drugs. Age-specific incidence of epilepsy peaks in youth and old age, with relatively low levels in the third and fourth decades. (p765)

Answer 44-5: C
The risk of later epilepsy in patients with febrile seizures is between 2% and 11% depending on the type of seizures. The remainder of the statements are true. (p765)

Answer 44-6: B.
Concordance among monozygotic twins is approximately 20-30%. The other statements are true. The risk of a primary relative developing MS is approximately 3-4%, in contrast to the general population prevalence of 0.1%. (p768)

Question 44-7:
Which of the following statements regarding epidemiology of AIDS are true?

1. There has been a progressive increase in AIDS mortality in the US.
2. 90% of HIV infections are in developing countries.
3. Late complications of HIV develop when CD4 counts increase to above 200 cells/mm^3.
4. Patients with HIV often have an asymptomatic period for 8-10 years before developing frank symptoms.

Select: A = 1, 2, 3. B = 1, 3. C = 2, 4. D = 4 only. E = All

Questions 44-8 through 44-10
Patients with HIV infection have early and late complications. The early complications occur when CD4 counts are greater than 200 cells/mm^3, whereas the late complications occur when CD4 counts are less than 200 cells/mm^3. For each of the following three questions, select the best answer from the following list:

A. Early complications of HIV infection
B. Late complications of HIV infection
C. Both early and late complications
D. Neither early nor late complications

Question 44-8:
Acute aseptic meningitis.

Question 44-9:
Chronic inflammatory demyelinating polyradiculoneuropathy.

Question 44-10:
Dementia.

Answer 44-7: C.
The vast majority of HIV infections are in developing countries, and patients are often asymptomatic for years. There has been a decline in AIDS mortality in the US recently, probably due to new combination therapy, but we do not know how long this decrement will be sustained. Patients typically develop late complications of HIV when their CD4 counts fall below 200 cells/mm3. (p769)

Answer 44-8: A.
Aseptic meningitis is an early complication. (p772)

Answer 44-9: C.
CIDP and AIDP are typically seen as an early complication but can occur late also. (p772)

Answer 44-10: B.
HIV dementia is a late complication. (p772)

Chapter 45: Clinical Neurogenetics

Questions 45-1 through 45-4:
Inheritance pattern can aid with diagnosis of a hereditary neurologic disease as well as predict who is at risk for having or carrying the disorder. Below are some important inheritance patterns encountered in neurology. For the following questions, select the best answer from this list.

A. Autosomal dominant
B. Autosomal recessive
C. X-linked inheritance
D. Mitochondrial inheritance
E. Sporadic

Question 45-1:
Siblings of an affected patient have a 25% chance of being homozygous for the disorder.

Question 45-2:
Transmission only from mother to children.

Question 45-3:
Inheritance of adrenoleukodystrophy.

Question 45-4:
Inheritance of Friedreich's ataxia.

Question 45-5:
Which of the following statements are true regarding X-linked inheritance?

1. It includes Duchenne's and Becker's muscular dystrophies.
2. Male and female children of carrier females can have an equal risk of developing the disease.
3. Affected males cannot pass the gene to sons.
4. Females cannot be affected.

Select: A = 1, 2, 3. B = 1, 3. C = 2, 4. D = 4 only. E = All

Question 45-6:
Which of the following statements regarding trinucleotide repeats are true?

1. Successive generations are often more severely affected
2. Trinucleotide repeats in the dystrophia myotonica protein kinase gene cause myotonic dystrophy.
3. Repeat size can be determined by polymerase chain reaction.
4. Patients with Fragile-X syndrome have increased trinucleotide repeats on the X chromosome.

Select: A = 1, 2, 3. B = 1, 3. C = 2, 4. D = 4 only. E = All

Answer 45-1: B.
Autosomal recessive disorders result in siblings with a 25% chance of being homozygous for the gene. (p779)

Answer 45-2: D.
Mitochondria are carried only in the eggs, so these disorders are only passed from mothers to children. (p779)

Answer 45-3: C.
ADL is usually inherited as X-linked recessive. (p779)

Answer 45-4: B.
Friedreich's ataxia and many related disorders are inherited as autosomal recessive. (p779)

Answer 45-5: A.
Females can be affected if the unaffected X-chromosome is inactivated, leaving the affected X-chromosome activated. Therefore, a few heterozygous females may be affected. In X-linked dominant, inheritance affected heterozygous females occur, although males are usually more severely affected. (p779-780)

Answer 45-6: E.
All of these statements are true. Successive generations are often affected earlier and more severely because of amplification of the repeat. An increased number of trinucleotide repeats cause myotonic dystrophy. PCR and southern hybridization can be used to identify these repeats. Patients with Fragile-X syndrome and myotonic dystrophy have trinucleotide repeat, but the exact mechanism of function of the disordered gene is unknown. (p789)

Chapter 46: Neuroimmunology

Question 46-1:
Which of the following statements regarding natural killer cells are true?

1. NK cells are large granulocytes.
2. NK cells normally represent less than 5% of peripheral blood lymphocytes.
3. NK cells lack the cell surface markers of B and T cells.
4. NK cells lack immunologic memory.

Select: A = 1, 2, 3. B = 1, 3. C = 2, 4. D = 4 only. E = All

Question 46-2:
Which of the following statements regarding immunoglobulins are true?

1. The carboxy terminus is important for binding to host cells and binding complement.
2. All immunoglobulin classes can activate the complement cascade.
3. Immunoglobulins bind to antigens via the variable regions distant from the Fc region.
4. IgM molecules have more light chains than heavy chains.

Select: A = 1, 2, 3. B = 1, 3. C = 2, 4. D = 4 only. E = All

Questions 46-3 through 46-5:
Below are listed some of the important cells of the immune system. For the following descriptions, select the cell type which most closely corresponds.

A. T lymphocytes
B. B lymphocytes
C. Natural killer (NK) cells
D. Macrophages

Question 46-3:
Precursors of antibody-producing cells.

Question 46-4:
Includes the subset of CD4 cells.

Question 46-5:
Important for killing bacteria and processing antigens.

Question 46-6:
Guillain-Barré syndrome has been associated with which of the following conditions?

1. Campylobacter jejuni
2. Mycoplasma pneumoniae
3. Herpes virus
4. HIV

Select: A = 1, 2, 3. B = 1, 3. C = 2, 4. D = 4 only. E = All

Question 46-7:
Which of the following statements regarding inflammatory muscle disease are true?

1. Polymyositis and inclusion body myositis are mediated by CD8+ T cells.
2. Cytokines play a role in generation of the inflammation of both polymyositis and inclusion body myositis.
3. IBM is less responsive to corticosteroid therapy than polymyositis.
4. IBM is associated with systemic neoplasm more commonly than with chance alone.

Select: A = 1, 2, 3. B = 1, 3. C = 2, 4. D = 4 only. E = All

Answer 46-1: E.
All of these statements are true. The exact function of the NK cells is poorly understood. (p807)

Answer 46-2: B.
The Fc (carboxy) terminus is important for binding to host cells and for activating complement. The Fab segment is distant from the Fc segment and is a variable region which binds to antigens. The only immunoglobulin classes which can activate the cascade are IgG, IgG1, and IgG3. (p807)

Answer 46-3: B.
B lymphocytes are the immediate precursors of antibody-producing cells. After antigen challenge, B cells differentiate with the assistance of T cells into plasma cells which produce antibody. (p807)

Answer 46-4: A.
T cells may express the CD4 and CD8 markers on their cell surfaces. (p806)

Answer 46-5: D.
Macrophages have bacterial destruction and digestion as a main function. (p807)

Answer 46-6: E.
All of these infections have been associated with GBS, and additional infections and even vaccinations have been implicated. (p819)

Answer 46-7: A.
Dermatomyositis is more commonly associated with systemic neoplasm than would be expected on the basis of chance alone. Inclusion body myositis does not have this strong association. The other statements are true. (p820).

Questions 46-8 through 48-10:
Below are some antibodies which have been implicated in important neurologic paraneoplastic syndromes. For each of the questions which follow, select the best answer from this list:

A. Anti-Hu
B. Anti-Yo
C. Anti-Ri
D. None of the above

Question 46-8:
Associated with ovarian cancer.

Question 46-9:
Implicated in opsoclonus-myoclonus.

Question 46-10:
Can produce sensory neuropathy.

Answer 46-8: B.
Anti-Yo antibody is associated with breast and ovarian cancer and produces a cerebellar ataxia due to degeneration of Purkinje cells. (p821)

Answer 46-9: C.
Anti-Ri antibody is implicated in opsoclonus-myoclonus and is associated with ovarian and breast cancer. (p821)

Answer 46-10: A.
Anti-Hu antibody is associated with small-cell lung cancer and has been implicated in producing sensory neuropathy and encephalomyelitis. (p821)

Chapter 47: Neurovirology

Questions 47-1 through 47-3:
Herpesviruses are implicated in many important neurologic diseases. For the following questions, select the best answer from the following list:

A. HSV-1
B. HSV-2
C. EBV
D. CMV
E. VZV
F. None of the above

Question 47-1:
Neonatal encephalitis.

Question 47-2:
Most common cause of aseptic meningitis.

Question 47-3:
Most common cause of acute radicular symptoms.

Question 47-4:
A 56-year-old female presents with headache, mental status changes, fever, and focal seizure activity. Which of the following are likely correct?

1. CSF PCR is positive for HSV-1.
2. CSF shows excess RBCs in the absence of a traumatic tap.
3. CSF protein is elevated.
4. Glucose is reduced.

Select: A = 1, 2, 3. B = 1, 3. C = 2, 4. D = 4 only. E = All

Question 47-5:
Acyclovir is indicated for treatment of which of the following encephalitides?

1. HSV-1
2. HSV-2
3. VZV
4. CMV

Select: A = 1, 2, 3. B = 1, 3. C = 2, 4. D = 4 only. E = All

Answer 47-1: B.
HSV-2 is the main cause of neonatal encephalitis. (p825)

Answer 47-2: F.
Herpesviruses are not the most common causes of aseptic meningitis, enteroviruses are. Among the herpesviruses, HSV-2 is the most likely to cause meningitis. (p823)

Answer 47-3: E.
Varicella zoster virus is by far the most likely to produce acute radicular symptoms due to ganglionitis. (p824)

Answer 47-4: A.
This is a typical presentation for HSV-1 encephalitis. CSF shows elevated protein, normal glucose, and often excess RBCs. There is a mild to moderate CSF pleocytosis with a prominent lymphocytic composition. (p825)

Answer 47-5: A.
Acyclovir is indicated for the treatment of patients with HSV and VZV infections, but CMV is usually treated with foscarnet. (p839)

Chapter 48: Neuroendocrinology

Question 48-1:
Beta-endorphins have been implicated in which of the following?

1. Activation of T and B lymphocytes
2. Thermoregulation
3. Learning and memory
4. Analgesic mechanisms

Select: A = 1, 2, 3. B = 1, 3. C = 2, 4. D = 4 only. E = All

Question 48-2:
A 23-year-old female with headache is also noted to have galactorrhea. Which of the following statements are likely to be true?

1. Serum prolactin is elevated.
2. MRI shows a pituitary tumor.
3. She has amenorrhea and infertility.
4. Growth hormone is elevated.

Select: A = 1, 2, 3. B = 1, 3. C = 2, 4. D = 4 only. E = All

Question 48-3:
Which of the following statements regarding acromegaly is not true?

A. GH is increased.
B. Carpal tunnel syndrome is common.
C. The patient may have a vertex headache.
D. Hypotension is common.
E. Proximal muscle weakness is common.

Question 48-4:
Which of the following statements regarding diabetes insipidis is not true?

A. The most common cause in clinical practice is head trauma.
B. Nephrogenic DI is does not respond to DDAVP.
C. Replacement of fluids should be with normal saline.
D. Lithium induces nephrogenic DI.

Question 48-5:
Which is the most appropriate treatment of a prolactin-secreting adenoma without other neurologic signs?

A. Transsphenoidal resection
B. External beam radiation therapy
C. Medical therapy with bromocriptine
D. Proton beam therapy

Question 48-6:
A 56-year-old man presents with episodes of headache, palpitations, diaphoresis, nausea, and vomiting. BP is markedly elevated during these episodes. Which of the following statements is likely true?

1. Treatment should be with sumatriptan.
2. Angiography may precipitate acute increase in BP.
3. 24-hour urine is positive for 5-HIAA.
4. Beta blockers may elevate BP.

Select: A = 1, 2, 3. B = 1, 3. C = 2, 4. D = 4 only. E = All

Answer 48-1: E.
All of these functions have been attributed to beta-endorphin. Analgesic function is the best known but this is clearly not the only function. (p842)

Answer 48-2: A.
The patient most likely has a prolactin-secreting pituitary tumor. GH would not be expected to be increased, and in fact would be expected to be normal or reduced. Amenorrhea is due to inhibition of LH and FSH production by the prolactin. (p850)

Answer 48-3: D.
Hypertension is common in patients with acromegaly rather than hypotension. All of the other statements are true. Vertex headache may be produced when the GH overproduction is due to a pituitary adenoma with some mass effect. Rarely, ectopic GH production can produce the same findings in the absence of headache. (p851)

Answer 48-4: C.
The high urine output of DI is hypo-osmolar fluid, so replacement is typically with D5W rather than NaCl, which can exacerbate the polyuria. The remainder of the statements are true. (p854-855)

Answer 48-5: C.
Bromocriptine produces regression of prolactin-secreting tumors and resection is often not necessary. Other types of pituitary tumors often require surgery. Transsphenoidal surgery is generally preferred over use of radiation for accessible lesions because of the risk of damage to the optic nerves and other surrounding structures. (p857)

Answer 48-6: C.
This is a typical presentation of pheochromocytoma. Patients with pheochromocytoma secrete catecholamines and other biogenic amines in increased quantities in their urine, but elevation of 5-HIAA would be more typical of carcinoid than pheochromocytoma. Marked elevation in BP suggests that this is not simple migraine; because of the doubt about the diagnosis of migraine and the elevation in blood pressure, triptans are contraindicated. Beta blockers may paradoxically increase BP in patients with pheochromocytoma. Angiography also may increase BP dramatically in patients with pheochromocytoma. (p858)

Chapter 49: Management of Neurological Disease

Question 49-1:
A 56-year-old man has a cardiac arrest and suffers severe anoxic encephalopathy. There is some brainstem function, but he never regains consciousness and is dependent on ventilator and tube feedings. He does not have an advanced directive. The family wants the life supports removed. Which is the appropriate medical approach?

A. Consult the Ethics committee.
B. Disconnect the life supports.
C. Continue the life supports.
D. Perform EEG for determination of cerebral death.
E. Have a court-appointed attorney make a substituted judgment.

Question 49-2:
Intractable pain from a peripheral nerve lesion would likely be managed best by which of the following approaches?

1. Tricyclic antidepressants
2. Anticonvulsants
3. SSRIs
4. Controlled doses of sustained-release narcotics

Select: A = 1, 2, 3. B = 1, 3. C = 2, 4. D = 4 only. E = All

Question 49-3:
Increased exercise is helpful to augment strength for which of the following conditions?

1. Hereditary neuropathy
2. ALS
3. Parkinson's disease
4. Myasthenia gravis

Select: A = 1, 2, 3. B = 1, 3. C = 2, 4. D = 4 only. E = All

Question 49-4:
A 58-year-old man with advanced ALS has elected to forego intubation and other means of ventilatory support. When his ventilatory failure is imminent and he suffers from the anxiety of air hunger, which is the best treatment strategy?

A. Intubate and ventilate despite the patient's wishes.
B. Use supportive care only. No sedatives are given because they may hasten death.
C. Use morphine or other sedative to lessen the anxiety and promote comfort even though it can hasten death.
D. Consult the Ethics committee.

Question 49-5:
A 25-year-old woman presents with her 4-year-old child, asking him to be tested for Huntington's disease. Her father has clearly documented Huntington's disease, but no one else in the family was known to be affected. Which clinical formulation would be the best?

A. Since no one else was affected, the woman's father had a sporadic occurrence and will not pass it to his children, hence no need to test the woman or her child.
B. Testing the child would have implications for the mother as well. Genetic and psychologic counseling prior to a decision on testing is indicated.
C. It is the obligation of the physician to test regardless of the implications, so the examination should be performed at once.

Answer 49-1: B.

In most states it is appropriate to disconnect the life supports. It would not be unreasonable to have an independent physician evaluate the patient to advise regarding prognosis so there can be more security on the part of the physician and family regarding prognosis. Consulting the Ethics committee is usually not necessary in these situations. There is no point in evaluation for brain death since the patient has some intact brainstem function. We should avoid involving court-appointed attorneys, if possible. (p865)

Answer 49-2: A.

Most physicians do not prescribe narcotics for nonmalignant pain, although there are a few vocal proponents of this regimen. Anticonvulsants are a cornerstone for treatment along with antidepressants. SSRIs and TCAs alone or in combination are commonly used. (p863)

Answer 49-3: A.

Exercise tends to exacerbate myasthenia gravis but can aid the other conditions. Although ALS and Parkinson's disease are progressive conditions, exercise can help re-establish some motor function, resulting in meaningful, though temporary, functional improvements. (p863)

Answer 49-4: C.

This patient is terminal and lessening suffering and anxiety with medications is the right approach even though there is substantial risk of it hastening death. The treatment is not causing death, since that outcome has already been determined. Choosing the Ethics committee consultation is less needed in this situation than others, but would not be unreasonable. Unfortunately, many members of Ethics committees lack the confidence to advise withholding and withdrawing of life supports or giving sedatives in this situation because of the fear of litigation. (p865)

Answer 49-5: B.

Counseling is indicated prior to these tests even if there is no child involved. Patients often jump to the conclusion that a test should be performed without considering the ramifications of the findings. Once the genetic, psychologic, and medical issues have been discussed, the mother could certainly be tested; testing of children is even more complicated and should be discouraged at this age. (p866)

Chapter 50: Principles of Neuropharmacology and Therapeutics

Question 50-1:
Which of the following statements regarding GABA and its receptors are true?

1. GABA is mainly inhibitory.
2. Benzodiazepines bind to GABA receptors.
3. Barbiturates bind to GABA receptors.
4. Baclofen binds to GABA receptors.

Select: A = 1, 2, 3. B = 1, 3. C = 2, 4. D = 4 only. E = All

Question 50-2:
Which of the following statements are true regarding glutamate and aspartate?

1. Glutamate is the most prevalent excitatory neurotransmitter.
2. Carbamazepine blocks some glutamate receptors.
3. Excess release of glutamate causes neuronal degeneration.
4. Aspartate is the main transmitter for neuronal projections from the brainstem to the spinal cord.

Select: A = 1, 2, 3. B = 1, 3. C = 2, 4. D = 4 only. E = All

Question 50-3:
Which of the following statements are true regarding acetylcholine receptors?

1. Sympathetic ganglion receptors are nicotinic.
2. Motor endplate receptors are muscarinic.
3. Patients with myasthenia have increased receptor turnover, causing fewer receptors to be available for binding with acetylcholine.
4. Botulinum toxin blocks binding of acetylcholine to the post-synaptic receptors.

Select: A = 1, 2, 3. B = 1, 3. C = 2, 4. D = 4 only. E = All

Question 50-4:
Which of the following agents are acetylcholinesterase inhibitors?

1. Edrophonium
2. Tacrine
3. Pyridostigmine
4. Donepezil

Select: A = 1, 2, 3. B = 1, 3. C = 2, 4. D = 4 only. E = All

Question 50-5:
Glutamate and NMDA are involved in which of the following conditions?

1. Memory
2. Neonatal glycine encephalopathy
3. Stroke
4. Migraine

Select: A = 1, 2, 3. B = 1, 3. C = 2, 4. D = 4 only. E = All

Question 50-6:
Parkinsonian symptoms would be produced by a drug which binds to which subset of the dopamine receptors?

A. D1
B. D2
C. D3
D. D4

Answer 50-1: E.
All of these are true, although these are not unique functions of the chemicals. Actions from binding to the GABA receptors may be only part of the pharmacologic action of some of these medications. (p870)

Answer 50-2: A.
There are no known purely aspartate synapses. Glutamate and aspartate are interconvertible and likely act at the same receptor. CBZ is only one of several AEDs which act at least partly at glutamate receptors; others include felbamate, topiramate, and phenobarbital. (p870)

Answer 50-3: B.
Sympathetic ganglion and motor endplate receptors are nicotinic, and many CNS receptors are both nicotinic and muscarinic. Most post-ganglionic parasympathetic receptors are muscarinic. Botulinum toxin binds to the presynaptic terminal to prevent release of transmitter. (p878)

Answer 50-4: E.
All of these agents are acetylcholinesterase inhibitors, although they differ substantially in clinical use. Edrophonium (Tensilon) is used as a diagnostic test for myasthenia gravis. Pyridostigmine (Mestinon) is used for symptomatic treatment of myasthenia. Tacrine (Cognex) and Donepezil (Aricept) are used for Alzheimer's disease. (p877)

Answer 50-5: E.
Glutamate is felt to be implicated in all of these conditions. NMDA is thought to be involved in long-term potentiation, an important experimental model of memory. Neonatal glycine encephalopathy presents with hypotonia, seizures, and a burst suppression pattern on EEG which is thought to be due to a deficit in a glycine-cleavage enzyme. Glutamate is thought to be partly responsible for augmenting the damage following stroke by its excitotoxic effect after release. MSG is a common precipitant of migraine. (p873)

Answer 50-6: B.
Binding to the D2 receptors is thought to induce parkinsonian findings. Atypical neuroleptics, which have a much lower frequency of inducing parkinsonian adverse effects, bind mainly to the D3 and D4 receptors. (p881)

Question 50-7:
Which of the following statements are true regarding the pharmacology of dopamine in the brain?

1. Metabolized by MAO-A
2. Metabolized by COMT
3. The action of dopamine is ended by enzymatic degradation at the receptor.
4. Reserpine depletes dopamine by preventing reuptake into storage vesicles.

Select: A = 1, 2, 3. B = 1, 3. C = 2, 4. D = 4 only. E = All

Question 50-8:
Which of the following statements are true regarding serotonin action and metabolism?

1. Migraine headache is preceded by increased free plasma 5-HT.
2. Serotonin is a precursor of melatonin.
3. Psychotic features of LSD exposure are thought to be due to binding to the 5-HT2 receptors.
4. Sumatriptan activates the 5-HT1D receptors.

Select: A = 1, 2, 3. B = 1, 3. C = 2, 4. D = 4 only. E = All

Answer 50-7: C.
Dopamine is metabolized by COMT and MAO-B, whereas MAO-A metabolizes norepinephrine and serotonin. Dopamine is subjected to reuptake before degradation rather than being degraded at the receptor. Reserpine does prevent reuptake of dopamine into storage vesicles and initially augments release, initiating the depletion. (p881)

Answer 50-8: E.
All of these statements are true. The psychotic features of Alzheimer's disease may also be related to reduction in 5-HT2 receptors. Serotonin's involvement in sleep is complex and includes its precursor status for the synthesis of melatonin, which aids regulation of circadian rhythm. (p887)

Chapter 51: Principles of Pain Management

Question 51-1:
Which of the following agents is least likely to be helpful for a patient with chronic pain secondary to traumatic nerve injury?

A. Gabapentin
B. Naproxen
C. Amitriptyline
D. Oxycodone
E. Carbamazepine

Question 51-2:
Which of the following statements is true regarding sympathetic involvement in chronic pain?

1. The edema and trophic changes are due to overactivity of sympathetic outflow.
2. Regional sympathetic blockade is effective for complex regional pain.
3. Sympathetic outflow to the affected region is increased in most patients.
4. Spread of the distribution of pain and sensory change is common and does not implicate a psychogenic etiology.

Select: A = 1, 2, 3. B = 1, 3. C = 2, 4. D = 4 only. E = All

Question 51-3:
The frequency of major depression in patients with chronic pain syndromes is approximately what percent?

A. 2%
B. 10%
C. 25%
D. 50%
E. 65%

Question 51-4:
What is the estimated proportion of patients with chronic back pain who are malingering?

A. 5%
B. 15%
C. 30%
D. 50%
E. 70%

Question 51-5:
A 52-year-old man with chronic neuropathic pain is admitted for pain control, since he cannot be managed on outpatient oral analgesics. During the initial treatment, he appears to have good relief of his pain from a saline infusion. The pain responds but then returns, responding a second time. Which clinical impression is the best founded in this case?

A. He has a psychogenic cause for his pain and should not be given more infusions or analgesics. Psychiatric counseling is warranted.
B. He responded to the placebo infusion with a common response but will need comprehensive pain management for his organic pain.
C. He is suffering from symptom amplification and should be treated with saline infusions until his pain has subsided to his level of baseline pain.

Question 51-6:
A 54-year-old woman with parkinsonism has chronic lumbosacral plexus pain from spread of ovarian cancer. She is already on carbamazepine and sustained-release morphine in addition to levo-dopa (Sinemet) and selegiline. Which of the following short-acting adjuncts would be the most likely to be helpful?

A. Meperidine (Demerol)
B. Short-acting morphine
C. Pentazocine (Talwin)
D. Fentanyl (Duragesic)

Answer 51-1: B.
Naproxen and other non-steroidal anti-inflammatory agents are unlikely to be helpful for chronic neuropathic pain. They have some minor analgesic effect in addition to the anti-inflammatory effect, but this is not major. The anticonvulsants and tricyclics are especially helpful for neuropathic pain. Oxycodone is avoided when possible but can be of benefit in patients with refractory neuropathic pain syndromes. Opiates are often also needed for patients with acute neuropathic pain syndromes such as herpetic neuralgia and acute bouts of trigeminal neuralgia. (p912)

Answer 51-2: D.
Only the last statement is correct. Spread of the area of pain may be secondary to change in receptive fields of neurons and not from psychogenic amplification. The edema and trophic changes are commonly present in the absence of sympathetic changes, and, in fact, sympathetic over-activity has not been documented in most patients. Other factors producing these changes can be local chemical changes and disuse. Regional sympathetic blockade has not been found effective for the majority of patients, although this procedure still has its advocates. (p905)

Answer 51-3: B.
Approximately 5-10% of patients with chronic pain meet criteria for major depression. However, the frequency of more mild affective disturbance is greater than this, perhaps as high as 50%. (p905)

Answer 51-4: A.
Most of us in a referral practice are surprised to learn that the proportion of patients with chronic back pain who are malingerers is 5% or less. A larger percentage than this will have symptom amplification, which, when detected by the physician, may trigger the erroneous conclusion that all of the complaints are factitious. (p905)

Answer 51-5: B.
The frequency of a placebo response is approximately equal for patients with psychogenic and nociceptive pain. The identification of some features which suggest a functional component should never be followed by the conclusion that all of the complaints are psychosomatic. (p907)

Answer 51-6: B.
Additional short-acting morphine is the best of these listed options for adjunctive treatment of the patient. Meperidine should be avoided because of the co-administration of selegiline, a MAOI. Pentazocine has mixed agonist-antagonist qualities and may precipitate acute withdrawal in patients who are dependent on chronic opiates. Fentanyl is another long-acting agent usually given by a transdermal delivery system, and would not be expected to be helpful as a short-acting adjunct. (p910)

Chapter 52: Principles of Neurointensive Care

Question 52-1:
Which of the following statements regarding airway pressures are correct?

1. PEEP should be kept below 15 cm H$_2$O to avoid impeding venous return and producing hypotension.
2. Sustained high PEEP may cause tension pneumothorax.
3. High respiratory rate in a patient with COPD may precipitate high airway pressures and subsequent hypotension.
4. PEEP is reserved for patients who have impaired oxygenation despite high FIO_2.

Select: A = 1, 2, 3. B = 1, 3. C = 2, 4. D = 4 only. E = All

Question 52-2:
Which of the following statements are true concerning patients with myasthenia gravis?

1. Intubation and mechanical ventilation should be anticipated when the vital capacity falls below 1L.
2. Ventilation should be discontinued as soon as the patient's vital capacity exceeds 1L.
3. Weaning usually requires disease intervention with corticosteroids, plasmapheresis, or intravenous immunoglobulin.
4. Early tracheostomy is often needed for patients in myasthenic crisis.

Select: A = 1, 2, 3. B = 1, 3. C = 2, 4. D = 4 only. E = All

Question 52-3:
Which of the following conditions are appropriate indications for intracranial pressure monitoring?

1. Cerebral edema from trauma
2. Subarachnoid hemorrhage
3. Acute obstructive hydrocephalus
4. Cerebral edema from hepatic encephalopathy

Select: A = 1, 2, 3. B = 1, 3. C = 2, 4. D = 4 only. E = All

Question 52-4:
Which of the following statements regarding EEG monitoring in the ICU is not true?

A. Monitoring should be performed in many patients with serious CNS insults because non-convulsive seizures are common.
B. A burst suppression pattern in a head trauma patient indicates non-convulsive seizure activity and should be treated with anticonvulsants.
C. Normal sleep patterns in a patient with head injury suggest a good prognosis for neurologic recovery.

Question 52-5:
Which of the following procedures should not be used as supportive evidence of brain death?

A. EEG
B. BAEP
C. VEP
D. Cerebral blood flow
E. All can be used.

Question 52-6:
Transcranial doppler is used for many purposes. For which of these clinical uses are TCD studies clinically valuable?

1. Spasm from subarachnoid hemorrhage
2. Cerebral steal
3. Intracranial carotid stenosis
4. Increased intracranial pressure

Select: A = 1, 2, 3. B = 1, 3. C = 2, 4. D = 4 only. E = All

Answer 52-1: A.

PEEP is used routinely by most critical care physicians and need not be reserved for those with high FIO_2 levels. A level of 5 cm H_2O is typically used. The other statements are true. The increased airway pressure in a patient with COPD is termed auto-PEEP and can be immediately diagnosed by temporarily disconnecting the ventilator, at which point the hypotension should abate quickly. (p921)

Answer 52-2: B.

Ventilation should be continued until the vital capacity is approximately 60% of the patient's predicted value and bulbar function is almost normal. Because of the fatigability, there should not be a rush to extubate as soon as some independent breaths can be taken. On the other hand, myasthenia often responds to hospital care relatively quickly, so tracheostomy is seldom needed. (p924)

Answer 52-3: E.

All of these are reasonable indications for intracranial pressure monitoring. Patients with hepatic encephalopathy may have a coagulopathy, so this may increase the risk of the surgical procedure. Not all patients with SAH, trauma, and hydrocephalus require monitoring, but this is indicated if critical increase in pressure is suspected and the information would help management. (p927)

Answer 52-4: B.

A burst suppression pattern suggests a poor prognosis for recovery but is not epileptiform. Therefore, anticonvulsants are typically not needed. The other statements are true. One series indicated that 35% of patients admitted to the neuro-ICU had seizures and 75% of those were non-convulsive. (p928)

Answer 52-5: C.

The visual evoked potential cannot be used because there is no certainty that the signal has been transduced in the eye and relayed to the brain. The other tests can provide supportive evidence of brain death but require the patient to meet clinical criteria. (p929)

Answer 52-6: E.

All of these are valuable uses for transcranial doppler. While TCD does not provide much truly unique information, much of this cannot be obtained without an invasive study (e.g. angiogram) or with a study which cannot be routinely performed on critically ill patients (e.g., MRI with MRA). (p930)

Chapter 53: Principles of Neurosurgery

Question 53-1:
Which one of the following statements regarding cerebellar stroke is true?

A. Cerebellar hemorrhage can be treated by ventriculostomy of the lateral ventricle to treat hydrocephalus.
B. The prognosis for good neurologic function for patients with cerebellar hemorrhage who require posterior fossa decompression is poor.
C. A patient with cerebellar ataxia who develops stupor with a gaze palsy and a facial palsy usually needs decompression.
D. A patient with cerebellar ataxia who has Horner's syndrome ipsilateral to the ataxia with ipsilateral facial sensory loss is likely to require cerebellar decompression.

Question 53-2:
A 24-year-old female presents with the acute onset of headache, nausea, vomiting, diplopia, and visual loss and eventually develops coma. Review of recent medical records indicates that she has recently complained to her gynecologist about amenorrhea and galactorrhea. Which of the following statements is likely to be true?

A. She has basilar migraine and these findings are not indicative of a worrisome lesion.
B. She has pituitary apoplexy in the setting of a prolactin-secreting pituitary adenoma.
C. She may have a binasal hemianopia and diplopia secondary to CN-6 palsy.

Question 53-3:
Which of the following are reasonable indications for emergent spinal cord decompression?

1. Spinal epidural hematoma following trauma which is compressing the cord
2. Intramedullary hemorrhage following trauma with progressive myelopathy
3. Epidural tumor producing myelopathy which has been resistant to radiotherapy and corticosteroids
4. Epidural tumor producing back pain without other deficit in a patient with known metastatic cancer

Select: A = 1, 2, 3. B = 1, 3. C = 2, 4. D = 4 only. E = All

Question 53-4:
Which of the following statements regarding lumbar spine disorders are true?

1. The prognosis of cauda equina compression is better than that of spinal cord compression.
2. Urinary incontinence in the absence of other findings is an indication for immediate surgical evaluation.
3. The most common cause of cauda equina compression is extrusion of the L4-L5 disc.
4. MRI is the first choice for evaluation of suspected cauda equina syndrome.

Select: A = 1, 2, 3. B = 1, 3. C = 2, 4. D = 4 only. E = All

Question 53-5:
A 52-year-old man is admitted with subarachnoid hemorrhage, grade 2, and has a CN-6 palsy. He is hemodynamically stable; however, he requires intravenous treatment for hypertension. Which would be the most appropriate clinical approach?

A. Early angiography and surgery if an accessible aneurysm is identified
B. Delay angiography for 10 days to allow the neurological deficit to clear, then proceed with studies
C. Early angiography for identification of the aneurysm then surgery 10-14 days later, after recovery from the acute episode

Answer 53-1: C.

The development of mental status changes with facial palsy and a gaze palsy following a cerebellar infarct suggests brainstem compression; evaluation for possible decompression is needed. The patient with Horner's syndrome and facial sensory loss likely has lateral medullary syndrome, so decompression should not be needed. Cerebellar hemorrhage is seldom treated with only a ventriculostomy for the resultant hydrocephalus because there is the possibility of upward herniation from the posterior fossa; suboccipital decompression is usually needed. A patient who has suboccipital decompression for cerebellar hemorrhage has a reasonable expectation for survival providing the patient does not become comatose prior to the procedure. (p933)

Answer 53-2: B.

She has a typical history for pituitary apoplexy, which is characterized by hemorrhage and/or infarction in the setting of a pituitary adenoma. The amenorrhea and galactorrhea suggest that she has a prolactin secreting tumor. Eye findings are typically a bitemporal hemianopia and partial CN-3 palsy. (p935)

Answer 53-3: A.

All of these are reasonable indications for spinal decompression except the last. Close observation during radiotherapy and corticosteroid administration may be all that is required. If the patient declines, surgical intervention may then be required. (p935)

Answer 53-4: E.

All of these are correct. Patients with cauda equina syndrome typically present with back pain, bladder dysfunction, and often leg symptoms including foot drop. MRI is the preferred method of evaluation, but it is not always available, so CT and occasionally myelography are often performed. (p935)

Answer 53-5: A.

The answer to this question will not be unanimous, but most clinicians advocate early angiography and surgery for patients with grade 1 and 2 SAH. Hemodynamic factors, presence of increased intracranial pressure, and location of the aneurysm may certainly influence this decision. (p936)

Question 53-6:
Which of the following is least likely to be helpful for management of vasospasm in patients with subarachnoid hemorrhage?

A. Plasma expansion with colloid
B. Lowering of blood pressure with labetolol
C. Nimodipine
D. Angioplasty
E. They are all appropriate treatments.

Question 53-7:
A 27-year-old woman with epilepsy is evaluated by a neurologist who finds a venous hemangioma in the right centro-temporal region. Interictal EEG is normal. Which is the most appropriate clinical formulation?

A. The venous angioma is likely an incidental finding and should not play a role in decision making regarding the seizure management.
B. The seizures may be arising from the venous angioma and it should be resected.
C. The seizures may be arising from the region of the venous angioma, but medical treatment should be attempted rather than surgical intervention.

Question 53-8:
A 30-year-old woman with seizures is found to have an AVM in the right parietal region. EEG shows polymorphic slow activity and some spikes in this region. Which of the following clinical approaches is most appropriate?

A. Surgical treatment with excision, radiosurgery, or embolization and medical management of the seizures.
B. Medical management of the seizures without treatment of the AVM unless the seizures are refractory.
C. Successive scans to evaluate the AVM to look for enlargement or bleeding before deciding on surgical treatment; treat the seizures medically.

Question 53-9:
Which of the following statements are true regarding extracranial carotid dissection?

1. Angioplasty with stent placement may be performed.
2. TIAs may develop from extracranial carotid dissection.
3. Horner's syndrome is common.
4. Anticoagulation is contraindicated.

Select: A = 1, 2, 3. B = 1, 3. C = 2, 4. D = 4 only. E = All

Answer 53-6: B.

Lowering blood pressure is helpful to lower the risk of rebleeding, but it increases the effects of vasospasm on cerebral perfusion. Plasma expansion typically increases the blood pressure, which in the setting of increased intracranial pressure is essential to increase perfusion pressure. Angioplasty is not widely used for vasospasm but is felt by many specialists to be a reasonable option when medical treatment has failed. (p937)

Answer 53-7: C.

Venous angioma should be considered a developmental anomaly and can contribute to generation of partial seizures with and without secondary generalization. However, the lesion is typically not progressive and has a low incidence of bleeding. Therefore, the seizures can be treated medically. Surgery can be performed but has a substantial risk of morbidity, so it should be avoided if possible. (p940)

Answer 53-8: A.

The risk of bleeding of an AVM is greater than that of an aneurysm, so if surgery is feasible, it should be performed. Following with successive scans is warranted for cryptic AVMs but not for true AVMs. (p941)

Answer 53-9: A.

Extracranial carotid dissection usually responds to anticoagulation, and surgery is rarely necessary. Angioplasty with stent placement has been used in many centers recently with success. TIAs and fixed neurologic deficit may develop from the dissection. Horner's syndrome develops from damage to the ascending sympathetic fibers. (p946)

Chapter 54: Principles of Neurological Rehabilitation

Question 54-1:
Which of the following is the greatest concern to caregivers of a patient with stroke in an inpatient rehabilitation unit?

A. DVT with subsequent PE
B. Repeat stroke
C. Skin ulcers
D. Dysphagia and aspiration causing pneumonia

Question 54-2:
Which of the following are used to assess patients with brain lesions and their overall level of functioning?

1. Barthel index
2. Glasgow outcome scale
3. Rankin disability scale
4. Ashworth scale

Select: A = 1, 2, 3. B = 1, 3. C = 2, 4. D = 4 only. E = All

Question 54-3:
Which of the following statements are true regarding cognitive changes with brain lesions?

1. A small proportion of patients over the age of 75 with cerebral infarct have subsequent cognitive deficits.
2. Hypotension at the time of traumatic brain injury augments the chance of poor cognitive outcome.
3. The major thrust of cognitive therapy is to train damaged neurons to work.
4. Urinary tract infections commonly exacerbate the cognitive performance of patients with brain damage from any cause.

Select: A = 1, 2, 3. B = 1, 3. C = 2, 4. D = 4 only. E = All

Question 54-4:
What is the most important outcome measure for rehabilitation?

A. Return to work rate
B. Nursing home placement rate
C. ADLs and independence
D. Level of improvement in motor power and coordination

Answer 54-1: A.
All of these are real concerns, but DVT has a high risk of developing and PE has a high mortality rate. The combination of immobility plus other medical conditions at the time of a stroke make DVT formation likely. Repeat stroke during the few weeks of rehabilitation is of certain concern, but since the transfer is usually past the initial phase of stroke, recurrence is not highly likely. Skin ulcers should be preventable with good nursing care. Dysphagia rapidly improves within the first few days to weeks in most stroke patients, but when present can be managed with tube feedings and preventative measures against aspiration. (p980)

Answer 54-2: A.
The first three are commonly used scales for evaluating patients with stroke and other cerebral lesions. They all concern the patient's responsiveness and ability to perform activities during the day. The Ashworth scale is a scale for evaluating spasticity, and while there will be a correlation between the score on this assessment and other scores, the measure is not of disability, per se. (p967, 983)

Answer 54-3: C.
The proportion of patients over the age of 75 who have cognitive changes subsequent to stroke is approximately 74%. Cognitive therapy mainly helps adaptation to the deficit and is secondary to the formation of alternative neuronal pathways for accomplishing tasks. (p989)

Answer 54-4: C.
Activities of daily living and independence are the most important factors in evaluating outcome from rehabilitation. The other measures will factor into this but are of secondary importance. (p997)

Question 54-5:
Which of the following statements is true regarding exercise programs and Parkinson's disease?

A. PD is a progressive disorder which cannot be helped by exercise and rehabilitative techniques.
B. PD is a progressive disorder which can be helped by exercise and retraining within the bounds of the patient's functional limitations.
C. Exercise and rehabilitation mainly have benefit on balance and tremor in patients with PD; associated bradykinesia and rigidity require medical therapy for improvement.

Answer 54-5: B.

PD has clearly been shown to improve with an exercise program and rehabilitative training. The improvements are mainly in the spheres of rigidity and bradykinesia. While balance may improve, tremor is not expected to make as great an improvement. Unfortunately, many insurance carriers have subscribed to choice A and fail to realize that programs to improve function can be helpful for PD and many other chronic degenerative disorders. (p999)

Chapter 55A: Neurological Complications of Systemic Disease: In Adults

Question 55A-1:
What is the approximate risk of stroke in patients undergoing coronary artery bypass surgery?

A. 0.1%
B. 1%
C. 5%
D. 10%

Question 55A-2:
A 58-year-old man has severe encephalopathy following CPR. He recovers after a few days to the point that he is only mildly confused and has mild ataxia. He then has progressive encephalopathy and motor deterioration. MRI is performed. Which is the most likely result of the MRI?

A. Subarachnoid hemorrhage
B. Demyelination of the white matter
C. Diffuse cerebral edema
D. Normal

Question 55A-3:
Which of the following statements are true regarding giant cell arteritis?

1. ESR may not be elevated.
2. Peripheral neuropathy may be a complication.
3. Treatment usually requires 18-24 months.
4. Corticosteroids are administered if the temporal artery biopsy shows inflammation.

Select: A = 1, 2, 3. B = 1, 3. C = 2, 4. D = 4 only. E = All

Question 55A-4:
Which of the following statements are true regarding nervous system complications of SLE?

1. The most common neurologic complication is peripheral neuropathy.
2. The presence of antineuronal antibodies does not correlate with CNS involvement by SLE.
3. Approximately 25% of patients with SLE have neurologic involvement.
4. The most common CNS complications are psychiatric.

Select: A = 1, 2, 3. B = 1, 3. C = 2, 4. D = 4 only. E = All

Question 55A-5:
Behçet's disease is a rare condition which presents with uveitis and oral and genital ulcers. Which of the following statements are true regarding neurologic involvement?

1. Mononeuropathy multiplex is uncommon but may occur.
2. Aseptic meningitis and meningoencephalitis are the most common findings.
3. Neurologic findings may include focal signs from cerebral ischemia.
4. CSF is usually normal.

Select: A = 1, 2, 3. B = 1, 3. C = 2, 4. D = 4 only. E = All

Question 55A-6:
Which of the following statements regarding neurologic complications of sarcoidosis are true?

1. Facial nerve palsy is the single most common symptom of neurologic involvement.
2. Visual involvement may be via optic neuritis or uveitis.
3. Weakness may develop from myopathy.
4. Neurologic involvement occurs in approximately 50% of patients with sarcoidosis.

Select: A = 1, 2, 3. B = 1, 3. C = 2, 4. D = 4 only. E = All

Answer 55A-1: C.
Approximately 5% of patients who have a coronary artery bypass and graft have stroke. The risk is increasing because older patients are being subjected to this surgery. (p1011)

Answer 55A-2: B.
Secondary demyelination develops 7-10 days following recovery from hypoxic encephalopathy. The MRI would show demyelinating changes. Cerebral edema would not be expected after a latent period, with interval improvement in function. Subarachnoid hemorrhage can be missed on MRI and would not be expected to develop after a latency. (p1011)

Answer 55A-3: A.
The ESR is not elevated in all patients, although it is elevated in most. Although uncommon, peripheral neuropathies can occur as a recognized complication. Corticosteroids are administered even prior to a temporal artery biopsy to lower the risk of blindness. Biopsies are not always positive, and awaiting results usually means a delay in treatment. (p1017)

Answer 55A-4: C.
CNS involvement by SLE is more common than PNS involvement. Approximately 75% of patients will have neurologic involvement at some course in their disease. The most common neurologic findings are affective and psychotic symptoms which may be difficult to differentiate from adverse effects of corticosteroids. (p1017)

Answer 55A-5: A.
Behçet's disease produces neurologic complications in approximately 20% of patients. CSF usually shows a mild pleocytosis and increased protein. (p1019)

Answer 55A-6: A.
Facial palsy is the most common neurologic finding in sarcoidosis. Neurologic involvement may occur in approximately 5% of patients with sarcoidosis. Myopathy can develop from granulomas in the muscle tissue. Visual changes may result from many types of attack, including optic neuritis, uveitis, or even papilledema from hydrocephalus. (p1020)

Question 55A-7:
Vitamin B12 levels are checked frequently in a search for causes of neurologic problems including dementia, neuropathy, weakness, and ataxia. Which one of the following statements is not true regarding B12 deficiency?

A. Patients with neurologic complications of vitamin B12 deficiency usually have no anemia.
B. Optic neuropathy may develop.
C. The most common cause of vitamin B12 deficiency is impaired absorption in the GI tract.
D. Failure of the neurologic symptoms to resolve with replacement indicates that the vitamin B12 deficiency was probably an incidental finding.

Question 55A-8:
The POEMS syndrome is associated with all of the following clinical features except which one?

A. Distal symmetric polyneuropathy
B. Association with lymphoma
C. Hepatosplenomegaly
D. Lymphadenopathy

Question 55A-9:
A 68-year-old woman with chronic renal failure from untreated hypertension has been on hemodialysis for several years. She develops confusion and a seizure following dialysis one day. Neurologic examination shows a diffuse encephalopathy and papilledema. Which is the most likely diagnosis?

A. Dialysis dementia
B. Dialysis dysequilibrium
C. Cryptococcal meningitis
D. Intracerebral hemorrhage

Question 55A-10:
A 50-year-old male is admitted because of encephalopathy. He is a long-time alcoholic, although alcohol level is currently zero. He has multiple electrolyte disorders including hyponatremia, hyperglycemia, hypocalcemia, and hypomagnesemia. These are treated and he initially responds but then develops spastic quadriparesis and increasing encephalopathy. Which is the most likely diagnosis?

A. Wernicke's encephalopathy
B. Subdural hematoma
C. Central pontine myelinolysis
D. Alcoholic rhabdomyolysis

Answer 55A-7: D.
Prolonged and profound vitamin B12 deficiency is often associated with incomplete improvement following replacement. The rest of the statements are true. Patients with clinically significant vitamin B12 deficiency often have no anemia, because folate in the diet masks the anemia. Optic neuropathy is not the most common neurologic manifestation but may occur. (p1021)

Answer 55A-8: B.
POEMS is polyneuropathy, organomegaly, endocrinopathy, M protein, and skin changes. This is associated with myeloma rather than lymphoma. The other listed features are typical of the condition. (p1023)

Answer 55A-9: B.
Dialysis dysequilibrium is characterized by headache, agitation, seizures, and other symptoms and typically develops after dialysis and subsequently abates. Papilledema is not a common finding but can develop. Dialysis dementia would be expected to produce progressive intellectual decline without an acute decline. Cryptococcal meningitis usually has a more insidious course. Intracerebral hemorrhage is possible, especially since patients are anticoagulated during hemodialysis, but with this presentation, dialysis dysequilibrium is the most likely diagnosis. Nevertheless, CT or MRI would be warranted with these symptoms. (p1028)

Answer 55A-10: C.
CPM is characterized by encephalopathy with quadriparesis which may be spastic or flaccid. By the time the patient is recovering from acute encephalopathy, thiamine should have been given, so Wernicke's encephalopathy should not occur. If thiamine had been overlooked, then Wernicke's encephalopathy could be precipitated, especially by the glucose administration. Alcoholic rhabdomyolysis should not produce spastic quadriparesis, but if the patient had flaccid weakness, this would have to be considered. (p1029)

Chapter 55B: Neurological Complications of Systemic Disease: In Children

Question 55B-1:
Which of the following statements are true for growth hormone deficiency?

1. Neonates are small for gestational age.
2. Most patients have non-functioning pituitary adenomas as a cause for the failure of growth hormone production.
3. Patients have delayed achievement of motor milestones.
4. Neonates may have hypoglycemic seizures.

Select: A = 1, 2, 3. B = 1, 3. C = 2, 4. D = 4 only. E = All

Question 55B-2:
Which of the following statements are true regarding valproate-induced hepatotoxicity?

1. The incidence is highest in the under-2-years age group than in any other group.
2. Elevations in serum transaminases of 2-3 fold suggest high risk for subsequent hepatotoxicity.
3. It usually develops within 6 months from beginning valproate therapy.
4. It is most common when used at high-therapeutic levels in monotherapy.

Select: A = 1, 2, 3. B = 1, 3. C = 2, 4. D = 4 only. E = All

Question 55B-3:
A 5-year-old boy presents with recurrent episodes of syncope followed by brief clonic activity. The episodes are described as loss of consciousness and pallor followed occasionally by 2-3 seconds of clonic activity. Fright or exertion may precipitate an event. Which is the most likely diagnosis?

A. Breath-holding spells
B. Long QT syndrome
C. Epilepsy
D. Familial benign syncope

Question 55B-4:
Cardiac surgery in children is associated with neurologic complications, just as it is with adults. Which of the following statements are true regarding neurologic sequelae of cardiac surgery?

1. Infants with post-operative seizures have increased chance of developmental delay.
2. MRI may be abnormal in 75% of patients undergoing surgery for congenital heart disease.
3. Focal infarcts are associated with less effect on later intellect than diffuse hypoxia.
4. Cardiac surgery results in lower IQ.

Select: A = 1, 2, 3. B = 1, 3. C = 2, 4. D = 4 only. E = All

Question 55B-5:
Which of the following statements regarding childhood diabetes mellitus are true?

1. Diabetes mellitus in children is usually due to insulin resistance.
2. Most complications from DM in children are acute rather than chronic.
3. Peripheral neuropathy is the most common neurologic complication of childhood DM.
4. Hyperglycemia from DM may exacerbate seizures in a child with epilepsy.

Select: A = 1, 2, 3. B = 1, 3. C = 2, 4. D = 4 only. E = All

Answer 55B-1: D.
Neonatal hypoglycemic seizures may occasionally develop when patients also have ACTH deficiency. Otherwise, neurologic development is normal. Neonates have normal bodies because intrauterine growth is independent of the child's own growth hormone production. The most common cause of growth hormone deficiency is decreased hypothalamic release of GH-releasing factor. (p1037)

Answer 55B-2: B.
Modest elevations in transaminases do not predict later development of toxicity. Hepatotoxicity is most likely with polytherapy rather than monotherapy. (p1041)

Answer 55B-3: B.
This history is typical for the Long-QT syndrome, which may produce syncope followed by brief clonic activity due to cerebral ischemia. They can be triggered as described. The initial loss of consciousness and pallor are the main clues to the identity of the spells. These findings would not be expected in patients with epilepsy. (p1036)

Answer 55B-4: A.
In the absence of complications, cardiac surgery does not lower later IQ. Studies in adults have shown cognitive changes in the absence of known complications, but this is not felt to be a common problem in children. Focal infarcts can result in motor impairment, but less of a chance of cognitive difficulty than in patients with global cerebral dysfunction, such as hypoxic encephalopathy. (p1036)

Answer 55B-5: C.
Diabetes in children is usually due to decreased insulin release rather than insulin resistance. Neuropathy is uncommon in children, and most of the complications are acute, relating to metabolic effects of hyperglycemia or hypoglycemia. Epilepsy may be aggravated by hyperglycemia and should be considered with a change in seizure pattern, even if the patient is not a known diabetic. (p1057)

Chapter 56A: Trauma of the Nervous System: Basic Neuroscience of Neurotrauma

Question 56A-1:
A 22-year-old man sustains a closed head injury in a motor vehicle accident. CT is initially normal. After an initial phase of improvement, he deteriorates, with decreasing mental status and decreased motor movements. Which of the following should be considered in the differential diagnosis?

1. Cerebral edema
2. Secondary deterioration from reperfusion injury
3. Epidural hematoma
4. Sepsis

Select: A = 1, 2, 3. B = 1, 3. C = 2, 4. D = 4 only. E = All

Question 56A-2:
A 58-year-old man who is a former boxer develops symptoms of dementia associated with psychomotor slowing. The symptoms did not develop until more than 10 years after cessation of the boxing. Which of the following clinical formulations is most likely to be at work?

A. He was unfortunate enough to develop dementia, which would have occurred independently of the prior history of cerebral trauma.
B. The repeated head injury initiated a degenerative cascade which resulted in the cognitive and motor declines.
C. The repeated head injury damaged many cells to the point that normal aging is ongoing with the patient having less neuronal reserve.

Question 56A-3:
Fever is common after closed head injury. Which one of these statements regarding post-traumatic fever is incorrect?

A. Fever following head injury suggests meningitis.
B. Fever following head injury exacerbates neuronal damage.
C. Fever following head injury should be aggressively treated.
D. Fever is significant following significant head injury.

Question 56A-4:
Experimental models of traumatic brain injury infrequently report selective damage to the CA1 area of the hippocampus, a region important for memory. What is felt to be the most likely precipitant for CA1 injury in trauma patients?

A. Previous brain injury sensitizing the neurons to the second injury
B. Hypotension or hypoxia producing ischemic injury in the setting of recent trauma
C. Non-convulsive seizure activity producing hippocampal damage

Question 56A-5:
Which of the following are potential mechanisms of delayed neuronal dysfunction after head injury?

1. Opening of the blood-brain barrier
2. Shearing injury of the axons
3. Excitotoxic effects on cerebral neurons
4. Hemorrhage

Select: A = 1, 2, 3. B = 1, 3. C = 2, 4. D = 4 only. E = All

Answer 56A-1: E.

All of these conditions should be tested for in the evaluation of patients with exacerbation of mental status following head injury. Cerebral edema can progress after initial improvement, resulting in reduction in increased intracranial pressure, reduction in cerebral perfusion pressure, and ischemia. Reperfusion injury is thought to have its foundations in inflammation and free radical formation. Epidural hematoma is commonly considered when a patient presents to the ER after a head injury but can develop days to even weeks after an acute injury. (p1051)

Answer 56A-2: B.

Dementia is of increased frequency in patients who have had repeated head injury, and there are some data to suggest that the development of injury correlates with success in the ring. Current thinking is that the head injury initiates a cascade which takes years to be clinically manifest. Patients with head injuries have a greater chance of being diagnosed with AD. The deterioration is not thought to be merely a byproduct of the normal aging process, although certainly there is less clinical reserve. (p1047)

Answer 56A-3: A.

Meningitis can develop in patients with penetrating brain injuries and in some patients with basilar skull fracture and should be considered in trauma patients with fever but this is not common. Fever is common after significant head injury and can exacerbate neuronal injury. Because of this, accepted practice is that fever should be aggressively lowered, and the use of hypothermia is currently under study. (p1051)

Answer 56A-4: B.

The concept of a second injury has recently been emphasized in experimental models which explain a clinical observation, which is that prominent memory damage is more likely if there is a second insult such as hypotension or hypoxia. Non-convulsive seizure activity can produce hippocampal dysfunction, but this is unusual. (p1048)

Answer 56A-5: B.

Opening of the blood-brain barrier results in edema, which develops over days after the injury. Excitotoxic effects of agents such as glutamate are also thought to have a major role at this time. Shearing injury is an acute process rather than a chronic process and should not be expected to produce delayed deterioration. Hemorrhage is also largely an acute process, although delayed damage can rarely occur. (p1051)

Chapter 56B: Trauma of the Nervous System: Craniocerebral Trauma

Question 56B-1:
Which of the following statements regarding hemorrhage from craniocerebral trauma are true?

1. Acute subdural hematoma is the most common hemorrhage following cerebral trauma.
2. All epidural hematomas are arterial blood.
3. Epidural hematoma develops more quickly than subdural hematomas.
4. All subdural hematomas are venous blood.

Select: A = 1, 2, 3. B = 1, 3. C = 2, 4. D = 4 only. E = All

Question 56B-2:
Which of the following statements regarding prognosis in head injury are true?

1. Hypotension upon presentation worsens prognosis for good neurologic outcome.
2. Low Glasgow Coma Scale score predicts a poor prognosis.
3. Hypoxia upon presentation predicts a poor outcome.
4. For patients with fluctuating neurologic status, the best response is a better predictor of outcome than the worst response.

Select: A = 1, 2, 3. B = 1, 3. C = 2, 4. D = 4 only. E = All

Question 56B-3:
Hypotension frequently complicates significant head injury. Which of the following clinical formulations is true?

A. Hypotension develops as a consequence of the brain injury and indicates a poor prognosis. Aggressive treatment is futile and should not be encouraged.
B. Hypotension is a cardiovascular effect of the head injury and will only correct when the intracranial pressure is reduced. Mannitol and Lasix are given. Surgery is done for an evacuable hematoma.
C. Hypotension is due to hypovolemia in most patients and needs to be treated initially with normal saline.

Question 56B-4:
Which of the following clinical features predict a better outcome for recovery after head injury?

1. Youth vs old age
2. Surgical procedure vs no surgery
3. Normal eye movements vs ocular motor deficits
4. Motor posturing

Select: A = 1, 2, 3. B = 1, 3. C = 2, 4. D = 4 only. E = All

Questions 56B-5 through 56B-8:
Below are some basic herniation syndromes which are encountered in trauma patients. For the following questions, pick the syndrome which is most likely to be associated.

A. Uncal
B. Cingulate
C. Central
D. Tonsillar
E. None of these

Questions 56B-5:
Ipsilateral CN-3 palsy.

Question 56B-6:
Result of a cerebellar hemorrhage.

Question 56B-7:
Best prognosis of these herniation syndromes.

Question 56B-8:
Results in a posterior cerebral artery infarction.

Answer 56B-1: B.
While epidural hematomas tend to be arterial blood and subdural hematomas tend to be venous blood, the opposite can occur. Subdural hematoma can arise from cortical arteries rather than bridging veins. Since epidural hematomas are frequently arterial blood, they develop more quickly than subdural hematomas. (p1058)

Answer 56B-2: E.
All of these are correct. A second insult, such as hypoxia or hypotension, worsens prognosis. Some patients fluctuate substantially on examination; however, the prognosis is best indicated by the response observed when the patient is doing the best rather than the worst. The Glasgow Coma Scale is not absolutely predictive, but there is a correlation between response and survival providing the decreased response is not due to sedatives or paralytic agents. (p1059-1060)

Answer 56B-3: C
Hypotension in trauma patients is usually due to hypovolemia from hemorrhage rather than an autonomic effect of the head injury. While there is debate about the exact fluid to use, initial treatment with normal saline is often begun, although subsequent blood or fluid administration depends on the clinical situation. (p1060)

Answer 56B-4: B.
Patients who require surgery have a much lower good-outcome rate and a much higher death rate, owing to the severity and type of injuries. Motor posturing is a poor prognostic sign rather than a good sign. The others are typical prognostic indicators. (p1061)

Answer 56B-5: A.
Uncal herniation typically produces ipsilateral CN-3 palsy because of compression on the edge of the tentorium. (p1063)

Answer 56B-6: D.
Posterior fossa mass lesions can produce displacement of the cerebellar tonsils through the foramen magnum, resulting in compression of the medulla and rostral spinal cord. Coma quickly develops. (p1063)

Answer 56B-7: B.
Cingulate herniation is often seen on CT in patients with expanding mass lesions but does not have a specific strong clinical correlate. Treatment of the mass lesion is often successful in relieving the pressure and allowing for recovery. While this is not a good prognostic sign, it is better than the other herniation syndromes. (p1063)

Answer 56B-8: A.
Uncal herniation can occlude the posterior cerebral artery resulting in infarction of the occipital and temporal lobes. Because of the clinical findings associated with this lesion, the deficit may not be noted by examiners until after recovery of the patient from the acute injury. (p1063)

Question 56B-9:
A 50-year-old man is evaluated in the ER because of a motor vehicle accident. Blood alcohol is zero. Metabolic parameters are not significantly abnormal. He has no focal findings and normal mental status, but has a left frontal bruise plus glass imbedded in his scalp. These superficial lesions are treated. His family is supportive and concerned. Which would be the best clinical approach for neurologic management?

A. Admit overnight to the hospital and keep on IV fluids. Schedule an MRI of the brain for the next morning.
B. Check skull films and, if they are normal, discharge into the care of his family with detailed post-injury instructions.
C. Check CT head and, if normal, discharge home in the care of the family with detailed post-injury instructions.
D. Check skull films and, if normal, observe overnight.

Question 56B-10:
A 27-year-old man is admitted because of a closed head injury. CT is normal. Three days later he is still markedly confused and lethargic, not deteriorated from initial examination but little improved. Which of the following imaging studies would be most helpful for re-evaluation?

A. Repeat CT
B. MRI
C. PET
D. TCD
E. No reevaluation is necessary

Question 56B-11:
Hematoma in which of the following regions has the greatest risk of developing tentorial herniation?

A. Frontal
B. Temporal
C. Parietal
D. Occipital

Question 56B-12:
A 30-year-old female sustains a severe head injury in a motor vehicle accident. CT four hours after the initial incident shows diffuse cerebral edema. An intracranial pressure monitor is placed and vigorous anti-edema therapy is initiated. ICP remains approximately 5 cm H_2O for several hours then climbs to 25 cm H_2O over two hours. Osmolarity is 320 mosm. Which is the most appropriate clinical formulation?

A. Increase the mannitol dose.
B. Initiate hyperventilation.
C. Repeat CT of the head.
D. Administer pressors to elevate cerebral perfusion.

Question 56B-13:
A 16-year-old man is admitted for closed head injury and is observed by paramedics to have a single generalized seizure. Which is the most appropriate clinical formulation?

A. Phenytoin should be given to prevent more early seizures then discontinued if seizure free after 10 days.
B. Phenytoin should be given to prevent more early seizures then discontinued if seizure free after 6 months.
C. The recurrence rate is so low that anticonvulsant treatment is not needed.

Answer 56B-9: C.
The CT is more valuable than the observation for evaluation of a patient with a head injury. Even though he has normal mental status, the significance of the head injury indicates that CT should be performed with bone windows. If this is normal and he has good supports at home, admission is not necessary. Choice D, skull films and admission, is only appropriate if CT is unavailable, and ERs without this capability should not be evaluating trauma patients. (p1064)

Answer 56B-10: B.
MRI is more sensitive than CT for traumatic brain damage such as non-hemorrhagic contusions and shearing injuries. PET does not yet have an established place in evaluating trauma patients. TCD is especially helpful for evaluation of patients with vasospasm from subarachnoid hemorrhage, but is not helpful for routine evaluation. Evaluation is indicated with failure to improve or deterioration because late structural sequelae can develop. (p1066)

Answer 56B-11: B.
Temporal hematoma has the greatest likelihood of producing tentorial herniation by virtue of the geometry of the temporal fossa and the ability of the tissue to expand only backwards. (p1068)

Answer 56B-12: C.
Repeat CT of the head is indicated for evaluation of patients with abrupt increases in ICP, since late development of hematoma can precipitate this rise. In reality, advancing edema is the most common finding when the CT is done. This may require hyperventilation. The dose of mannitol should not be increased with the osmolarity of 320 mosm. (p1069)

Answer 56B-13: A.
Recurrent early seizures should be prevented because they can cause increased edema or secondary insult from resultant hypoxia or hypotension. However, in the absence of a recurrence, the chance of having recurrent seizures is low enough that treatment beyond 10 days is not warranted. (p1076)

Chapter 56C: Trauma of the Nervous System: Spinal Cord Trauma

Question 56C-1:
Which of the following statements are true regarding spinal shock following acute spinal cord injury?

1. Motor manifestations of spinal shock usually abate within a few hours after the injury.
2. Autonomic manifestations of spinal shock may last months.
3. Sensory manifestations of spinal shock improve within hours after injury.
4. Reflex changes of spinal shock may last days.

Select: A = 1, 2, 3. B = 1, 3. C = 2, 4. D = 4 only. E = All

Question 56C-2:
A 23-year-old man presents after a motor vehicle accident with quadriplegia and anesthesia from C1-C4, plus respiratory arrest and hypotension. Sensory loss is also demonstrated on the face, sparing the perioral region. Which is the most likely anatomic explanation for the deficit?

A. Upper cervical lesion producing the quadriparesis and respiratory deficits plus functional facial sensory loss.
B. Cervicomedullary lesion from injury at the craniocervical junction producing cervical and medullary dysfunction.
C. Tandem lesions in the upper cervical cord and posterior fossa from multifocal trauma.

Question 56C-3:
A 74-year-old man presents with arm weakness after a rear-end collision. He has severe neck pain. Examination shows arm weakness with diminished biceps reflexes, but preserved strength in the legs. Which is the most likely clinical formulation?

A. He has cervical spondylosis which was exacervated by the trauma producing a central cord syndrome.
B. He has suffered an acutely ruptured cervical disk with cord compression.
C. The deficit does not suggest a neurologic lesion, and functional weakness should be considered.

Question 56C-4:
Which of the following clinical features would *not* be expected in patients with Brown-Séquard's syndrome?

A. Ipsilateral motor loss
B. Contralateral proprioceptive sensation loss
C. Contralateral pain sensation loss
D. Contralateral temperature sensation loss

Question 56C-5:
Which of the following statements are true regarding patients with traumatic cauda equina lesions?

1. Incomplete lesions are more likely to spare sensory function than spare motor function.
2. Prognosis for motor recovery is poorer than with central cord syndromes.
3. Most injuries causing cauda equina damage are at or below the L1-L2 level.
4. Bowel and bladder incontinence occurs only with complete or near-complete lesions.

Select: A = 1, 2, 3. B = 1, 3. C = 2, 4. D = 4 only. E = All

Answer 56C-1: E.
All of these statements are true. Motor and sensory findings improve within a few hours after the injury, although reflex and autonomic dysfunction may last muh longer, depending on the severity of injury and level of the lesion. (p1093)

Answer 56C-2: B.
This is a classic presentation of cervicomedullary syndrome, which is characterized by dysfunction of the medulla and upper cervical cord, producing this constellation of clinical findings. (p1094)

Answer 56C-3: A.
Central cervical cord syndrome may present with weakness which is most prominent in the arms with preservation of the leg function, owing to the different location of segmental motor systems and descending projections. In this age, the existence of cervical spondylosis is more likely that acute cord compression from disk herniation. (p1095)

Answer 56C-4: B.
The proprioceptive sensory loss in patients with Brown-Séquard's syndrome ipsilateral rather than contralateral. (p1097)

Answer 56C-5: B.
Prognosis for motor recovery is generally better for patients with cauda equina lesions than central cord lesions because the lower motor neurons have greater resilience and regenerative capacity than the upper motor neurons. Sphincter disturbance is common with cauda equina lesions even in patients with preservation of leg motor function. (p1098)

Chapter 56D: Trauma of the Nervous System: Peripheral Nerve Trauma

Question 56C-1:
Peripheral nerve damage following high-velocity missile injury usually involves which pathophysiological process?

A. Nerve section from direct missile injury
B. Shock waves from missile movement through body tissues
C. Vascular damage with nerve infarction

Question 56C-2:
A 23-year-old female with left arm numbness following a motor vehicle accident is shown to have normal sensory nerve action potentials (SNAPs) during routine nerve conduction study. Which is the most likely clinical formulation?

A. The patient has injury to the dorsal roots proximal to the ganglion, such that the peripheral connections of the sensory nerve survive.
B. The patient is an unreliable reporter of sensory loss and may be malingering.
C. The sensory nerve study was performed incorrectly, not examining proximal conduction.

Question 56C-3:
A 15-year-old man presents with weakness of the ulnar-innervated intrinsic muscles of the left hand. The injury was from a bike accident approximately 1 week ago; there were no lacerations or fractured identified. There is no function of these muscles on clinical examination and no motor units elicited on EMG. Which would be the most appropriate clinical course?

A. Follow the patient over subsequent weeks and months with clinical examination and EMG
B. Refer the patient for exploration of the brachial plexus
C. Refer the patient for ulnar nerve transposition at the elbow

Answer 56C-1: B.
The most common method of nerve damage is from pressure waves through the tissues. Direct missile injury and secondary vascular injury can occur, but are less likely. (p1116)

Answer 56C-2: A.
Avulsion of the nerve roots with injury proximnal to the dorsal root ganglia produces sensory loss with preservation of the SNAPs, as opposed to peripheral nerve lesions, which would be associated with loss of SNAPs with time after injury. (p1116)

Answer 56C-3: A.
This type of injury is more likely to produce damage stretch injury than nerve section. Therefore, the nerve is in continuity. Surgery is not likely to be of benefit. Without documented focal entrapment, transposition of the ulner nerve would be inappropriate. (p1116)

Chapter 57A: Vascular Diseases of the Nervous System: Ischemic Cerebrovascular Disease

Question 57A-1:
Which of the following are nonmodifiable risk factors for ischemic stroke?

1. Age
2. First-degree relative with stroke
3. Black versus white race
4. Increased fibrinogen

Select: A = 1, 2, 3. B = 1, 3. C = 2, 4. D = 4 only. E = All

Question 57A-2:
Which of the following statements are true regarding estrogens and stroke?

1. High-estrogen oral contraceptive pills have a lower risk of stroke than low-estrogen OCPs.
2. Estrogen replacement in postmenopausal women reduces the risk of stroke.
3. The age-adjusted risk of cerebral infarction is doubled during pregnancy.
4. The risk of pregnancy-associated stroke is highest in the 6 weeks after delivery.

Select: A = 1, 2, 3. B = 1, 3. C = 2, 4. D = 4 only. E = All

Question 57A-3:
What proportion of patients with ischemic stroke have a preceding TIA?

A. < 5%
B. 10-15%
C. 30-40%
D. 50%

Question 57A-4:
Which is the most frequent site of atherosclerotic plaque formation?

A. Aorta
B. Carotid bifurcation
C. Femoral arteries
D. Coronary arteries

Question 57A-5:
Which of the following features would not be expected in a patient with TIA?

A. Abrupt onset of a hemiparesis
B. Focal weakness which clears over 20 minutes
C. Progression of weakness up the arm over 10 minutes
D. Loss of monocular vision

Question 57A-6:
A 54-year-old man presents with abrupt onset of right hemiparesis and Broca's aphasia. The weakness is most prominent in the face and arm, although the leg is affected to a lesser extent. Language comprehension is preserved. Which is the most likely site of vascular occlusion?

A. Upper division of the middle cerebral artery
B. Lower division of the middle cerebral artery
C. Stem of the middle cerebral artery
D. Internal carotid artery distal to the carotid bifurcation

Question 57A-7:
Which of the following clinical findings is least likely in a patient with infarction in the distribution of the left anterior choroidal artery?

A. Right hemiparesis
B. Right hemisensory loss
C. Right hemianopia
D. Aphasia

Question 57A-8:
Which of the following statements is not true regarding the dysarthria–clumsy hand syndrome?

A. Lacunar infarction is likely present in the basis pontis.
B. Central face weakness is common.
C. Babinski's sign is absent.
D. Dysphagia may accompany the dysarthria.

Answer 57A-1: A.
Age, family history, and race all are nonmodifiable risk factors, whereas increased fibrinogen is a modifiable risk factor. Elevated fibrinogen levels are associated with other risk factors such as smoking, obesity, hypertension, and diabetes. (p1126-1127)

Answer 57A-2: C.
Low-estrogen OCPs have lowered the risk of OCP-related thrombosis. In contrast, estrogen replacement in post-menopausal women has reduced the incidence of stroke. The risk of stroke is increased after delivery, but not during pregnancy itself. (p1127)

Answer 57A-3: B.
Approximately 10-15% of patients with stroke have a preceding TIA. (p1127)

Answer 57A-4: A.
The aorta is the first and most frequent site of formation of plaque. (p1127)

Answer 57A-5: C.
TIAs typically have weakness which begins abruptly and does not evolve over time. The other statements are typical of TIA. (p1129)

Answer 57A-6: A.
The expressive difficulty and more prominent involvement of the face and arm than leg suggests the upper division of the MCA has been affected. Preservation of comprehension indicates that the lower division of the MCA is preserved, which makes proximal MCA or ICA occlusion unlikely. (p1131)

Answer 57A-7: D.
Some language abnormalities can develop in patients with dominant-hemisphere infarctions in the distribution of the anterior choroidal artery, but prominent aphasia is not expected. The other clinical findings are typical with this lesion. (p1131)

Answer 57A-8: C.
Babinski's sign is common in patients with the dysarthria–clumsy hand syndrome. This is often due to lacunar infarction in the basis pontis. Dysphagia, dysarthria, and central facial weakness are typical clinical features. (p1132)

Questions 57A-9 through 57A-12:
The following four questions concern vertebrobasilar system stroke syndromes. For each of the mini-vignettes, select the primary vessel of involvement from the following list:

A. Superior cerebellar artery
B. Anterior inferior cerebellar artery
C. Posterior inferior cerebellar artery
D. Penetrating branches of the posterior cerebral artery

Question 57A-9:
A 76-year-old male with nausea, vomiting, nystagmus, cerebellar ataxia, right Horner's syndrome, loss of pain and temperature on the right side of the face and on the left side of the body, and pharyngeal muscle weakness.

Question 57A-10:
A 76-year-old male with right facial weakness and numbness, difficulty with conjugate right gaze, deafness, tinnitus, and ataxia.

Question 57A-11:
A 50-year-old female with right hemiplegia involving face, arm, and leg, left oculomotor paresis with mydriasis.

Question 57A-12:
A 70-year-old female with left hemiataxia, gait ataxia, left Horner's syndrome, left intention tremor, and right pain and temperature loss.

Question 57A-13:
What is the major cause of cardiogenic emboli in older adults?

A. Rheumatic atrial fibrillation
B. Non-valvular atrial fibrillation
C. Patent foramen ovale
D. Atrial myxoma

Question 57A-14:
Which of the following statements regarding treatment of cervicocephalic artery dissections is not true?

A. Risk factors include trauma, fibromuscular dysplasia, and syphilitic arteritis.
B. Initial treatment to prevent intracranial extension of carotid dissections is with heparin, usually followed by anticoagulation with coumadin.
C. Dissection may produce subarachnoid hemorrhage.
D. Horner's syndrome may develop from carotid dissection.

Question 57A-15:
Which is the most appropriate treatment for most patients with fibromuscular dysplasia involving the carotid vessels?

A. Warfarin (Coumadin)
B. Antiplatelet agents
C. Angioplasty
D. Carotid surgery

Question 57A-16:
Which of the following statements are true regarding Behçet's syndrome?

1. Carotid aneurysms may form.
2. Arterial occlusive disease is more common than venoocclusive disease.
3. Many patients have a history of uveitis.
4. It is most common in patients of African origin.

Select: A = 1, 2, 3. B = 1, 3. C = 2, 4. D = 4 only. E = All

Question 57A-17:
Headache is least likely in which of the following?

A. Giant cell arteritis
B. Lacunar infarction
C. Subarachnoid hemorrhage
D. Moyamoya

Answer 57A-9: C.
　The PICA is the vessel involved in producing the lateral medullary syndrome, although the most common direct cause is occlusion of the intracranial portion of the vertebral artery. This clinical presentation is typical. (p1134)

Answer 57A-10: B.
　Infarction in the distribution of the anterior inferior cerebellar artery can produce the lateral inferior pontine syndrome which is described in the mini-vignette. (p1134)

Answer 57A-11: D.
　This is Weber's syndrome, which is due to midbrain infarction from involvement of penetrating branches of the PCA. (p1132)

Answer 57A-12: A.
　Infarction in the distribution of the superior cerebellar artery can produce the dorsal cerebellar syndrome along with the midbrain signs described in the vignette. Patients may additionally have nystagmus. (p1132)

Answer 57A-13: B.
　NVAF is the most common cause of cardioembolic infarcts in older adults. PFO is more a problem in younger patients than elderly patients. Rheumatic atrial fibrillation confers a marked increase in the incidence of stroke, but is a smaller proportion of total strokes. Atrial myxomas are rare at any age. (p1139)

Answer 57A-14: B.
　Intracranial dissections carry a substantial risk of subarachnoid hemorrhage, so anticoagulation should be withheld in these patients. The other statements are true. (p1140)

Answer 57A-15: B.
　FMD is a relatively benign condition for most patients, so antiplatelet agents are indicated for most patients rather than more aggressive anticoagulants or surgery. (p1144)

Answer 57A-16: B.
　Venous occlusive disease is more common than arterial occlusive disease in patients with Behçet's disease. This disorder is most common in many patients of Mediterranean or East Asian origin. A history of uveitis is common, plus oral and genital ulcers. (p1145)

Answer 57A-17: B.
　Headache may be seen in patients with many types of stroke but is unlikely in patients with lacunar infarction. The other listed conditions are frequently associated with headache. (p1146)

Question 57A-18:
Which of the following are potential causes of stroke in patients with SSLE?

1. Nonbacterial endocarditis
2. Antiphospholipid antibody syndrome
3. Non-inflammatory vasculopathy
4. Immune-mediated vasculitis

Select: A = 1, 2, 3. B = 1, 3. C = 2, 4. D = 4 only. E = All

Questions 57A-19 through 57A-24:
The following group of questions is true/false. Select the best response for each statement.

Question 57A-19:
Antithrombin-III deficiency, protein C deficiency, and protein S deficiency all have autosomal dominant inheritance.

Question 57A-20:
Antiphospholipid antibodies should be suspected in a female with recurrent miscarriages.

Question 57A-21:
Patients with antiphospholipid antibodies have an increased incidence of mitral and aortic vegetations.

Question 57A-22:
Afibrinogenemia presents with increased risk of intracranial and systemic hemorrhage.

Question 57A-23:
Stroke with tumors is usually hemorrhagic with solid tumors and infarction with leukemias.

Question 57A-24:
The most common cause of stroke in patients with malignancy is low-grade DIC and secondary fibrinolysis.

Question 57A-25:
Nephrotic syndrome predisposes to which of the following stroke syndromes?

1. Arterial thrombosis
2. Subarachnoid hemorrhage
3. Venous thrombosis
4. Intracerebral hemorrhage

Select: A = 1, 2, 3. B = 1, 3. C = 2, 4. D = 4 only. E = All

Question 57A-26:
Which of the following are considered relative contraindications to the use of oral contraceptives?

1. Arterial hypertension
2. Post-partum period
3. Smoking
4. Age older than 35 years

Select: A = 1, 2, 3. B = 1, 3. C = 2, 4. D = 4 only. E = All

Question 57A-27:
Paroxysmal nocturnal hemoglobinuria predisposes to which of the following cerebrovascular conditions?

A. Arterial thrombosis
B. Arterial dissection
C. Venous thrombosis
D. Aneurysm formation and rupture

Question 57A-28:
Which of the following statements are true regarding heparin-induced thrombocytopenia?

1. Low-molecular-weight heparanoids are contraindicated in affected patients.
2. Hemorrhagic complications are common.
3. The disorder is a direct effect of the heparin on platelets.
4. Treatment consists of immediate discontinuation of heparin.

Select: A = 1, 2, 3. B = 1, 3. C = 2, 4. D = 4 only. E = All

Answer 57A-18: E.

All of these are potential causes of stroke in patients with SLE. Immune-mediated vasculitis is much less common than non-inflammatory vasculopathy in patients with SLE, although it can occur. (p1145)

Answer 57A-19: True.

These three conditions which predispose to stroke all have autosomal dominant inheritance, although homozygotes and heterozygotes or the Protein C and Protein S deficiencies have different presentations. (p1149)

Answer 57A-20: True.

Recurrent fetal loss is common in patients with antiphospholipid antibodies. (p1150)

Answer 57A-21: True.

Patients with antiphospholipid antibodies have an increased risk of stroke not only from vasculopathy but also from cardiac valvular disease. (p1150)

Answer 57A-22: True.

Afibrinogenemia is probably inherited as an autosomal recessive disorder and presents with increased risk especially of intracranial and GI hemorrhage. (p1150)

Answer 57A-23: False.

The exact opposite is true. Solid tumors, carcinomas, and lymphomas predispose to infarctions while leukemias predispose to hemorrhages. (p1150)

Answer 57A-24: False.

The most common cause of stroke in patients with malignancy is still atherosclerotic disease, although low-grade DIC and secondary fibrinolysis are tumor-related factors that make stroke more likely. (p1151)

Answer 57A-25: B.

Nephrotic syndrome has a complex effect on coagulation to predispose to both arterial and venous thromboses. The risk of primary hemorrhage is not increased; in fact, because of the possibility of infarction, anticoagulation is often necessary. (p1152)

Answer 57A-26: E.

Although none of these are absolute contraindications to the use of OCPs, all of these are relative contraindications. The risk is especially increased when multiple risk factors are in combinations, e.g., smoking plus age greater than age 35 years. (p1152)

Answer 57A-27: C.

PNH predisposes especially to cerebral venous thrombosis and portal vein thrombosis. (p1153)

Answer 57A-28: D.

When heparin-induced thrombocytopenia is diagnosed, the heparin is immediately discontinued. If anticoagulation is required, low-molecular-weight heparanoids may be used. The risk of hemorrhagic complications is low, and the disorder is characterized by arterial and venous thrombosis. The disorder is immune-mediated rather than a direct effect of the heparin on the platelets; there are increased levels of platelet-associated IgG and IgM. (p1153)

Question 57A-29:
A 49-year-old male presents with a mild left hemiparesis which was present upon awakening. He is a smoker and has a history of hypertension that is currently untreated. He is on no medications. There is no pain or headache. There is no neglect or visual field defect. Examination is stable, showing no substantial improvement or deterioration. CT head is normal. Which of the following clinical approaches is most appropriate?

A. Admission to the hospital, heparin administration IV
B. Admission to the hospital, antiplatelet agent
C. Administration of antiplatelet agent and discharge from the emergency department
D. Admission to the hospital, administration of t-PA

Question 57A-30:
Which of the following statements is true regarding depression in patients with stroke?

1. Depression is most likely with left-hemisphere infarcts.
2. Depression is mainly situational.
3. Depression is present in about 25% of patients with stroke.
4. Antidepressants should be avoided in patients with stroke.

Select: A = 1, 2, 3. B = 1, 3. C = 2, 4. D = 4 only. E = All

Question 57A-31:
A 24-year-old female presents with headache, nausea, and vomiting, and has a generalized seizure. Examination reveals mild confusion and papilledema. She is 2 weeks postpartum. What is the most likely diagnosis?

A. Carotid dissection
B. Cardiogenic emboli
C. Venous thrombosis
D. Meningitis

Answer 57A-29: B.
When the patient presents with a small stable infarction, administration of heparin is not of proven benefit. A case can be made for use of heparin IV when patients have presumed cardiogenic emboli, carotid dissection, or hypercoagulable states. Therefore, administration of an antiplatelet agent would be appropriate. T-PA would not be appropriate in this situation because the time of onset of the stroke cannot be determined; according to current guidelines, t-PA must be administered within three hours of the onset of symptoms. In addition, uncontrolled hypertension is a contraindication to t-PA treatment, depending on the exact measurements. A patient with acute stroke has a risk of worsening and development of other complications, so inpatient management is most appropriate. (p1156-1158,1162)

Answer 57A-30: B.
Depression is most common with patients with left-hemisphere infarcts, especially of the frontal lobe. The frequency is about 25% overall. The depression is not all situational, being part of the cerebral dysfunction, and may be related to disorder of catecholamine-mediated pathways. Antidepressants are often effective, and should not be withheld just because the depression is caused by a stroke. (p1163)

Answer 57A-31: C.
Cerebral venous thrombosis is the most likely diagnosis in this patient with seizure and signs of increased intracranial pressure in the immediate post-partum period. The other listed diagnoses are possible but less likely. (p1164)

Chapter 57B: Vascular Diseases of the Nervous System: Intracerebral Hemorrhage

Question 57B-1:
Which is the greatest single risk factor in development of intracerebral hemorrhage?

A. Hypertension
B. Family history
C. Obesity
D. Lipid profile

Question 57B-2:
Which of the following statements are true regarding anticoagulant use and intracerebral hemorrhage (ICH)?

1. Oral anticoagulants increase the risk of ICH approximately 10-fold.
2. Older age increases the relative risk of ICH while using oral anticoagulants.
3. Previous cerebral infarction increases the relative risk of ICH while using oral anticoagulants.
4. ICH in patients on oral anticoagulants progresses at a slower pace than ICH in patients with severe hypertension.

Select: A = 1, 2, 3. B = 1, 3. C = 2, 4. D = 4 only. E = All

Question 57B-3:
Which of the following statements are true regarding cerebral amyloid angiopathy (CAA)?

1. CAA may be associated with pathological changes of Alzheimer's disease in some patients.
2. ICH due to CAA is predominantly a problem of middle age.
3. Hemorrhages are usually lobar.
4. Episodes of transient neurologic deficit preceding a lobar hemorrhage suggest hemorrhagic infarction rather than CAA.

Select: A = 1, 2, 3. B = 1, 3. C = 2, 4. D = 4 only. E = All

Question 57B-4:
Which of the following features would not be expected in ICH related to sympathomimetic use?

A. Beaded appearance of intracranial arteries on angiography
B. Marked hypertension at the time of presentation
C. Multiple simultaneous subcortical and deep hemorrhages
D. Onset of symptoms delayed days from last use of the agent

Question 57B-5:
Hemorrhagic infarction would be least likely in which of the following conditions?

A. Embolic infarction
B. Lacunar infarction
C. Venous thrombosis

Question 57B-6:
Which is the most likely cause of caudate hemorrhage?

A. AVM
B. Aneurysm
C. Hypertension
D. Hemorrhagic transformation of infarction

Question 57B-7:
A 57-year-old female presents with decreased responsiveness, horizontal gaze palsy, pinpoint pupils, and decerebrate posturing. Which would be the most likely etiology?

A. Mesencephalic hemorrhage
B. Pontine hemorrhage
C. Cerebellar hemorrhage
D. Thalamic hemorrhage

Answer 57B-1: A.
Hypertension is by far the most important risk factor in development of intracerebral hemorrhage. All of the other factors play a role, plus the presence of vascular malformations, coagulation disorders, trauma, and other factors. (p1167)

Answer 57B-2: E.
All of these statements are true. Other factors which increase the relative risk of ICH in a patient on oral anticoagulants include excessive prolongation of the prothrombin time and trauma. (p1170)

Answer 57B-3: B.
CAA is associated with pathological changes of AD more frequently than might be expected by chance alone, so patients may develop progressive dementia during the period when ICH may develop. Hemorrhages are usually lobar, although localized subarachnoid hemorrhages are common, as well. CAA is mainly a problem of advanced age, with ICH due to this pathology seldom occurring prior to the age of 55 years. Episodes of transient neurologic deficit may precede the development of a clinically apparent lobar hemorrhage; these probably represent small hemorrhages for which the symptoms resolve quickly. They may be easily mistaken for TIAs or seizures. (p1172)

Answer 57B-4: D.
The onset of symptoms is usually shortly after the administration of the drug rather than delayed. The other features would be expected in patients with sympathomimetic-associated ICH. (p1172)

Answer 57B-5: B.
Lacunar infarction is unlikely to be associated with hemorrhagic transformation. Venous thrombosis and embolic stroke is most likely to be associated with hemorrhage. (p1172)

Answer 57B-6: C.
Hypertension is the most common cause of caudate hemorrhage, and of most hemorrhages. AVM or aneurysm is unusual in this area. Also, hemorrhagic transformation of a small vessel infarction producing caudate infarction would not be expected. (p1176)

Answer 57B-7: B.
This clinical presentation is typical of pontine hemorrhage. Damage to pontine gaze centers, reticular formation, and corticospinal tracts will produce most of these symptoms. Cerebellar hemorrhage can produce brainstem compression and these findings but usually not as an initial presentation. (p1178)

Question 57B-8:
Surgery for relief of intracranial hemorrhage is most likely to be necessary for patients with which of the following conditions?

A. Subarachnoid hemorrhage
B. Putaminal hemorrhage
C. Lobar hemorrhage
D. Cerebellar hemorrhage

Question 57B-9:
Which of the following are true of thalamic hemorrhage?

1. The major prognostic sign is size of the hematoma.
2. Ventricular extension signifies a poor prognosis for survival.
3. Hydrocephalus signifies a poor prognosis for recovery.
4. The thalamus is the most common location of intracranial hemorrhage.

Select: A = 1, 2, 3. B = 1, 3. C = 2, 4. D = 4 only. E = All

Question 57B-10:
Which of the following statements are true regarding intracerebral hemorrhage in patients treated with t-PA for acute myocardial infarction?

1. Hemorrhage is usually early, often during the drug infusion.
2. Most hemorrhages are lobar.
3. Prognosis is generally poor for hemorrhage associated with t-PA administration.
4. The risk of intracerebral hematoma in patients currently treated with t-PA for AMI is less than 1%.

Select: A = 1, 2, 3. B = 1, 3. C = 2, 4. D = 4 only. E = All

Answer 57B-8: D.
Cerebellar hemorrhage frequently requires surgery to prevent deterioration. Most patients with the other conditions do not require surgery, although occasional patients with lobar hemorrhage will require surgery as a life-saving maneuver. (p1182)

Answer 57B-9: B.
Size is the most important prognostic sign for a thalamic hematoma with hydrocephalus indicating a poor prognosis. Ventricular extension does not correlate with prognosis. (p1177)

Answer 57B-10: E.
All of these statements are true. Using current recommendations for t-PA administration for AMI, the risk of cerebral hemorrhage is approximately 0.5-0.6%. The mortality rate for patients with intracerebral hemorrhage with t-PA for AMI is at least 44%. (p1170)

Chapter 57C: Vascular Diseases of the Nervous System: Intracranial Aneurysms and Subarachnoid Hemorrhage

Question 57C-1:
A 27-year-old male presents with the abrupt onset of headache, which abates during the next 24 hours. Brain CT is normal including with contrast. CSF shows 3 WBCs/ul, no RBCs, normal glucose and protein. Which of the following statements is not true?

A. Aneurysm may still be present despite these findings, although migraine is the most likely diagnosis.
B. Recurrent localized pain may be due to aneurysm despite the absence of meningeal symptoms.
C. The normal CT and CSF rule out aneurysmal rupture, securing the diagnosis of migraine.
D. Sentinel headaches occur in about half of patients with aneurysmal rupture.

Question 57C-2:
A patient with subarachnoid hemorrhage presents with headache, nausea, vomiting, and mild left hemiparesis and is drowsy but responsive to stimuli, and does follow commands appropriately. Which is the grade of the SAH according to the Hunt and Hess scale?

A. Grade 1
B. Grade 2
C. Grade 3
D. Grade 4
E. Grade 5

Question 57C-3:
A patient presents with limitation of movement of one eye and ipsilateral peri-orbital headache, and has ipsilateral numbness of the upper face. Which is the most likely location of an aneurysm which would produce these symptoms?

A. Anterior communicating artery
B. Posterior communicating artery
C. Basilar artery
D. Intracavernous portion of the internal carotid artery

Questions 57C-4 through 57C-7:
For each of the following questions, select the appropriate aneurysm location from the following list:

A. Anterior communicating artery
B. Posterior communicating artery
C. Basilar artery
D. Internal carotid artery
E. Middle cerebral artery

Question 57C-4:
Junctional scotoma.

Question 57C-5:
Carotid cavernous fistula.

Question 57C-6:
Isolated third nerve palsy

Question 57C-7:
Aphasia and right arm weakness.

Question 57C-8:
CT is sensitive for detection of SAH, but it has certain limitations. Which of the following statements is true regarding CT in SAH?

A. CT performed 72 hours after SAH is more sensitive than CT within 24 hours.
B. Modern CT is able to detect SAH in at least 90% of patients within 24 hours.
C. Modern CT is sufficiently sensitive that LP is seldom necessary if the CT is normal.
D. If CT suggests SAH, LP is done for confirmation.

Answer 57C-1: C.
The normal CT and CSF are reassuring but cannot completely rule out the diagnosis of intracranial aneurysm. Hemorrhage within the walls of the vessel may produce headache with acute aneurysmal enlargement without the CSF findings. (p1185)

Answer 57C-2: C.
Grade 3 is drowsiness with mild deficit. The presence of the hemiparesis takes this patient out of grade 2, which would have no neurologic deficit except perhaps a cranial nerve palsy. The responsiveness would keep this patient currently out of grade 4. (p1186)

Answer 57C-3: D.
Aneurysm of the intracavernous portion of the internal carotid artery may produce compression of the third, fourth, fifth, and sixth cranial nerves. Posterior communicating artery aneurysm produces third nerve palsy, but fifth nerve dysfunction would not be expected. (p1186)

Answer 57C-4: A.
Aneurysm of the anterior communicating artery may produce compression of the optic chiasm, resulting in a junctional scotoma. (p1187)

Answer 57C-5: D.
Aneurysm of the internal carotid artery may produce a carotid cavernous fistula within the cavernous sinus. (p1186)

Answer 57C-6: B.
Aneurysm of the posterior communicating artery may produce oculomotor nerve compression, with diplopia and mydriasis. (p1186)

Answer 57C-7: E.
Aneurysm of the middle cerebral artery is most likely to produce focal cortical signs, including aphasia and right arm weakness, with a left-sided lesion. These focal signs may indicate intracranial hematoma complicating a MCA aneurysm. (p1186)

Answer 57C-8: B.
Modern CT is able to detect 90-95% of subarachnoid hemorrhages, but this sensitivity declines by 72 hours. If CT is positive, there is little diagnostic utility for LP, so it usually does not need to be performed. However, if CT is negative in a patient with appropriate clinical history, LP should be performed to look for blood. (p1187)

Question 57C-9:
Predisposition to intracranial aneurysms occurs with which of the following conditions?

A. Autosomal dominant polycystic kidney disease
B. Neurofibromatosis type I
C. Cigarette smoking
D. First-degree relative with aneurysmal SAH
E. All of the above

Question 57C-10:
All of the following statements regarding prognosis after SAH are true except which?

A. The most common cause of death in patients surviving 6 months after nonoperative management of a single ruptured aneurysm is rebleeding.
B. The majority of patients who have craniotomy for SAH have abnormalities on neuropsychological testing.
C. Surgery has not been proven to lower the risk of delayed bleeding.
D. Operative intervention should be done early after hemorrhage in patients with good functional status for the best prognosis.

Question 57C-11:
Which of the following statements are true regarding vasospasm in patients with subarachnoid hemorrhage?

1. Nimodipine reduces the frequency of infarction in patients with SAH.
2. The benefit of nimodipine in SAH is due to its marked reduction in vasospasm.
3. Other calcium channel blocking agents have been shown to also reduce ischemic events.
4. Angioplasty is contraindicated in patients with ischemia associated with SAH.

Select: A = 1, 2, 3. B = 1, 3. C = 2, 4. D = 4 only. E = All

Answer 57C-9: E.
All of the listed disorders predispose to intracranial aneurysms. In addition, Ehlers-Danlos syndrome, Marfan's syndrome, and hypertension should be added to this list. Cigarette smoking is a greater risk factor than hypertension. (p1189)

Answer 57C-10: C.
Surgery has been proven to reduce the frequency of late bleeding from aneurysmal hemorrhage. The other statements are true. (p1191)

Answer 57C-11: B.
The benefits of nimodipine and some other calcium channel blocking agents is proven, but the reduction in ischemic events is more prominent than would be expected on the basis of angiographic findings. Angioplasty can open vessels which have undergone spasm, and is not contraindicated if the practitioners are experienced in the techniques. (p1195)

Chapter 57D: Vascular Diseases of the Nervous System: Arteriovenous Malformations

Question 57D-1:
Which of the following statements is true regarding cavernous malformations?

A. Cavernous malformations do not hemorrhage.
B. Cavernous malformation will not form cryptic malformations.
C. Familial cavernous malformations are usually multiple.
D. Most patients are diagnosed in childhood.

Question 57D-2:
Which of the following statements is true for arteriovenous malformations?

A. Seizures are rare in patients with AVMs.
B. Seizures in a patient with AVM indicate that surgery should be performed.
C. Stereotactic radiosurgery has little or no role in treatment of AVMs.
D. High output heart failure can develop due to AVM in infancy.

Question 57D-3:
Which is the most common vascular malformation?

A. Arteriovenous malformation
B. Cavernous malformation
C. Venous angioma
D. Telangiectasia

Question 57D-4:
A 27-year-old man is found to have a small AVM with signs of bleeding surrounding it. Neurologic examination is normal. In counseling the patient, which of the following statements would not be true?

A. Seizures may occur and if present would be treated with conventional anticonvulsants.
B. Small AVMs are less likely to bleed than large AVMs.
C. Hypertension will increase the likelihood of re-bleeding.
D. The incidence of re-bleeding is less than 10% per year.

Question 57D-5:
Surgical vs medical management of AVMs is a controversial area, and decisions have to be individualized based on many clinical features. Which of the following factors would favor surgical treatment?

1. Young age of the patient
2. Large lesion
3. Location outside a clinically crucial area
4. Multiple feeding vessels and draining veins

Select: A = 1, 2, 3. B = 1, 3. C = 2, 4. D = 4 only. E = All

Answer 57D-1: C.
A cavernous malformation typically shows signs of hemorrhage. Cavernous malformations account for 25-50% of cryptic malformations. Familial malformations are usually multiple. Most patients are diagnosed in the second to fourth decade. (p1203)

Answer 57D-2: D.
The so-called "Vein of Galen aneurysm" is really an AVM which can produce high-output heart failure in infancy. Seizures are common in patients with AVM, with more than 50% of patients with AVM having at least one seizure by the age of 30. Stereotactic radiosurgery is a very useful tool for treatment of AVMs, although not for all patients because of physical characteristics of the lesion. Seizures should be managed medically, if possible. Decisions on surgery are generally made independently of the presence of seizures. (p1204, 1209-1210)

Answer 57D-3: C.
Venous angiomas are the most common vascular malformation, although they are almost always clinically silent. (p1201)

Answer 57D-4: B.
Small AVMs are more likely to bleed than large AVMs because of the differences in pressures and flow patterns. The frequency of rebleeding after hemorrhage from an AVM is approximately 6% in the first year and 4% in subsequent years. Hypertension will increase the likelihood of rebleeding. (p1205-1206)

Answer 57D-5: B.
Young patients have their entire lifetime to experience the increase in risk of bleeding of an unoperated AVM, so surgical therapy would be entertained more aggressively in a young patient than in an elderly individual. Large lesions are less likely to bleed and more likely to have surgical complications than small lesions, so smaller lesions would favor surgical treatment. Likewise, multiple feeding vessels make surgery more difficult and potentially hazardous. New surgical techniques have been used to approach difficult areas, but in general, a favorable location would make surgery more attractive. (p1210)

Chapter 57E: Vascular Diseases of the Nervous System: Stroke in Childhood

Question 57E-1:
Which of the following statements regarding stroke in children versus adults are true?

1. Hemorrhage is a greater proportion of strokes in children than in adults.
2. Congenital causes of stroke are more common in children than adults.
3. Children have a greater likelihood of having seizures with acute stroke than adults.
4. Fluent aphasia develops commonly with dominant hemisphere strokes in children and adults.

Select: A = 1, 2, 3. B = 1, 3. C = 2, 4. D = 4 only. E = All

Question 57E-2:
A 10-year-old female is brought in to the hospital with aphasia and right hemiparesis. The child is afebrile. CT 3 hours after the event shows no abnormalities. Laboratory studies are normal except for the CBC, which is remarkable for mild anemia, low platelets, plus increased WBCs at 86,000/μl. Which of the following is the most likely diagnosis?

A. Right-to-left shunt with resultant cerebral emboli
B. Septic emboli from endocarditis
C. Thrombosis due to leukemia
D. Meningitis with secondary vasculopathy

Question 57E-3:
Which of the following conditions are associated with increased risk of stroke in childhood?

1. Homocystinuria
2. Fabry's disease
3. Leigh disease
4. HDL-deficiency

Select: A = 1, 2, 3. B = 1, 3. C = 2, 4. D = 4 only. E = All

Question 57E-4:
Which is the most common cause of intracerebral hemorrhage in children?

A. AVMs
B. Coagulopathies
C. Trauma
D. Aneurysm

Questions 57E-5 through 57E-8:
The following questions are True/False. Select the best answer.

Question 57E-5:
Cerebral infarction from arterial occlusion is more common in premature infants than term infants.

Question 57E-6:
Maternal use of cocaine in the prepartum period predisposes to cerebral infarction in neonates.

Question 57E-7:
Children with unilateral strokes have normal intellect.

Question 57E-8:
HIV infection predisposes to cerebral hemorrhagic and non-hemorrhagic infarcts.

Answer 57E-1: A.
Hemorrhage is a greater proportion of the strokes in children than in adults. In children, 45% of strokes are hemorrhages. Congenital abnormalities are a much greater proportion of the etiologies of stroke in children than in adults. Seizures are much more common with strokes in children than in adults, and in acute hemiplegia of childhood, 80% of patients have seizures. Fluent aphasia is uncommon in children; mutism is a more common presentation of dominant hemisphere stroke. (p1215)

Answer 57E-2: C.
Cerebral thrombosis associated with acute leukemia is the most likely diagnosis in this patient. The degree of elevation in WBC would be unexpected for infectious illnesses. The anemia and reduction in platelets would also be common findings in leukemia. (p1219)

Answer 57E-3: E.
All of these metabolic disorders increase the risk of stroke in childhood. Leigh disease is one of a number of mitochondrial disorders which cause stroke syndromes. Homocystinuria produces an increased frequency of stroke by intimal thickening and fibrosis and increased platelet adhesiveness. (p1220)

Answer 57E-4: C.
Trauma is the most common cause of intracranial hemorrhage in children, followed by coagulopathies and AVMs. Aneurysms are uncommon in children. (p1221)

Answer 57E-5: False.
Arterial occlusion resulting is cerebral infarction is more common in term infants than premature infants. (p1222)

Answer 57E-6: True.
Cocaine may produce vasoconstriction and cerebral infarction in neonates. (p1222)

Answer 57E-7: False.
Children with even strictly unilateral strokes typically have measurably reduced IQs. (p1223)

Answer 57E-8: True.
HIV infection in children predisposes to both hemorrhagic and non-hemorrhagic infarcts. (p1219)

Chapter 57F: Vascular Diseases of the Nervous System: Spinal Cord Vascular Disease

Question 57F-1:
Which of the following can produce spinal cord infarction?

1. Cross-clamping of the aorta
2. Hypotension
3. Aortic dissection
4. Venous occlusion

Select: A = 1, 2, 3. B = 1, 3. C = 2, 4. D = 4 only. E = All

Question 57F-2:
Which of the following statements are true regarding subarachnoid hemorrhage of spinal cord origin?

1. The most common cause of SAH of spinal origin is spinal angioma.
2. Spinal origin accounts for approximately 10% of all SAH.
3. Spinal SAH may present as acute onset of back pain.
4. Papilledema does not develop with spinal SAH.

Select: A = 1, 2, 3. B = 1, 3. C = 2, 4. D = 4 only. E = All

Question 57F-3:
Which of the following statements are true regarding the artery of Adamkiewicz?

1. It supplies blood to the posterior 2/3 of the thoracic and lumbar cord.
2. Occlusion typically causes paraparesis.
3. The only other blood supply is via the anterior spinal artery from branches of the vertebral artery.
4. It follows one of the lower thoracic or upper lumbar nerve roots into the spinal column.

Select: A = 1, 2, 3. B = 1, 3. C = 2, 4. D = 4 only. E = All

Question 57F-4:
A 58-year-old male presents with three episodes of transient leg weakness and numbness. The duration is 15-20 minutes. One of these occurred with walking, but the others occurred at rest. Which is the most likely diagnosis?

A. Spinal stenosis
B. Spinal cord transient ischemic attack
C. Multiple sclerosis
D. Devic's disease
E. Iliac artery insufficiency

Question 57F-5:
A 68-year-old female presents with onset of severe pain over the lower thoracic spine associated with leg weakness and loss of bowel and bladder control. The symptoms develop over about 6 hours. She recently had an epidural injection for chronic back pain. Which is the most likely diagnosis?

A. Transverse myelitis
B. Spinal epidural hematoma
C. Spinal epidural abscess
D. Spinal cord infarction

Answer 57F-1: E.

All of these are potential causes of spinal cord ischemia. In patients with hypotension, cerebral symptoms usually eclipse spinal cord symptoms, but signs of cord damage can occur. (p1227)

Answer 57F-2: B.

Spinal angioma is the most common cause of SAH of spinal origin. Less than 1% of SAH are due to spinal causes. Papilledema may develop with SAH of spinal origin, just as it can develop from SAH of intracranial vessels. (p1229)

Answer 57F-3: C.

The artery of Adamkiewicz is a major vessel which supplies blood to the lower thoracic and upper lumbar cord. Infarction typically results in paraparesis with some sensory findings, as well. Although this is a very important vessel, there are other radicular arteries which supply blood to the cord. (p1225-1226)

Answer 57F-4: B.

Spinal TIA is uncommon but can occur. Patients typically have brief episodes of leg weakness and numbness, which totally resolve. Demyelinating disease would produce symptoms of longer duration. (p1228)

Answer 57F-5: B.

Spinal epidural hematoma typically presents with back pain at about the level of the lesion associated with myelopathy or cauda equina lesion. Transverse myelitis would not be expected to produce symptoms over a short period of time. Spinal cord infarction would not be expected to produce symptoms which develop over such a long period of time, and would not be expected to be a complication of epidural injection. Abscess is a potential complication of epidural hematoma but would not be expected to develop over such a short time. (p1230)

Chapter 57G: Vascular Diseases of the Nervous System: Central Nervous System Vasculitis

Question 57G-1:
Which of the following statements regarding isolated CNS vasculitis are not true?

A. Headache and confusion are the most common presenting features.
B. Most patients have abnormalities in CSF.
C. Most patients have a markedly elevated erythrocyte sedimentation rate.
D. Angiography may be normal in pathologically confirmed cases.

Question 57G-2:
Which of the following treatment regimens is currently used first-line for treatment of patients with isolated CNS vasculitis?

A. High-dose prednisone
B. Prednisone plus cyclophosphamide
C. Plasma exchange plus azathioprine
D. Intravenous immunoglobulin

Questions 57G-3 through 57G-6:
The following statements are true or false. Select the best answer for each statement.

Question 57G-3:
Hodgkin's disease is associated with an increased likelihood of developing isolated CNS vasculitis.

Question 57G-4:
Wegener's granulomatosis may affect the PNS but not the CNS.

Question 57G-5:
CNS angiitis presenting as stroke syndrome usually is a manifestation of intracerebral hemorrhage.

Question 57G-6:
Angiography is of no value in the diagnosis of isolated CNS angiitis.

Answer 57G-1: C.
ESR is elevated in some patients, but is frequently normal. When elevated, the degree of increase is less prominent than is typically seen in temporal arteritis. The other statements are true. (p1231-1232)

Answer 57G-2: B.
High-dose prednisone plus cyclophosphamide is the most commonly used treatment for initial treatment of patients with isolated CNS vasculitis. IVIG has been tried in a few patients with reported success, but there is insufficient clinical experience for this treatment to supplant traditional therapy. (p1232-1233)

Answer 57G-3: True.
Hodgkin's disease is the most common lymphoma to be associated with development of isolated CNS vasculitis. Some of these cases have been associated with development of disseminated herpes zoster infection, although certainly not all. (p1233)

Answer 57G-4: False.
Wegener's granulomatosis is a systemic vasculitis which can affect the CNS. (p1231)

Answer 57G-5: True.
Isolated CNS angiitis is more likely to present with a stroke syndrome due to hemorrhage than infarction or TIA. (p1231)

Answer 57G-6: False.
Angiography may be normal in pathologically confirmed cases of isolated CNS angiitis, but it still has value. The angiographic findings can be supportive of a clinical diagnosis, differentiating this disorder from some other disorders with which it can be confused. (p1232)

Chapter 58: Primary and Secondary Tumors of the Central Nervous System

Question 58-1:
The most prevalent tumors in the CNS are which?

A. Neuroendocrine tumors
B. Metastases of systemic neoplasm
C. Malignant gliomas
D. Benign glial tumors

Question 58-2:
Which of the following statements is not true?

A. Early diagnosis is important for treatment of most malignant brain tumors.
B. MRI is superior to CT for identification of brain tumors.
C. The blood-brain barrier is an impediment to delivery of chemotherapeutic agents to brain tumors.
D. Complete resection of most tumors is impossible without jeopardizing normal neural tissue.

Answer 58-1: B.
Metastases of systemic neoplasms are the most common CNS tumors. Up to 25% of patients with systemic neoplasms are found to have CNS metastases at time of autopsy. (p1235)

Answer 58-2: A.
Unfortunately, early diagnosis is not helpful for diagnosis of most malignant brain tumors. The remainder of the statements are true. Complete resection is frequently impossible since there is interdigitation of tumor cells within normal brain tissue. The blood-brain barrier is an important impediment to chemotherapy, even when the tumor has resulted in damage to the barrier; many tumor cells are still within the protected regions of the brain, relatively protected from delivery of many drugs. (p1235)

Chapter 58A: Primary and Secondary Tumors of the Central Nervous System: Pathology of Nervous System Tumors

Question 58A-1:
Glial fibrillary acidic protein best identifies which of the following tumor types?

A. Astrocytoma
B. Primitive neuroectodermal tumor (PNET)
C. Oligodendroglioma
D. Meningioma

Question 58A-2:
Which of the following statements about the NF-1 gene is not true?

A. The gene is on chromosome 17.
B. NF-1 is a tumor suppressor gene.
C. Neurofibromatosis type 1 is due to expansion of the region coding for NF-1.
D. NF-2 is not directly related to the NF-1 gene

Question 58A-3:
The S-100 protein is a marker for which of the following tumors?

A. Meningioma
B. Astrocytoma
C. Oligodendroglioma
D. Schwannoma

Question 58A-4:
Which of the following statements is not true regarding histological grading system for patients with astrocytomas?

A. The differentiation between anaplastic astrocytoma and glioblastoma is the presence of necrosis in the latter.
B. Anaplastic astrocytoma is the most common of the astrocytic tumors.
C. Pseudopalisading is more prominent in glioblastoma than in astrocytomas and anaplastic astrocytomas.
D. Amplification of the epidermal growth factor receptor gene is most prominent in glioblastoma.

Questions 58A-5 through 58A-9:
The following questions concern pathological and pathophysiological features of CNS tumors. Select the best answer from the following list:

A. Astrocytoma
B. Anaplastic astrocytoma
C. Glioblastoma
D. Oligodendroglioma
E. Ependymoma
F. Choroid plexus papilloma
G. Primitive neuroectodermal tumor

Question 58A-5:
Excessive CSF production.

Question 58A-6:
"Fried-egg" appearance of tumor cell nuclei.

Question 58A-7:
Medulloblastoma.

Question 58A-8:
Obstructive hydrocephalus.

Question 58A-9:
Retinoblastoma.

Question 58A-10:
Which of the following statements regarding medulloblastoma are true?

1. Most common PNET of the CNS
2. Most common in childhood
3. May produce distant metastases
4. Origin in the midline, usually anterior to the hypothalamus

Select: A = 1, 2, 3. B = 1, 3. C = 2, 4. D = 4 only. E = All

Answer 58A-1: A.
GFAP is an immunohistochemical marker especially for astrocytomas. PNET and oligodendroglioma may also occasionally stain, but this is not typical. Meningiomas have essentially GFAP immunoreactivity. (p1239)

Answer 58A-2: C.
NF-1 is due to a loss of the NF-1 gene, a tumor suppressor gene on chromosome 17. Many disorders are due to expansion of trinucleotide repeats, but that does not apply in NF-1. (p1240)

Answer 58A-3: D.
The S-100 protein is a marker for schwannoma but is not highly useful in clinical practice. Astrocytomas and oligodendrogliomas react only weakly positively for S-100 protein. (p1239)

Answer 58A-4: B.
Glioblastoma is the most common primary brain tumor in adults, and certainly the most common of the tumors in the astrocytic line. There are several differences between anaplastic astrocytomas and glioblastomas, but the cardinal feature is the presence of necrosis. Amplification of the EGF-receptor gene is common in GBM, and an adjunct to diagnosis. (p1243)

Answer 58A-5: F.
Choroid plexus papillomas can make CSF at an excessive rate, resulting in hydrocephalus. (p1246)

Answer 58A-6: D.
The "fried-egg" appearance of tumor cell nuclei is the most distinctive pathological feature of oligodendrogliomas. (p1244)

Answer 58A-7: G.
PNETs in the CNS include medulloblastoma, neuroblastoma, and pineoblastoma. (p1247)

Answer 58A-8: E.
Almost any tumor can ultimately cause obstructive hydrocephalus, but ependymomas are the most likely of these to cause hydrocephalus because of their location in the ventricle and the propensity for their infratentorial location. (p1245)

Answer 58A-9: G.
PNETs outside of the CNS include adrenal neuroblastoma and retinoblastoma. (p1247)

Answer 58A-10: A.
Medulloblastomas originate from the cerebellum, usually in the midline. The other statements are true. Medulloblastomas are prone to CSF metastases and distant metastases. More than 50% occur in children younger than 10 years of age. (p1247)

Question 58A-11:
Which of the following statements are true regarding meningiomas?

1. Most are associated with abnormalities of chromosome 22.
2. Posterior fossa is the most common location for meningiomas in adults.
3. Multiple meningiomas suggest neurofibromatosis type 2.
4. Estrogen and progesterone receptors rarely occur on meningiomas.

Select: A = 1, 2, 3. B = 1, 3. C = 2, 4. D = 4 only. E = All

Questions 58A-12 through 58A-15:
The following questions concern CNS involvement with lymphoma. For each question, select the best answer from the following list.

A. Primary CNS lymphoma
B. Systemic lymphoma
C. Both
D. Neither

Question 58A-12:
Increased incidence in immunodeficient patients.

Question 58A-13:
B-cell tumors.

Question 58A-14:
Commonly infiltrate the meninges.

Question 58A-15:
Parenchymal involvement.

Question 58A-16:
What is the most likely location of germ cell tumors in the CNS?

A. Third ventricle
B. Fourth ventricle
C. Pineal region
D. Subthalamic region

Answer 58A-11: B.
Adults usually have meningiomas over the cerebral convexity; posterior fossa meningiomas are more common in children. About 50% of meningiomas have progesterone receptors, and about 20% of mengiomas have estrogen receptors. (p1248)

Answer 58A-12: C.
Both primary CNS lymphoma and systemic lymphoma are more likely in patients with immunodeficiency. (p1250)

Answer 58A-13: C.
Both primary CNS lymphomas and systemic lymphomas are commonly B-cell tumors. (p1250)

Answer 58A-14: B.
Systemic lymphomas commonly infiltrate the meninges, while primary CNS lymphoma extends into the CSF in only 25% of cases. (p1250)

Answer 58A-15: A.
Primary CNS lymphoma commonly originates in the parenchyma, as opposed to systemic lymphomas, which rarely cause parenchymal involvement. (p1250)

Answer 58A-16: C.
The pineal region is the most common area for germ cell tumors to affect the CNS. (p1250)

Chapter 58B: Primary and Secondary Tumors of the Central Nervous System: Molecular Biology of Nervous System Tumors

Question 58B-1:
Expression of which of the following growth factors is increased in patients with gliomas, compared to normal brain tissue?

1. TGF-alpha
2. Basic FGF
3. EGF
4. PDGF

Select: A = 1, 2, 3. B = 1, 3. C = 2, 4. D = 4 only. E = All

Question 58B-2:
Which of the following tumor types are associated with the NF-2 gene?

1. Meningioma
2. Acoustic neuroma
3. Pheochromocytoma
4. Retinoblastoma

Select: A = 1, 2, 3. B = 1, 3. C = 2, 4. D = 4 only. E = All

Question 58B-3:
Which of the following statements are true regarding neurofibromatosis types 1 and 2?

1. Both genes are on chromosome 17.
2. The protein produce of both is neurofibromin.
3. Both genes are tumor promotors.
4. NF-1 and NF-2 both have autosomal dominant inheritance.

Select: A = 1, 2, 3. B = 1, 3. C = 2, 4. D = 4 only. E = All

Question 58B-4:
Transcription and translation of enzymes required for DNA synthesis occurs during which phase of the cell cycle?

A. S
B. G1
C. G2
D. M

Question 58B-5:
Separation of the chromosomes into equal compartments occurs during which part of the cell cycle?

A. S
B. G1
C. G2
D. M

Answer 58B-1: E.
Expression of all of these growth factors is increased in gliomas. In addition, TGF-alpha and acidic FGF are also increased. (p1256)

Answer 58B-2: A.
Retinoblastoma is related to the tumor suppressor gene RB, whereas the other three are associated with NF-2 gene on chromosome 22. (p1258)

Answer 58B-3: D.
The NF-1 gene is on chromosome 17, whereas NF-2 is on chromosome 22. The protein product of NF-1 is neurofibromin, whereas the protein product of NF-2 is merlin. These are felt to be tumor suppressor genes. (p1259)

Answer 58B-4: B.
Manufacture of the enzymes required for DNA synthesis occurs during the late G1 part of the cell cycle, which is between the M and S phases. (p1254)

Answer 58B-5: D.
During the mitosis phase of the cell cycle, the duplicate chromosomes condense and there is spindle attachment and chromosomal segregation. (p1254-1255)

Chapter 58C: Primary and Secondary Tumors of the Central Nervous System: Clinical Presentation and Therapy of Nervous System Tumors

Question 58C-1:
Which of the following statements regarding headache in brain tumor is not true?

A. Headache is present in the majority of patients at some time in the course of the disease.
B. Headache may be contralateral to the tumor.
C. Most headaches with brain tumors are due to increased intracranial pressure.
D. Early morning headache is present in a minority of patients with brain tumor.

Question 58C-2:
A 12-year-old female is found to have a cerebellar lesion which has the appearance suggestive of a cystic astrocytoma. Which is the most appropriate clinical approach?

A. Resection without other treatment
B. Resection followed by radiation therapy
C. Resection followed by radiation and chemotherapy
D. Stereotactic biopsy followed by radiation therapy
E. Stereotactic biopsy followed by radiation and chemotherapy

Question 58C-3:
All of the following indicate a poor prognosis for patients with malignant astrocytoma except which?

A. Large amounts of residual tumor
B. Necrosis
C. Adult vs. child
D. Presence of seizures
E. Short duration of symptoms

Question 58C-4:
Which of the following statements best represents the current consensus regarding radiotherapy for patients with malignant gliomas?

A. Stereotactic radiosurgery should be used where available for primary treatment of malignant brain tumors.
B. Stereotactic radiosurgery has not been proven to be more effective for treatment of malignant gliomas.
C. Stereotactic radiotherapy has the most benefit for patients with large tumor volumes.

Question 58C-5:
Which of the following statements are true regarding brain tumors in children under the age of 6 months?

1. Infratentorial tumors are more common than supratentorial tumors.
2. Meningeal dissemination of tumors is common early in the course.
3. Seizures are uncommon with tumors in infancy.
4. Very young children have an increased susceptibility to radiation-induced neurotoxicity.

Select: A = 1, 2, 3. B = 1, 3. C = 2, 4. D = 4 only. E = All

Question 58C-6:
Which is the most common tumor in children with neurofibromatosis type 2?

A. Glioma
B. Optic glioma
C. Acoustic neuroma
D. Germ cell tumors

Answer 58C-1: C.
Increased intracranial pressure and pressure waves may be a contributing factor to headache in some patients but is not thought to be the major factor since the frequency of headache does not differ depending on whether the patient has increased intracranial pressure. (p1264)

Answer 58C-2: A.
Surgery is frequently curative for children with cerebellar astrocytomas. Most other primary brain tumors need adjunctive therapy for long-term survival. (p1266)

Answer 58C-3: D.
Seizures signify a better prognosis in that they indicate a lesion has been present for a longer time. The other findings are all indicative of a poorer prognosis. (p1267)

Answer 58C-4: B.
Stereotactic radiotherapy has been studied extensively, but has not yet supplanted conventional external beam radiotherapy for most patients with malignant gliomas. The potential for acute radiation toxicity increases with treatment of larger lesions, such that this treatment is used predominantly for patients with smaller lesions. (p1268)

Answer 58C-5: C.
Supratentorial tumors are more common than infratentorial tumors for children less than 6 months of age. Seizures are common in infants with brain tumors. (p1276)

Answer 58C-6: B
Optic glioma is the most common tumor in children with neurofibromatosis type 2. Screening with CT scanning may be necessary. (p1276)

Question 58C-7:
Which of the following statements are true regarding ependymomas?

1. Most ependymomas are in the posterior fossa.
2. Ependymomas may occur in the parenchyma distant from the ventricular surface.
3. Treatment is typically debulking followed by radiation therapy.
4. Peak frequency is in children less than 5 years of age.

Select: A = 1, 2, 3. B = 1, 3. C = 2, 4. D = 4 only. E = All

Questions 58C-8 through 58C-12:
The following questions are true/false. Select the best answer.

Question 58C-8:
Nitrosoureas have good blood-brain barrier penetrance which makes them attractive as chemotherapy for brain tumors.

Question 58C-9:
Cyclical vomiting and occipital headache suggest a cerebellar tumor.

Question 58C-10:
Most primary brain tumors are benign.

Question 58C-11:
Cerebral PNETs are usually localized and require local radiation after surgery.

Question 58C-12:
Surgical resection of vestibular schwannomas results in facial paralysis and hearing loss in virtually all patients.

Answer 58C-7: E.
All of these statements are true. The highest frequency is between birth and 4 years of age. About 2/3 are in the posterior fossa. Although we typically think of ependymomas as arising from the ventricular surface, they can occur in the parenchyma, distant from the ventricular surface. (p1271)

Answer 58C-8: True.
Nitrosoureas such as BCNU and CCNU have better penetrance through the blood-brain barrier than most other agents, which makes them used widely for patients with malignant brain tumors. (p1268)

Answer 58C-9: True.
Cerebellar tumors commonly produce vomiting and occipital headache, although these symptoms are not specific. (p1265)

Answer 58C-10: False.
The majority of primary brain tumors are malignant. (p1267)

Answer 58C-11: False.
Cerebral PNETs have a propensity to metastasize within the CSF, so total neuraxis radiation is indicated following surgery. (p1272)

Answer 58C-12: False.
With current state-of-the-art techniques, facial nerve is preserved in 86% of patients and cochlear function is preserved in 26% of patients. (p1274)

Chapter 58D: Primary and Secondary Tumors of the Central Nervous System: Clinical Presentation and Therapy for Spinal Tumors

Question 58D-1:
A 54-year-old male presents with thoracic myelopathy and is found to have tumor extending through the intravertebral foramen. Which is the most likely tumor type?

A. Small-cell lung cancer
B. Breast cancer
C. Colon cancer
D. Lymphoma

Question 58D-2:
A 56-year-old man with myeloma presents with myelopathy and is found on MRI to have epidural cord compression with tumor extending from the vertebral body. He has back pain but is ambulatory. High-dose corticosteroids are immediately administered. Which clinical approach is most appropriate?

A. Immediate resection of the tumor and replacement of the vertebral body, followed by radiation therapy
B. Chemotherapy to start immediately with close monitoring of response of the tumor
C. Immediate radiation therapy
D. Decompressive laminectomy followed by radiation therapy

Question 58D-3:
Leptomeningeal metastases are most common with which of the following tumor types?

A. Breast cancer
B. Myeloma
C. Non-Hodgkin's lymphoma
D. Leukemia

Question 58D-4:
Which imaging modality would be best performed for documentation of leptomeningeal metastases?

A. Myelogram and post-myelogram CT
B. Gadolinium-enhanced MRI
C. Contrast-enhanced spine CT
D. PET scan

Question 58D-5:
Which is the most appropriate treatment for patients with leptomeningeal metastases from breast cancer?

A. Local irradiation to symptomatic areas with intrathecal chemotherapy
B. Whole neuraxis radiation
C. Systemic chemotherapy with local irradiation
D. Whole neuraxis radiation with intrathecal chemotherapy

Question 58D-6:
A 30-year-old man presents with a malignant astrocytoma in the lower thoracic spine. Which of the following associated findings can develop?

1. Paresthesias in the legs
2. Syrinx
3. Back pain
4. CSF seeding

Select: A = 1, 2, 3. B = 1, 3. C = 2, 4. D = 4 only. E = All

Answer 58D-1: D.
Lymphoma is the most likely tumor to grow through the intravertebral foramen into the spinal canal. Radicular symptoms are typical, but cord compression can develop. (p1281)

Answer 58D-2: C.
Myeloma and a few other tumors tend to be radiosensitive, so that resection is often not needed, especially since the surgery, if done, would entail replacement of the involved vertebral body. Chemotherapy is not likely to be effective fast enough to be effective for treatment of epidural spinal cord compression. (p1284)

Answer 58D-3: D.
Up to 70% of patients with leukemia develop leptomeningeal metastases. Among solid tumors, adenocarcinomas are the most likely to produce leptomeningeal metastases, but the frequency is less than that of leukemia, in general. (p1285)

Answer 58D-4: B.
Enhanced MRI is the best test for visualization of leptomeningeal metastases, although CSF analysis is the gold standard for documentation of tumor cells. (p1286)

Answer 58D-5: A.
Local irradiation is performed because total spine radiation would result in myelosuppression. Intrathecal chemotherapy is typically used, in addition, since systemic chemotherapy does not penetrate the CSF in sufficient amounts to be able to eradicate the CSF tumor. (p1287)

Answer 58D-6: E.
All of these can develop in patients with malignant astrocytomas of the spinal cord. CSF seeding and the possible presence of other tumor sites makes evaluation for these possibilities essential before deciding on treatment options. (p1290)

Chapter 58E: Primary and Secondary Tumors of the Central Nervous System: Clinical Presentation and Therapy of Peripheral Nerve Tumors

Question 58E-1:
Neurofibromatosis type 2 predisposes to which of the following tumors?

A. Bilateral acoustic schwannomas
B. Meningiomas
C. Gliomas
D. Peripheral neurofibromas
E. All of the above

Question 58E-2:
Most neurofibromas fall into which one of the following categories?

A. NF-1
B. NF-2
C. Solitary neurofibromas

Questions 58E-3 through 58E-5:
The following questions concern lesions of peripheral nerves. For each question, select the best answer from the following list:

A. Schwannoma
B. Neurofibroma
C. Morton's neuroma
D. Nerve sheath ganglion
E. Malignant peripheral sheath tumor

Question 58E-3:
Histologic type of acoustic nerve lesion in NF-2.

Question 58E-4:
Mucin-filled cyst on the perineurium.

Question 58E-5:
Fibrosing process of the plantar digital nerve.

Answer 58E-1: E.
Bilateral acoustic schwannomas are characteristic of NF-2, but all of these may occur. (p1296)

Answer 58E-2: C.
About 90% of neurofibromas are solitary, whereas neurofibromatosis accounts for patients with multiple neurofibromas. Solitary neurofibromas are usually on cutaneous nerves. (p1296)

Answer 58E-3: A.
Bilateral acoustic schwannomas are typically seen in NF-2. (p1296)

Answer 58E-4: D.
Nerve sheath ganglion is a mucin-filled cyst on the perineurium which may resemble peripheral nerve tumor in presentation. (p1294)

Answer 58E-5: C.
Morton's neuroma is a fibrosing process of the plantar digital nerve which produces pain between the third and fourth metatarsals. (p1294)

Chapter 58F: Primary and Secondary Tumors of the Central Nervous System: Paraneoplastic Syndromes

Question 58F-1:
Paraneoplastic syndromes are thought to be due predominantly to which of the following causes?

A. Autoimmune attack
B. Nutritional deficiency
C. Chemotherapy
D. Radiation therapy

Question 58F-2:
A 45-year-old female with ovarian cancer presents with cerebellar ataxia. MRI shows no significant abnormalities. CSF shows 15 WBCs, all mononuclear cells. Cytology is negative. Which of the following is most likely?

A. The patient has paraneoplastic cerebellar degeneration and serum is likely positive for anti-Yo antibodies.
B. The patient most likely has paraneoplastic encephalomyelitis and serum is likely positive for anti-Hu antibodies.
C. The patient has carcinomatous meningitis despite the negative cytology. Repeat CSF sampling and analysis is indicated.

Question 58F-3:
Limbic encephalitis is associated most commonly with which of the following tumors?

A. Ovarian cancer
B. Small-cell lung cancer
C. Colon cancer
D. Hodgkin's disease
E. Non-Hodgkin's lymphoma

Questions 58F-4 through 58F-6:
The following questions concern antibodies found in patients with paraneoplastic syndromes. For each of the syndromes, select the most likely associated antibody.

A. Anti-Yo
B. Anti-Hu
C. Anti-Ri
D. Anti-VGCC

Question 58F-4:
Patient with small-cell lung cancer and the Lambert-Eaton myasthenic syndrome.

Question 58F-5:
Male with small-cell lung cancer and cerebellar ataxia with opsoclonus.

Question 58F-6:
Male with small-cell lung cancer and encephalomyelitis.

Answer 58F-1: A.
True paraneoplastic conditions are not related to therapy or other metabolic derangements of the cancer patient. Most, if not all, of these conditions are thought to be autoimmune. (p1299)

Answer 58F-2: A.
Paraneoplastic cerebellar degeneration typically develops in patients with ovarian cancer. Anti-Yo antibody is the most common associated mediator, which reacts with Purkinje cells. (p1302)

Answer 58F-3: B.
Small-cell lung cancer is the associated neoplasm in about 70% of patients with limbic encephalitis, although the tumor may not be diagnosed for up to 2 years following development of the symptoms. (p1305)

Answer 58F-4: D.
LEMS is associated with antibodies to the voltage-gated calcium channel in some patients with small-cell lung cancer. (p1300)

Answer 58F-5: C.
Anti-Ri is associated with cerebellar ataxia and opsoclonus in patients with SCLC as well as gynecological and breast cancers. Anti-Yo is typically seen in patients with gynecological and breast cancer with cerebellar degeneration. (p1300)

Answer 58F-6: B.
Anti-Hu is the most common antibody associated with encephalomyelitis and sensory neuropathy in patients with small-cell lung cancer. (p1300)

Chapter 58G: Primary and Secondary Tumors of the Central Nervous System: Quality of Life and Late Effects of Treatment

Question 58G-1:
Intellectual decline is common in children who are survivors of cancer treatment. Which of the following is thought to be the greatest contributor to this decline?

A. Chemotherapy
B. Radiation therapy
C. Hydrocephalus
D. Residual tumor

Question 58G-2:
Which of the following statements regarding CNS-irradiation–induced growth hormone deficiency in children is not true?

A. Irradiation-induced growth hormone deficiency is the most common endocrine complication of CNS irradiation.
B. For most patients, the suppression of GH production is transient, resolving after 2-3 months.
C. There is a dose-effect relation between amount of irradiation and suppression of GH production.
D. The locus of damage causing irradiation-induced GH deficiency is thought to be the hypothalamus.

Question 58G-3:
Which of the following are thought to contribute to short stature in patients who receive cranio-spinal irradiation in childhood?

1. Growth hormone deficiency
2. Hypothyroidism
3. Decreased vertebral body height
4. Precocious puberty

Select: A = 1, 2, 3. B = 1, 3. C = 2, 4. D = 4 only. E = All

Question 58G-4:
Hypothyroidism is common in patients who have received radiation for brain tumors, especially children. All of the following statements are true for this condition except which?

A. The most common cause is pituitary damage due to cranial irradiation.
B. Treatment may not be lifelong since some patients may have improvement in thyroid function.
C. Chemotherapy given in addition to radiotherapy increases the risk of hypothyroidism.
D. Failure to treat hypothyroidism may lead to an increased risk of subsequent thyroid carcinoma.

Answer 58G-1: B.
Radiation therapy is thought to be the greatest contributor to progressive intellectual decline in children who are long-term survivors of cancer. The decline is progressive over years, even though the exposure to brain radiation is remote. (p1309)

Answer 58G-2: B.
For most patients the suppression of GH production is not transient and can be demonstrated 8-10 years following treatment. (p1310)

Answer 58G-3: E.
All of these are thought to be important factors for producing short stature in children exposed to cranio-spinal irradiation. (p1310)

Answer 58G-4: A.
The most common cause is direct thyroid damage due to cervical irradiation. Chemotherapy augments the risk of hypothyroidism. Failure to treat the hypothyroidism may result in overproduction of TSH, which can later produce thyroid carcinoma. (p1311)

Chapter 59A: Infections of the Nervous System: Bacterial Infections

Question 59A-1:
A 24-year-old male presents with headache, nausea and vomiting and fever and has meningeal signs on examination. Examination shows moderate confusion but is otherwise normal. Which is the most appropriate clinical approach?

A. Lumbar puncture followed by administration of intravenous antibiotics
B. CT head then lumbar puncture if the CT is normal, followed by intravenous antibiotics
C. Administration of intravenous antibiotics and urgent CT scanning. Lumbar puncture if the CT is normal.
D. Administration of intravenous antibiotics until MRI can be performed

Question 59A-2:
Which of the following is the most common pathogen in acute bacterial meningitis?

A. *Haemophilus influenzae*
B. *Streptococcus pneumoniae*
C. *Neisseria meningitidis*
D. None of these

Questions 59A-3 through 59A-6:
The following four questions pertain to antibiotic selection for patients with bacterial meningitis. For each organism, select the best empiric antibiotic from the following list.

A. Penicillin G
B. Ampicillin
C. Cephalosporin
D. Vancomycin
E. Aminoglycoside
F. C plus D
G. B plus E
H. C plus E

Question 59A-3:
Gram-positive cocci.

Question 59A-4:
Gram-positive bacilli.

Question 59A-5:
Gram-negative cocci.

Question 59A-6:
Gram-negative bacilli.

Question 59A-7:
Which of the following are complications of bacterial meningitis?

1. Subdural effusion
2. Seizures
3. Hemiparesis
4. Cranial neuropathies

Select: A = 1, 2, 3. B = 1, 3. C = 2, 4. D = 4 only. E = All

Question 59A-8:
Which of the following should be considered in the differential diagnosis of a patient with fever, headache, confusion, and left hemiparesis?

1. Brain abscess
2. Meningitis
3. Septic emboli
4. Subdural empyema

Select: A = 1, 2, 3. B = 1, 3. C = 2, 4. D = 4 only. E = All

Answer 59A-1: C.

The clinical presentation is of a patient with probable acute bacterial meningitis. CT is necessary in the presence of focal findings or increased intracranial pressure; however, the delay in initiating treatment may have tragic consequences for the patient. Therefore, if CT has to be performed prior to the LP, antibiotics should be given immediately. Antibiotics do not sterilize the culture for several hours following administration, and counterimmune-electrophoresis (CIE) can be performed to identify the organism even if the culture is negative. (p1318)

Answer 59A-2: B.

S. pneumoniae is the most common cause of meningitis now, with *N. meningitidis* close behind. *H. influenzae* used to be the most common pathogen; however, with widespread vaccination, this pathogen is much less common, although it is increasing in some patients with HIV. (p1318)

Answer 59A-3: F.

Cephalosporin plus vancomycin is used for patients with Gram-positive cocci on smears. These will usually be *S. pneumoniae*. (p1320)

Answer 59A-4: G.

Ampicillin or penicillin G plus an aminoglycoside antibiotic is used for patients with Gram-positive bacilli in the CSF. (p1320)

Answer 59A-5: A.

Penicillin G is the drug of choice for Gram-negative cocci such as *Neisseria meningitidis*. (p1320)

Answer 59A-6: H.

A broad-spectrum cephalosporin plus an aminoglycoside is used for gram negative bacilli. (p1320)

Answer 59A-7: E.

All of these are potential complications of bacterial meningitis. Subdural effusion is particularly likely with *H. influenzae* or other gram negative meningitis. Focal deficits may develop from infarction or cerebritis. Seizures can develop from cerebritis and other causes of focal cortical damage. CN-6 palsy is common with increased intracranial pressure, but other cranial nerves may be affected, as well. (p1323)

Answer 59A-8: E.

All of these should be considered in a patient with a febrile illness with diffuse and focal neurologic signs. Meningitis may produce focal signs by arteritis, thrombophlebitis, or cerebritis. Subdural empyema commonly produces encephalopathy, but focal signs are also common. (p1325)

Question 59A-9:
A patient with fever, confusion, and focal signs is found to have a 5 cm-diameter ring-enhancing mass lesion in the right temporal lobe on CT, consistent with abscess. Which is the best approach for subsequent clinical management?

A. Antibiotic treatment should be started with metronidazole plus penicillin followed by stereotactic aspiration for stains and cultures.
B. Antibiotic treatment should be started with metronidazole plus ceftazidime, followed by stereotactic aspiration for stains and cultures.
C. Antibiotic treatment should be started with metronidazole plus ceftazidime. If the patient fails to respond to treatment, surgical excision of the abscess should be performed.

Question 59A-10:
A 54-year-old man presents with fever and back pain and is found on MRI to have an enhancing epidural lesion consistent with abscess. Which is the most appropriate clinical approach?

A. Stereotactic aspiration and antibiotics
B. Surgical drainage and antibiotics
C. Antibiotics and close follow-up with serial MRIs

Question 59A-11:
Which of the following findings would not be expected in a patient with tuberculous meningitis and would suggest an alternative diagnosis?

A. CSF pleocytosis of 300 WBC/μl with a polymorphonuclear predominance
B. CSF protein of 200 mg/dl
C. Normal opening pressure
D. CSF glucose of less than 10 mg/dl
E. All would be compatible with the diagnosis.

Question 59A-12:
Which of the following statements are true regarding use of corticosteroids in patients with meningitis?

1. Corticosteroids may reduce the frequency of neurologic complications from acute bacterial meningitis.
2. Corticosteroids may reduce the CSF penetrance of some antibiotics.
3. Corticosteroids may reduce the frequency of neurologic complications from tuberculous meningitis.
4. Corticosteroids are contraindicated for patients with tuberculous meningitis.

Select: A = 1, 2, 3. B = 1, 3. C = 2, 4. D = 4 only. E = All

Questions 59A-13 through 59A-15:
The following questions pertain to neurologic complications of leprosy. For each of the questions, select the disorder most closely associated from the following list.

A. Lepromatous leprosy
B. Tuberculoid leprosy
C. Borderline (dimorphous)
D. All of the above

Question 59A-13:
Patients with impaired cellular immunity are most likely to develop which form of leprosy?

Question 59A-14:
Which form has a predilection for distal neural involvement?

Question 59A-15:
Patients witth which type are likely to present with a syndrome resembling mononeuritis multiplex?

Answer 59A-9: B.
Patients with frontal lobe abscesses should have penicillin added to the metronidazole, whereas with temporal and cerebellar abscesses ceftazidime is added. Needle aspiration is indicated for patients with large abscesses, especially in the non-dominant hemisphere. Small lesions, lesions in the dominant hemisphere, and areas of cerebritis without abscess formation are usually not subjected to aspiration. (p1326)

Answer 59A-10: B.
Immediate antibiotics and surgical drainage should be performed. Delay in decompression of the spinal cord may result in irreversible myelopathy. Antibiotic coverage should be sufficient to treat *S. aureus* and gram-negative bacilli until more definitive diagnosis can be established. (p1328)

Answer 59A-11: E.
Elevated CSF protein and reduced CSF glucose are typical of tuberculous meningitis although not specific. The pleocytosis is also typical, although a mononuclear pleocytosis is more common; polymorphonuclear pleocytosis can be present early in the infection. Opening pressure is usually increased, although it may be normal. (p1330)

Answer 59A-12: A.
Corticosteroids may reduce the frequency of neurologic complications in patients with acute bacterial and tuberculous meningitis, although they are more prominently used for patients with TB meningitis than acute bacterial meningitis. There is concern that CSF penetrance of some antibiotics may be impaired since they depend on CSF inflammation for passage. Corticosteroids are not contraindicated for patients with tuberculous meningitis and in fact are routinely given, especially in patients with increased intracranial pressure, tuberculomas with edema, complicated meningitis with arachnoiditis, hydrocephalus, or vasculitis, in patients with very high CSF protein and impending spinal block, and in a few other clinical situations. (p1320, 1323, 1331-1332)

Answer 59A-13: A.
Patients with impaired cellular immunity are most likely to develop lepromatous leprosy, while patients with good resistance are most likely to develop tuberculoid leprosy. Borderline leprosy is an intermediate form between these two. (p1333)

Answer 59A-14: D.
All forms of leprosy are associated with a predilection for distal tissues, because of the preference of the organism for temperatures lower than core temperature. (p1333)

Answer 59A-15: B.
Patients with tuberculoid leprosy are most likely to have multiple mononeuropathies, whereas patients with lepromatous leprosy have diffuse neural involvement which would have more the appearance of a polyneuropathy. Borderline leprosy also may have the presentation of a polyneuropathy. (p1333)

Question 59A-16:
This question and the following two questions refer to a single case. Answer each question on the basis of the information provided in order.

A 54-year-old man presents with a several-month history of progressive dementia, apathy, dysarthria, tremor, and myoclonus. Which of the following diagnoses should be considered?

1. Creutzfeldt-Jakob disease
2. Alzheimer's disease
3. Neurosyphilis
4. Frontotemporal dementia

Select: A = 1, 2, 3. B = 1, 3. C = 2, 4. D = 4 only. E = All

Question 59A-17:
The above patient has no specific abnormalities identified on neuroimaging but has a positive RPR. CSF shows positive VDRL, 15 WBC/μl all mononuclears, and protein of 85 mg/dl. Which is the best clinical formulation?

A. The patient has the encephalitic form of neurosyphilis.
B. The patient probably has a degenerative condition and the abnormal CSF findings are nonspecific.
C. The patient may have neurosyphilis but diagnosis should be confirmed by CSF FTA-ABS.

Question 59A-18:
Diagnosis of the above patient is confirmed to be general paresis, and treatment is begun. Which of the following is the best regimen for management?

A. Aqueous penicillin G 3-4 million units IV q4h for 10-14 days
B. Procaine benzyl penicillin 2.4 million units IM daily with probenecid 500 mg po qid, for 10-14 days
C. Doxycycline 200 mg PO bid for 4 weeks
D. All of the above are reasonable treatment regimens

Question 59A-19:
Which of the following are recognized early neurologic complications of Lyme disease?

1. Guillain-Barré syndrome
2. Facial palsy
3. Meningitis
4. Optic neuritis

Select: A = 1, 2, 3. B = 1, 3. C = 2, 4. D = 4 only. E = All

Question 59A-20:
Which of the following statements regarding Lyme disease are true?

1. Absence of the erythema chronicum migrans rash makes the diagnosis of Lyme disease extremely unlikely.
2. Meningitis is usually associated with a polymorphonuclear pleocytosis.
3. Encephalopathy with normal CSF findings is not due to Lyme disease.
4. Ceftriaxone is effective for treatment of CNS involvement of Lyme disease.

Select: A = 1, 2, 3. B = 1, 3. C = 2, 4. D = 4 only. E = All

Question 59A-21:
What is the mechanism of action of botulism toxin?

A. Binding to acetylcholine receptors with subsequent internalization of the receptor complexes
B. Binding to acetylcholine receptors with allosteric blockade of binding of acetylcholine to the active site
C. Prevention of release of acetylcholine from the terminal motor axons

Question 59A-22:
Which of the following findings would be least expected in patients with botulism?

A. Diplopia
B. Ptosis
C. Distal paresthesias
D. Symmetric limb weakness
E. Depressed tendon reflexes

Answer 59A-16: B.
CJD and the encephalitic form of neurosyphilis would be the only realistic differential diagnoses of this list. AD and FTD would not typically present with dysarthria, tremor, and myoclonus. (p1335)

Answer 59A-17: A.
The patient has a typical clinical presentation of the encephalitic form of neurosyphilis and the laboratory studies are supportive. The positive CSF VDRL is strongly suggestive of neurosyphilis and is more likely to be positive in patients with general paresis and meningovascular syphilis than in asymptomatic patients or patients with tabes dorsalis. FTA-ABS is best performed on serum rather than CSF. (p1336)

Answer 59A-18: D.
All of these are reasonable treatments, although the doxycycline is typically reserved for patients with penicillin allergy. However, even in penicillin-allergic patients, skin testing and desensitization should be considered. (p1336)

Answer 59A-19: E.
All of these are potential neurologic complications of Lyme disease early in the clinical course. GBS and opic neuritis are much less common than the other complications, however. (p1337)

Answer 59A-20: D.
Ceftriaxone is used IV for patients with CNS involvement with Lyme disease; penicillin is an alternative. Tetracycline and chloramphenicol are used for penicillin- or cephalosporin-allerigic patients. The erythema chronicum migrans rash is present in 60-80% of patients with Lyme disease, so its presence is strongly supportive of the diagnosis, but its absence does not rule out the diagnosis. Meningitis is associated with a lymphocytic predominance in both its acute and chronic forms. Encephalopathy with normal CSF may occur, although CSF findings are more commonly present. (p1337)

Answer 59A-21: C.
Botulinum toxin acts at the nerve terminal to prevent release of acetylcholine, thereby impairing neuromuscular transmission. The other choices are mechanisms of actions of other agents. (p1339)

Answer 59A-22: C.
Sensory symptoms are not expected in patients with botulism. The remainder of the findings are expected in patients with botulism. (p1339)

Question 59A-23:
Which of the following is least useful for confirmation of the diagnosis of botulism?

A. Toxin bioassay
B. Culture of *C. botulinum*
C. NCV with repetitive stimulation
D. All of these can confirm the diagnosis

Question 59A-24:
A neonate with poor umbilical care is most likely to develop which of the following?

A. Tetanus
B. Botulism
C. Neither of these

Question 59A-25:
Which is thought to be the mechanism of action of tetanospasmin in producing neurologic effects?

A. Increase in release of glutamate and aspartate
B. Inhibition of release of GABA and glycine
C. Inhibition of monoamine reuptake
D. Inhibition of breakdown of acetylcholine

Question 59A-26:
Which is the most common pathogen associated with subsequent development of Guillain-Barré syndrome?

A. *Mycoplasma pneumoniae*
B. *Chlamydia pneumoniae*
C. *Rickettsia rickettsii*
D. *Camplylobacter jejuni*

Answer 59A-23: C.
NCV with repetitive stimulation can eliminate many other causes of weakness but is unable to confirm the diagnosis since the findings are not specific for the disorder. The mouse bioassay and culture can be confirmatory, although treatment begins with clinical diagnosis and cannot wait for confirmation by these studies. (p1340)

Answer 59A-24: A.
Umbilical stump infection may produce neonatal tetanus. Infantile botulism is due to gut infection. (p1339-1340)

Answer 59A-25: B.
Tetanospasmin is thought to act by inhibition of release of GABA and glycine, two important inhibitory transmitters in the brainstem and spinal cord. The other listed mechanisms are thought to play roles in other disorders and with actions of certain drugs but are not involved in tetanus. (p1340)

Answer 59A-26: D.
Campylobacter jejuni is the most common pathogen associated with the subsequent development of GBS. *Rickettsia rickettsii* is the causative organism in Rocky Mountain spotted fever. *Mycoplasma pneumoniae* may be associated with GBS, but this is uncommon. *Chlamydia pneumoniae* is unassociated with this complication. (p1345, 1347-1348)

Chapter 59B: Infections of the Nervous System: Viral Infections

Question 59B-1:
Which is the most common cause of aseptic meningitis?

A. Enterovirus
B. Rickettsia
C. Myoplasma
D. HIV

Question 59B-2:
Which of the following is the *least* likely pathogen in an adult patient with viral encephalitis in New Jersey?

A. HSV-1
B. Arbovirus
C. Enteroviruses
D. Japanese encephalitis

Question 59B-3:
A 27-year-old male presents with fever, headache, confusion, and expressive speech difficulty and has a generalized seizure. Uncontrasted CT head is normal. CSF shows normal glucose, increased protein, 150 WBCs/μl with a lymphocytic predominance, 130 RBCs/μl. EEG cannot be obtained. Which is the best clinical formulation and approach?

A. The most likely diagnosis is herpes encephalitis. Treatment should begin with acyclovir while further analysis of the CSF is pending including cultures and PCR.
B. The most likely diagnosis is herpes encephalitis. Brain biopsy should be performed since EEG cannot be obtained and the CT does not show temporal lobe abnormalities.
C. The most likely diagnosis is arbovirus encephalitis. Treatment is supportive. When available, EEG and MRI should be performed for the possibility of herpes encephalitis.

Question 59B-4:
Which of the following regimens is considered first-line treatment for patients with herpes simplex virus type I encephalitis?

A. Acyclovir 10 mg/kg IV q8h for 10-14 days
B. Acyclovir 800 mg PO 5x/day for 10 days
C. Vidarabine 15 mg/kg IV per day for 14 days
D. Ganciclovir 4-6 mg/kg IV q12h for 6 weeks

Questions 59B-5 through 59B-7:
The following questions concern some important viruses and their neurologic complications. For each of the neurologic conditions, select the virus with which it is most associated.

A. CMV
B. EBV
C. HSV-1
D. HSV-2
E. VZV

Question 59B-5:
Post-herpetic neuralgia.

Question 59B-6:
Neonatal encephalitis.

Question 59B-7:
Hearing loss beginning in childhood.

Question 59B-8:
Which of the following may be caused by Epstein-Barr virus infection?

1. Aseptic meningitis
2. Optic neuritis
3. Guillain-Barré syndrome
4. Small-fiber sensory neuropathy

Select: A = 1, 2, 3. B = 1, 3. C = 2, 4. D = 4 only. E = All

Answer 59B-1: A.
Enteroviruses are the most common etiologic agents in aseptic meningitis, although all of the listed agents have been implicated. Some other important causes are arbovirus, mumps, herpesvirus, and lymphocytic choriomeningitis virus. (p1353-1354)

Answer 59B-2: D.
JE is the most common cause of focal encephalitis in Asia but is an uncommon cause in the United States. The others are all likely pathogens for encephalitis. HSV-1 is the most common cause of focal encephalitis in the United States. (p1354)

Answer 59B-3: A.
The potential for adverse effects of acyclovir in a patient with non-herpes encephalitis is less than the lost opportunity for treatment in these patients. Acyclovir should be begun with suspicion and should not await confirmation of diagnosis. (p1355)

Answer 59B-4: A.
Acyclovir is used IV for first-line treatment of HSV-1 encephalitis. Patients who relapse may be given a higher dose than indicated here. Ganciclovir is used mainly for CMV infection. Vidarabine is used for patients who cannot take acyclovir or for strains of virus resistant to acyclovir. (p1359, 1361)

Answer 59B-5: E.
VZV is the typical cause of postherpetic neuralgia. (p1360)

Answer 59B-6: D.
HSV-2 is the most common cause of neonatal encephalitis. (p1359)

Answer 59B-7: A.
CMV is the most common nonheritable cause of hearing loss in the United States. (p1360)

Answer 59B-8: E
All of these are potential neurologic complications of EBV infection. Other important disorders are transverse myelitis, cranial neuropathies other than optic, autonomic neuropathy, and encephalitis. (p1361)

Question 59B-9:
A 32-year-old female is admitted with a history of rapidly progressive confusion and marked agitation progressing to coma. She has a history of recent bite by an unknown forest animal. The provisional diagnosis of rabies is made. Which would be the best way(s) to confirm the diagnosis?

1. Intracerebral innoculation of mice with patient's saliva
2. CSF rabies titres
3. Search for rabies antigen from the skin near the hairline
4. Neutralizing antibody titres in the blood

Select: A = 1, 2, 3. B = 1, 3. C = 2, 4. D = 4 only. E = All

Question 59B-10:
Which of the following statements are true regarding management of potential rabies exposures?

1. Human diploid vaccine is preferable to animal-derived vaccines.
2. Veterinarians and other animal handlers should be vaccinated against rabies.
3. Post-exposure administration of antirabies immunoglobulin is reserved for patients who have not been vaccinated.
4. Rabies vaccine is administered to non-immunized patients following demonstration of lack of infection from immediate exposure.

Select: A = 1, 2, 3. B = 1, 3. C = 2, 4. D = 4 only. E = All

Question 59B-11:
Which is the most likely clinical manifestation of poliovirus infection?

A. Asymptomatic infection
B. Aseptic meningitis
C. Paralytic illness
D. None of these

Question 59B-12:
A 34-year-old female presents with headache, meningeal signs, and asymmetric paralysis of the limbs, and is given the provisional diagnosis of polio. CSF shows 100 WBC/μl with a mononuclear predominance. CSF protein is also elevated at 150 mg/dl. Which other conditions should be considered in the differential diagnosis?

1. Guillain-Barré syndrome
2. CMV infection
3. Tick paralysis
4. Carcinomatous meningitis

Select: A = 1, 2, 3. B = 1, 3. C = 2, 4. D = 4 only. E = All

Question 59B-13:
Which of the following features suggest St. Louis encephalitis rather than herpes simplex virus encephalitis?

1. Lack of focal findings
2. More rapid evolution of neurologic findings
3. Absence of seizures
4. Absence of a cellular response in the CSF

Select: A = 1, 2, 3. B = 1, 3. C = 2, 4. D = 4 only. E = All

Question 59B-14:
Subacute sclerosing panencephalitis (SSPE) is a late complication of which of the following infections?

A. HSV
B. Mumps
C. Rubella
D. Measles
E. None of these

Question 59B-15:
Which of the following has been implicated in direct causation of progressive multifocal leukoencephalopathy?

1. HIV
2. SV-40 virus
3. EBV
4. JC virus

Select: A = 1, 2, 3. B = 1, 3. C = 2, 4. D = 4 only. E = All

Answer 59B-9: B.

Intracerebral inoculation and examination of skin from near the hairline for the presence of rabies antigen are the typical methods of confirming the diagnosis of rabies. Rabies should be considered in any patient with a picture of rapidly-progressive encephalitis, especially when the patient lives in an endemic area. (p1362)

Answer 59B-10: A.

Human diploid vaccine has a lower incidence of development of Guillain-Barré syndrome and acute disseminated encephalomyelitis than the animal vaccines. Veterinarians and many other animal handlers should be vacinated because blood, CSF, and other body fluids are highly infectious. Post-exposure antirabies immunoglobulin is given to patients who have not been immunized. Rabies vaccine is given to patients who have not been immunized immediately rather than waiting until infection has been ruled out. (p1362)

Answer 59B-11: A.

Most patients are asymptomatic, whereas approximately 8% develop aseptic meningitis and about 1% develop the paralytic form of the illness. (p1363)

Answer 59B-12: C.

CMV infection and carcinomatous meningitis may produce these symptoms plus the CSF findings. Tick paralysis and Guillain-Barré syndrome would not be expected to produce the CSF findings, and frank meningeal signs would not be expected. (p1363)

Answer 59B-13: B.

HSV encephalitis is more likely to be associated with focal findings and seizures than St. Louis encephalitis, but the clinical course is usually more rapid. Both conditions typically have a cellular response in the CSF; although the CSF formulae may differ between the two encephalitides, this difference is not helpful for differential diagnosis. (p1364)

Answer 59B-14: D.

SSPE is an uncommon late complication of measles infection and is characterized by behavioral or personality change progressing to cognitive changes, myoclonus, spasticity, movement disorders, and eventually severe encephalopathy progressing to coma. A similar disorder may follow rubella infection, but there are a number of clinical and electrophysiological differences between the two disorders. (p1367)

Answer 59B-15: C.

Most cases of PML are due to the JC virus, although a few patients have been due to the SV-40 virus. PML is of increased frequency in patients with AIDS, but the HIV virus has not been implicated in direct causation. (p1370)

Chapter 59C: Infections of the Nervous System: Fungal Infections

Question 59C-1:
Which of the following tests is of greatest clinical utility in identification of patients with cryptococcal meningitis?

A. Fungus culture of CSF
B. Fungus smears of CSF
C. Cryptococcal polysaccharide antigen assay of CSF
D. India ink preparation of CSF

Question 59C-2:
What is the most common cause of chronic meningitis?

A. *Cryptococcus*
B. Adenovirus
C. Tuberculosis
D. Neurosyphilis

Question 59C-3:
Which of the following clinical presentations can develop from *Cryptococcus neoformans*?

A. Progressive dementia
B. Chronic meningitis
C. Brain abscess
D. Any of the above

Question 59C-4:
Which is standard first-line treatment for Cryptococal meningitis in immunocompetent patients?

A. Amphotericin IV monotherapy
B. Amphotericin IV plus flucytosine PO
C. Fluconazole PO
D. None of these

Question 59C-5:
What is the most likely clinical consequence of *Histoplasma capsulatum* infection?

A. Basilar meningitis
B. Cerebral granulomatosis
C. Acute pulmonary histoplasmosis
D. Asymptomatic infection

Question 59C-6:
Fluconazole is indicated for primary therapy for which of the following infections in the immunocompetent patient?

A. *Cryptococcus*
B. *Coccidioides*
C. *Histoplasma*
D. *Candida*
E. *Aspergillus*

Answer 59C-1: C.
Cryptococcal antigen assay is abnormal in about 90% of patients with cryptococcal meningitis, whereas the India ink preparation is abnormal in only about 50% of patients. Fungus cultures are the definitive test, but treatment cannot await the days to weeks required for cultures to become positive. Fungus smears are supportive to the diagnosis but are not highly sensitive. (p1376)

Answer 59C-2: C.
TB is the most common cause of chronic meningitis. Adenovirus may produce an acute syndrome, but chronic infection is not expected. (p1376)

Answer 59C-3: D.
All of these are potential clinical presentations of *Cryptococcus neoformans*. The development of progressive dementia without other signs of meningitis is uncommon but can occur. (p1377)

Answer 59C-4: B.
Standard treatment for cryptococcal meningitis is with amphotericin IV and flucytosine PO. Fluconazole PO has been advocated, but efficacy in non-AIDS patients has not been well established. (p1378)

Answer 59C-5: D.
Asymptomatic infection is the most common result of initial *H. capsulatum* infection. Neurologic complications may include basilar meningitis, cerebritis, and granuloma formation, but these complications are unusual. (p1379)

Answer 59C-6: B.
Fluconazole is primary treatment for *Coccidioides immitus* infection. Initial treatment of *Cryptococus neoformans* and *Candida albicans* is with amphotericin B plus flucytosine. *Histoplasma capsulatum* is treated with amphotericin B. *Aspergillus fumigatus* is treated with amphotericin B followed by itraconazole. (p1382-1383)

Chapter 59D: Infections of the Nervous System: Parasitic Infections

Questions 59D-1 through 59D-3:
The following questions concern a single patient with presumed malaria. Select the best answer for each question in order.

A 26-year-old male with recent exposure in an endemic area presents with malaise, myalgias, headache, and chills, then develops recurrent fevers to 105°F about every third day. He also develops nausea, vomiting, abdominal pain, and tachypnea and is found to have hepatomegaly on examination.

Question 59D-1:
Which of the following would be neurologic findings which may develop in this patient?

1. Seizures
2. Aphasia
3. Confusion
4. Muscle necrosis

Select: A = 1, 2, 3. B = 1, 3. C = 2, 4. D = 4 only. E = All

Question 59D-2:
Which would be the most appropriate approach to confirmation of the diagnosis of malaria?

A. Giemsa stain of CSF
B. Giemsa stain of blood
C. Wright's stain of CSF
D. Wright's stain of blood
E. None of these

Question 59D-3:
What is the most appropriate treatment for the patient described above?

A. Chloroquine
B. Quinine dihydrochloride
C. Quinidine gluconate
D. Artemeter

Question 59D-4:
Which is the expected organism in amoebiasis acquired from fresh water swimming?

A. *Acanthamoeba*
B. *Balamuthia*
C. *Naegleria*
D. None of these

Questions 59D-5 through 59D-7:
For each of the following questions, select the best answer from the following list of associated conditions:

A. Primary amebic meningoencephalitis
B. Granulomatous amebic encephalitis
C. Both
D. Neither

Question 59D-5:
Causes seizures.

Question 59D-6:
Chronic meningitis.

Question 59D-7:
Fulminant meningoencephalitis in patients recently swimming in warm water.

Question 59D-8:
What disorder is caused by *Trypanosoma cruzi*?

A. American trypanosomiasis
B. African trypanosomiasis
C. Sleeping sickness
D. None of these

Answer 59D-1: E.
Any of these can develop. Muscle necrosis with pain and weakness may develop because of lack of skeletal muscle perfusion from hyperviscosity or capillary obstruction. Seizures, aphasia, and other focal signs are typical of neurologic involvement. Confusion is common with focal deficits as well as increased intracranial pressure. (p1387-1388)

Answer 59D-2: B.
Giemsa stain of blood is used to establish the diagnosis of malaria and determine the type. If initial smears are negative but the diagnosis is suspected, repeat smears are performed at intervals of 6-8 hours. (p1388)

Answer 59D-3: B.
The clinical vignette suggests falciparum malaria. Quinine dihydrochloride is the first-line treatment for patients with falciparum malaria in most regions of the world, because of the prevalence of chloroquine-resistant malaria. Quinidine is used if IV quinine is not available. Artemeter is used for multidrug-resistant falciparum malaria. (p1388)

Answer 59D-4: C.
Naegleria is the expected organism acquired from swimming in fresh water, usually heated. *Acanthamoeba* is widely spread. (p1389)

Answer 59D-5: C.
Both PAM and GAE are associated with seizures. (p1389)

Answer 59D-6: B.
GAE is a subacute or chronic meningitis whereas PAM is an acute fulminating encephalitis. (p1389)

Answer 59D-7: A.
PAM is an acute encephalomyelitis which is typically caused by *N. fowleri* after swimming in warm water. (p1389)

Answer 59D-8: A.
T. cruzi produces American trypanosomiasis. African trypanosomiasis is caused by *T. brucei gambiense* and *T. b. rhodesiense*. Sleeping sickness is another term for African trypanosomiasis. (p1390-1391)

Questions 59D-9 through 59D-12:
The following questions are true or false statements. For each, select the best answer.

Question 59D-9:
Toxoplasma gondii is carried in birds and cats.

Question 59D-10:
Cysticercosis is caused by the pork tapeworm.

Question 59D-11:
Echinococcus is usually acquired in the household by close contact with dogs.

Question 59D-12:
Neurologic complications of trichinosis are usually due to direct muscle involvement.

Answer 59D-9: True.
T. gondii is carried by birds, which has given the organism a worldwide distribution. In the household, cats harbor the organism in the gut. (p1393)

Answer 59D-10: True.
Cysticercosis is the most common neurologic infection in the world, and is caused by the pork tapeworm *T. solium*. (p1394-1395)

Answer 59D-11: True.
Dogs are the most proximate contact in the household for most patients. (p1396)

Answer 59D-12: True.
Patients with trichinosis typically present with fever, periorbital edema, and myalgia and may progress to the muscle invasive phase with pain, swelling, and weakness which begins proximally and in extraocular muscles and becomes more extensive. CNS involvement occurs in approximately 10% of cases and is a meningoencephalitis. (p1398)

Chapter 59E: Infections of the Nervous System: Neurological Manifestations of Human Immunodeficiency Virus Infection

Question 59E-1:
Which is the least likely cause of focal cerebral deficit in a patient with HIV infection?

A. Progressive multifocal leukoencephalopathy
B. Primary central nervous system lymphoma
C. Cerebral toxoplasmosis
D. Cryptococcal meningitis

Question 59E-2:
A 27-year-old male with AIDS is evaluated for a ring-enhancing lesion in the left central region on CT. MRI shows this lesion, some surrounding edema, and a second lesion in the right frontal region. Which is the most appropriate clinical formulation?

A. The patient most likely has toxoplasmosis, but other etiologies should be considered. Stereotactic biopsy of the left frontal lesion should be performed prior to initiating therapy.
B. The patient most likely has toxoplasmosis and should be treated for this. Clinical examination and imaging will determine whether the patient responds, and further diagnostic study will be needed if there is no response to this treatment.
C. The most likely diagnosis is primary central nervous system lymphoma. If CSF cytology is normal, them empiric treatment for toxoplasmosis should be administered.

Question 59E-3:
A 24-year-old male presents with progressive cognitive decline, motor slowing, and personality change. The patient has AIDS. Brain MRI shows no mass lesions or areas of demyelination. CSF shows a mild lymphyocytic pleocytosis, elevated protein, and normal glucose. Which is the most likely diagnosis?

A. Progressive multifocal leukoencephalopathy
B. HIV dementia
C. Cryptococcal meningitis
D. Primary CNS lymphoma
E. None of these

Question 59E-4:
Which of the following statements are true regarding cryptococcal meningitis?

1. CSF WBC count less than $20/\mu l$ is a good prognostic sign.
2. Altered mental status at presentation is a poor prognostic sign.
3. Cryptococcal antigen is not helpful for diagnosis in patients with AIDS and very low CD4 counts.
4. MRI seldom shows signs of inflammation in cryptococcal meningitis.

Select: A = 1, 2, 3. B = 1, 3. C = 2, 4. D = 4 only. E = All

Question 59E-5:
Which of the following statements are true regarding diagnosis and treatment of syphilis in patients with AIDS?

1. CSF VDRL is not sensitive for diagnosis of syphilis in AIDS patients.
2. Treatment of syphilis in AIDS is essentially the same as in patients without AIDS.
3. Treatment failures with syphilis are more common in AIDS patients.
4. CSF lymphocytic pleocytosis and elevated protein suggests neurosyphilis.

Select: A = 1, 2, 3. B = 1, 3. C = 2, 4. D = 4 only. E = All

Answer 59E-1: D.
Cryptococcal meningitis is common in patients with HIV infection; however, it is the least of these diagnoses to produce focal cerebral deficits. (p1408)

Answer 59E-2: B.
Toxoplasmosis is the most likely diagnosis, but imaging cannot be certain about the differential diagnosis. While there is controversy about timing of cerebral biopsy, initiation of anti-toxoplasma treatment for 10-14 days is justified, providing there is close neurologic follow-up to assess for early signs of failure to respond. (p1412)

Answer 59E-3: B.
HIV dementia is the most likely cause of the mental status changes. The CSF findings might suggest cryptococcal meningitis or PCNSL, but the CSF findings described can be seen in AIDS patients independent of these other conditions and would be consistent with the diagnosis of HIV dementia. (p1415-1416)

Answer 59E-4: C.
MRI may show specific abnormalities in cryptococcal meningitis but more often shows no abnormalities. Low CSF WBC counts are a poor prognostic sign, rather than a good prognostic sign, reflecting the immune suppression. Cryptococcal antigen is a highly sensitive test for cryptococcal meningitis even in patients with immune suppression since this is an antigen test rather than an antibody titer. (p1418)

Answer 59E-5: A.
CSF VDRL is specific for the diagnosis of syphilis in AIDS patients but not highly sensitive. This fact plus the frequency of nonspecific abnormalities in the CSF in AIDS makes the diagnosis of syphilis in AIDS difficult. Treatment failure is more common in patients with AIDS, requiring close monitoring. CSF lymphocytic pleocytosis is common in patients with AIDS such that this cannot be used to support the diagnosis of syphilis. (p1419)

Question 59E-6:
What is the most common cause of spinal cord dysfunction in patients with AIDS?

A. HTLV-1
B. CMV
C. VZV
D. Vacuolar myelopathy

Question 59E-7:
Which is the most common neuropathy in patients with AIDS?

A. Distal sensory polyneuropathy
B. Guillain-Barré syndrome
C. CIDP
D. Mononeuropathy multiplex

Question 59E-8:
Which of the following statements are true regarding differentiation between distal sensory polyneuropathy and nucleoside neuropathy?

1. Nucleoside neuropathy develops more rapidly than DSP.
2. Nucleoside neuropathy is painless whereas DSP is painful.
3. Nucleoside neuropathy improves after discontinuation of the offending drugs.
4. NCV findings differentiate DSP from nucleoside neuropathy.

Select: A = 1, 2, 3. B = 1, 3. C = 2. 4. D = 4 only. E = All

Questions 59E-9 through 59E-12:
The following statements are true or false. Select the best answer for each.

Question 59E-9:
Patients with CIDP and HIV often have a lymphocytic pleocytosis in the CSF.

Question 59E-10:
Corticosteroids should be given to all patients with HIV-associated inflammatory myopathy.

Question 59E-11:
Zidovudine myopathy is due to mitochondrial dysfunction.

Question 59E-12:
Guillain-Barré syndrome is usually an early complication of HIV infection.

Answer 59E-6: D.
Vacuolar myelopathy is the most common cause of spinal cord dysfunction in patients with AIDS. The listed viruses can also cause spinal cord dysfunction in this clinical setting, although to a lesser extent than vacuolar myelopathy. (p1419)

Answer 59E-7: A.
DSP is the most common neuropathy in patients with AIDS. GBS and CIDP can both develop. Mononeuropathy multiplex is a rare manifestation of HIV infection. (p1419-1420)

Answer 59E-8: B.
Nucleoside neuropathy develops over weeks, in contrast to DSP, which develops over months to years. Nucleoside neuropathy is due to the effects of several antiretroviral drugs, and discontinuation produces improvement in the following months. NCV cannot differentiate these conditions. Both nucleoside neuropathy and DSP are painful, and they can appear clinically similar. (p1420)

Answer 59E-9: True.
Patients with CIDP and HIV often have a lymphocytic pleocytosis in their CSF, as opposed to patients without HIV. (p1420)

Answer 59E-10: False.
Not all patients with HIV-associated inflammatory neuropathy have to be treated. Long-term use of corticosteroids may exacerbate the immunosuppression, so they should be avoided if possible. (p1423)

Answer 59E-11: True.
Zidovudine causes a toxic mitochondrial myopathy which can be clinically similar to inflammatory myopathy. (p1421)

Answer 59E-12: True.
GBS and CIDP are usually early complications of HIV infection, as opposed to many of the other neuromuscular disorders which develop later in infection. (p1420)

Chapter 59F: Infections of the Nervous System: Transmissible Spongiform Encephalopathies

Question 59F-1:
Which of the following symptoms would not be expected in a patient with kuru?

A. Ataxia
B. Dysarthria
C. Motor weakness
D. Choreoathetosis

Question 59F-2:
Which is the most common cause of Creutzfeldt-Jakob disease?

A. Neurosurgical instrumentation
B. Ingestion of contaminated meat
C. Inheritance
D. Spontaneous mutation

Question 59F-3:
Which of the following features would not be expected in fatal familial insomnia (FFI)?

A. Autosomal dominant inheritance
B. Tremor
C. Myoclonus
D. Memory loss
E. All can be found in FFI

Answer 59F-1: C.
Motor weakness, sensory loss, and cranial nerve palsies are not expected in patients with kuru. The other symptoms are typical, although not found at all stages of the disease process. (p1423)

Answer 59F-2: D.
Spontaneous mutation is responsible for about 90% of cases of CJD. Most of the remaining cases are inherited, with only a small proportion due to neurosurgical procedures. Ingestion of contaminated meat is not known t be a method of transfer. (p1424)

Answer 59F-3: E.
All of these features are typical of FFI. Memory loss is common, although frank dementia may not occur. Motor symptoms besides tremor and myoclonus may include ataxia and hyperreflexia. (p1429)

Chapter 60: Multiple Sclerosis and Other Inflammatory Demyelinating Disorders of the Central Nervous System

Question 60-1:
Which of the following visual deficits is MS least likely to produce?

A. Bilateral loss of vision
B. Unilateral loss of vision
C. Bitemporal hemianopia
D. Homonymous hemianopia

Question 60-2:
Bilateral internuclear ophthalmoplegia can be caused by which of the following disorders?

1. Multiple sclerosis
2. Wernicke's encephalopathy
3. Stroke
4. Arnold-Chiari malformation

Select: A = 1, 2, 3. B = 1, 3. C = 2, 4. D = 4 only. E = All

Questions 60-3 through 60-7:
The following questions present some clinical findings encountered with structural disorders of the brain. For each, select the associated disorder(s).

A. Multiple sclerosis
B. Vascular disease
C. Both
D. Neither

Question 60-3:
Internuclear ophthalmoplegia.

Question 60-4:
Dementia early in the disorder.

Question 60-5:
Dysarthria.

Question 60-6:
Aphasia.

Question 60-7:
Lhermitte's sign.

Question 60-8:
MRI in MS shows areas of increased signal intensity in T2-weighted images, but these findings are not specific. Which of the following are alternative diagnoses?

1. Sjögren's syndrome
2. Normal aging
3. Behçet's disease
4. Lupus cerebritis

Select: A = 1, 2, 3. B = 1, 3. C = 2, 4. D = 4 only. E = All

Question 60-9:
Patient characteristics have an effect on the course and prognosis of MS. Which of the following features suggest a relatively good prognosis?

1. Female rather than male
2. Age less than 29 rather than older
3. Relapsing rather than progressive
4. Predominantly sensory symptoms rather than motor symptoms

Select: A = 1, 2, 3. B = 1, 3. C = 2, 4. D = 4 only. E = All

Answer 60-1: C.
Bitemporal hemianopia is more suggestive of a peri-chiasmatic structural lesion than demyelinating disease. Homonymous hemianopia is uncommon in MS, but can develop with substantial demyelination in the optic radiations. Bilateral loss of vision is rarely acute but is usually sequential in one eye and then the other. (p1439)

Answer 60-2: E.
All of these are potential causes of bilateral INO. The most common causes are MS and stroke. (p1439)

Answer 60-3: C.
Both can produce INO, although it is more commonly seen in MS. (p1441)

Answer 60-4: B.
Memory deficit and frank cognitive decline is more prominent in CVA than in MS. Late in the course of MS, with advanced plaque formation, dementia can develop. (p1441)

Answer 60-5: C.
Dysarthria can develop in either MS or stroke. Other forms of speech disorder can develop in patients with MS also. (p1441)

Answer 60-6: B.
Aphasia is not expected in MS, but will develop in patients with stroke in the dominant hemisphere. (p1440)

Answer 60-7: A.
Lhermitte's sign is an electric sensation which runs down the arms when the neck is flexed. This finding is seen most frequently in MS, but can also be seen with cervical spondylosis. (p1440)

Answer 60-8: A.
Lupus cerebritis produces changes which extend through the cortex, and should be distinguishable from MS plaques. The other disorders can all produce abnormal signal patterns resembling MS. (p1442)

Answer 60-9: E.
All of these features suggest a relatively good prognosis, compared with alternatives. (p1445)

Question 60-10:
Transverse myelitis can be an isolated entity or develop into multiple sclerosis. What is the chance of a patient with acute complete transverse myelitis subsequently developing MS?

A. 5-10%
B. 25-30%
C. 50%
D. 70%

Question 60-11:
What proportion of patients with partial transverse myelitis will have areas of abnormal signal intensity on T2-weighted images suggestive of plaque?

A. 10%
B. 25%
C. 40%
D. greater than 50%

Question 60-12:
A 38-year-old man with progressive myelopathy has a normal MRI of the brain and spine. Progressive myelopathy as a variant of MS is the provisional diagnosis. Which of the following differential diagnoses should also be considered?

1. HIV
2. Adrenomyeloneuropathy
3. HTLV-1
4. Vitamin B12 deficiency

Select: A = 1, 2, 3. B = 1, 3. C = 2, 4. D = 4 only. E = All

Answer 60-10: A.
Only 5-10% of patients with complete transverse myelitis subsequently develop MS, whereas a greater proportion of patients with partial myelitis will develop MS. (p1445)

Answer 60-11: D.
More than 50% of patients with partial transverse myelitis will have abnormal areas on MRI. Many of these will subsequently develop MS, but the presence of the signal abnormalities alone do not make the diagnosis. (p1445)

Answer 60-12: E.
All of these are potential causes of progressive myelopathy. Prognosis for recovery is poor, and treatment is difficult. (p1452)

Chapter 61: Anoxic and Ischemic Encephalopathies

Question 61-1:
A 60-year-old man with anoxic encephalopathy following cardiopulmonary arrest begins to regain responsiveness and is noted to have a left hemiparesis. What is the most likely cause of the focal deficit?

A. Right MCA infarct resulting in arrhythmia and cardiac arrest
B. Watershed infarction
C. Hemorrhage from anticoagulants given during the resuscitative procedure
D. Patchy cerebral edema

Question 61-2:
Which of the following features would be consistent with the persistent vegetative state?

1. Smiling, crying
2. Sleep-wake cycles
3. Blink to visual threat
4. Follow no verbal or visual commands.

Select: A = 1, 2, 3. B = 1, 3. C = 2, 4. D = 4 only. E = All

Questions 61-3 through 61-5:
The following questions deal with criteria for brain death and are based on the published guidelines for adults and children. For each of the mini-vignettes, select the appropriate observation and evaluation. More than one choice may be correct. Assume for each that complete brain death examinations have been performed, and that physiologic parameters were appropriate for the examination and period of observation.

A. Observation for 24 hours without a confirmatory test
B. Observation for 12 hours without a confirmatory test
C. Observation for 6 hours without a confirmatory test
D. Observation for 24 hours with an isoelectric EEG
E. Observation for 12 hours with an isoelectric EEG
F. Observation for 6 hours with an isoelectric EEG
G. Observation for 48 hours with two isoelectric EEGs
H. None of these

Question 61-3:
A 74-year-old man with intracerebral hematoma.

Question 61-4:
A 3-day-old female with intraventricular hemorrhage.

Question 61-5:
A 56-year-old female with coma following cardiac arrest.

Question 61-6:
Which of the following EEG patterns suggest a poor prognosis for good neurologic recovery, assuming the absence of sedatives?

1. Burst-suppression pattern
2. Periodic triphasic waves
3. Alpha coma
4. Mixed frequency invariant pattern

Select: A = 1, 2, 3. B = 1, 3. C = 2, 4. D = 4 only. E = All

Answer 61-1: B.
Hypotension resulting in anoxic encephalopathy can result in focal infarction mainly in watershed zones. This may produce focal signs which are not appreciated immediately but may be more obvious during the phase of recovery. At that time, a second insult is often considered when it actually occurred at the time of the arrest. Focal infarction may also be more likely when the patient has a focal stenosis of one cerebral artery which can result in a predisposition to infarction. (p1468)

Answer 61-2: E.
All of these can be seen in the persistent vegetative state. The blink to threat, when a hand is thrust in front of the patient's eyes, and the facial expressions are often interpreted by families as indicative of cognition; however, they are patterned responses generated by subcortical centers. (p1469)

Answer 61-3: B or F.
Either 12 hours of observation or 6 hours with an isoelectric EEG are sufficient to establish brain death when the cause is known and it is not anoxia. (p1471)

Answer 61-4: H.
There are currently no established criteria for determination of brain death in children younger than 7 days. (p1471)

Answer 61-5: A or E.
Either 24 hours of observation or 12 hours with a confirmatory test are required for determination of brain death when the cause is anoxia. The discrepancy between anoxia and other causes is because of the potential for improvement being better for a given level of unresponsiveness. (p1471)

Answer 61-6: A.
All of these patterns suggest a poor prognosis for good neurologic recovery except for the mixed-frequency background. The presence of burst-suppression pattern or alpha coma more than 24 hours after an event suggests that family counseling regarding poor prognosis is appropriate. (p1472)

Question 61-7:
A 54-year-old female has a cardiac arrest and resultant severe encephalopathy. CT shows massive edema. Which of the following treatments are effective for management of the edema?

1. Mannitol
2. Lasix
3. Corticosteroids
4. Hyperventilation

Select: A = 1, 2, 3. B = 1, 3. C = 2, 4. D = 4 only. E = All

Question 61-8:
Which of the following agents are used in treating myoclonus following hypoxia?

1. Clonazepam
2. Valproate
3. Lorazepam
4. Morphine

Select: A = 1, 2, 3. B = 1, 3. C = 2, 4. D = 4 only. E = All

Answer 61-7: D.
No anti-edema treatment will be particularly effective in post-anoxic edema, since the edema is due to brain necrosis. Of the listed mechanisms, hyperventilation can reduce intracranial vascular volume, temporarily reducing intracranial pressure. Osmotic agents are of no value because they will leak out of the vessels into damaged brain and have little effect on removing fluid volume. (p1473)

Answer 61-8: E.
All of these agents are used for treatment of post-anoxic myoclonus. In addition, some patients who have severe myoclonus which interferes with mechanical ventilation will require neuromuscular paralysis. (p1473)

Chapter 62: Toxic and Metabolic Encephalopathies

Question 62-1:
Toxin hypersensitivity is a characteristic of which of the following conditions?

A. Uremic encephalopathy
B. Hepatic encephalopathy
C. Phenytoin administration
D. Alzheimer's disease

Question 62-2:
What is the presumed mechanism of action of lactulose on hepatic encephalopathy?

A. Acidification of the bowel contents preventing ammonia absorption
B. Prevention of protein absorption via binding and decreasing transit time
C. Acts as substrate for bacteria which use ammonia

Questions 62-3 through 62-5:
The following questions concern uremic and hepatic encephalopathy. For each question, select the best association from the following list.

A. Hepatic encephalopathy
B. Uremic encephalopathy
C. Both
D. Neither

Question 62-3:
Diffuse disorganized slowing in the theta range.

Question 62-4:
Produce a mild encephalopathy which can be mistaken for degenerative dementia.

Question 62-5:
Disorder of GABA neurotransmission implicated in the pathogenesis of the encephalopathy.

Question 62-6:
A 58-year-old female is admitted because of severe encephalopathy to the point of being comatose. She is breathing and has no focal neurologic findings. Head CT is normal. Routine laboratory studies are remarkable for a glucose of 1100. Which of the following initial clinical treatments is appropriate?

A. Give DDAVP.
B. Give 2L normal saline immediately followed by more fluids and insulin as dictated by laboratory data.
C. Give furosamide (Lasix).
D. Insert a Swan-Ganz catheter before deciding on fluid balance.

Questions 62-7 through 62-10:
The following questions concern disorders of calcium. For the findings listed in the questions, select the calcium disorder(s) with which they are associated.

A. Hypercalcemia
B. Hypocalcemia
C. Both
D. Neither

Question 62-7:
Hyperparathyroidism.

Question 62-8:
Papilledema.

Question 62-9:
Mental status change.

Question 62-10:
Parkinsonism.

Answer 62-1: B.
Patients with all of these conditions may have heightened sensitivity to drugs and toxins, but this is especially true for patients with hepatic failure. Patients frequently have a mild encephalopathy which is punctuated by episodes of more severe confusion due to subtle metabolic changes or toxin or medication exposure. (p1480)

Answer 62-2: C.
Lactulose is used as a substrate by bowel bacteria, which then use ammonia, thereby preventing availability for absorption. (p1481)

Answer 62-3: C.
EEG in both can show slowing in the theta range. Persistent triphasic waves are often thought of as being typical in hepatic encephalopathy, but are not specific, and depending on the stage are not always present. (p1477)

Answer 62-4: C.
Both hepatic and uremic encephalopathy can be associated with cognitive changes in the absence of disturbance of consciousness, which may be mistaken for degenerative dementia. Additional physical signs and routine laboratory studies suggest the diagnosis. While there is a correlation between ammonia levels and encephalopathy for hepatic encephalopathy, there are other chemicals involved, as well. (p1484)

Answer 62-5: C.
Both hepatic and uremic encephalopathies have GABA implicated in the pathogenesis of the mental status changes, although the magnitude of information indicating correlation is greater for the former. (p1480, 1483)

Answer 62-6: B.
This is a typical clinical presentation of a patient with nonketotic hyperosmolar coma. This may be the initial presentation of their diabetes. The osmotic effect of the hyperglycemia results in diuresis and hypovolemia. Initial fluid replacement is indicated followed by additional fluids and insulin as dictated by lab results. A Swan-Ganz catheter may be required but should not preclude initial fluid administration. (p1487)

Answer 62-7: A.
Hyperparathyroidism is the most common cause of hypercalcemia. (p1491)

Answer 62-8: B.
Papilledema can develop as a complication of hypocalcemia with increased intracranial pressure. (p1491)

Answer 62-9: C.
Both hypercalcemia and hypocalcemia can produce mental status change, although of different types. Hypercalcemia produces confusion and weakness. Hypocalcemia can produce seizures and increased intracranial pressure. (p1491)

Answer 62-10: B.
Hypocalcemia can produce extrapyramidal signs which have a parkinsonian appearance. (p1491)

Chapter 63: Deficiency Diseases of the Nervous System

Question 63-1:
Which of the following features are seen with vitamin B12 deficiency?

1. Paresthesias of the hands and feet
2. Depression
3. Ataxia
4. GI distress

Select: A = 1, 2, 3. B = 1, 3. C = 2, 4. D = 4 only. E = All

Question 63-2:
Which is the most likely cause of vitamin B12 deficiency?

A. Dietary deficiency of vitamin B12
B. Deficiency of intrinsic factor
C. Drug administration interfereing with vitamin absorption
D. Short-bowel syndrome

Question 63-3:
Vitamin E deficiency has been implicated in which of the following conditions?

A. Myelopathy
B. Myopathy
C. Peripheral neuropathy
D. All of the above

Question 63-4:
Which of the following is the most common clinical presentation of folate deficiency?

A. Dementia
B. Peripheral neuropathy
C. Corticospinal tract signs
D. Normal neurologic function

Question 63-5:
Bassen-Kornzweig syndrome is associated with a deficiency of which of the following vitamins?

A. Vitamin E
B. Vitamin D
C. Folate
D. Pyridoxine

Answer 63-1: E.
All of these are potential clinical manifestations of vitamin B12 deficiency. GI symptoms may include dyspepsia, flatulence, and altered bowel habits. The ataxia may be on the basis of central or peripheral dysfunction. (p1496)

Answer 63-2: B.
Deficiency of intrinsic factor accounts for most cases of B12 deficiency. Causes of the deficiency may include autoantibodies and gastrectomy. (p1497)

Answer 63-3: D.
All of these are potential clinical manifestations of vitamin E deficiency. (p1499)

Answer 63-4: D.
The majority of patients with low folate levels have no neurologic symptoms secondary to the deficiency. Many patients with folate deficiency have other disorders which contribute to development of neurologic symptoms. (p1499)

Answer 63-5: A.
Bassen-Kornzweig syndrome is a rare familial form of fat malabsorption which causes vitamin E deficiency. Vitamin E supplementation can halt or even reverse the progression of neurologic symptoms in some patients. (p1500)

Chapter 64A: Effects of Toxins and Physical Agents on the Nervous System: Effects of Occupational Toxins on the Nervous System

Question 64A-1:
A 32-year-old female is admitted with severe encephalopathy. She was found asleep in her car at a rest area on the highway. CT was normal. Laboratory studies showed no diagnostic abnormalities. She gradually improved to the point that she was speaking and moving well, although with mild confusion. Several days later she worsens to the point of being unresponsive and becomes vegetative. Which is the most likely clinical formulation?

A. The initial insult was most likely carbon monoxide poisoning which resulted in an improving encephalopathy. Now she is developing late deterioration.'
B. The initial insult was heat stroke and is now followed by delayed demyelination.
C. The patient had a cardiac arrest and now suffers from delayed deterioration from anoxic encephalopathy.

Question 64A-2:
Which of the following intoxicants are typically associated with peripheral neuropathy?

1. Lindane
2. Methyl bromide
3. Styrene
4. Organophosphate

Select: A = 1, 2, 3. B = 1, 3. C = 2, 4. D = 4 only. E = All

Question 64A-3:
Which of the following statements are true regarding lead neuropathy?

1. Responds to chelation
2. Is a demyelinating neuropathy
3. May occur with acute lead exposure
4. May resemble ALS

Select: A = 1, 2, 3. B = 1, 3. C = 2, 4. D = 4 only. E = All

Question 64A-4:
Which of the following intoxicants may produce optic neuropathy?

1. Thallium
2. Methyl bromide
3. Toluene
4. n-Hexane

Select: A = 1, 2, 3. B = 1, 3. C = 2, 4. D = 4 only. E = All

Question 64A-5:
Minamata disease was recognized in Japan in the 1950s, but the same pathophysiological process is seen worldwide. What is the cause of Minamata disease?

A. Lead
B. Arsenic
C. Methyl mercury
D. Elemental mercury

Answer 64A-1: A.
This is a typical presentation for a patient subjected to carbon monoxide poisoning. The clinical presentation is essentially anoxia with initial improvement. Patients may develop late deterioration as patients with more typical anoxic encephalopathy will. Cardiac arrest would not be expected to allow the patient to drive to a rest stop, whereas CO poisoning would be expected because of the presumption of the patient taking a nap with the car on for air conditioning. (p1513)

Answer 64A-2: C.
Methyl bromide and organophosphate intoxication is typically associated with peripheral neuropathy. Lindane and styrene have had some adverse effects attributed to them, but neuropathy is not an accepted adverse effect. (p1514)

Answer 64A-3: D.
Chronic lead poisoning often produces an axonal neuropathy with predominantly motor findings. This may resemble ALS, although corticospinal tract signs are not typically present and tendon reflexes are decreased or absent. Unfortunately, lead neuropathy does not respond to chelation. Only chronic exposure is associated with neuropathy. (p1518)

Answer 64A-4: E.
All of these agents may produce optic neuropathy, although other neurologic complications can develop, as well. (p1513-1519)

Answer 64A-5: C.
Minamata disease was due to intoxication with organic mercury in the form of methyl mercury. The mercury was from industrial waste that was assimilated by the fish in Minamata Bay. (p1518)

Chapter 64B: Effects of Toxins and Physical Agents on the Nervous System: Effects of Drug Abuse on the Nervous System

Question 64B-1:
Overdose of which of the following is least likely to produce respiratory suppression?

A. Benzodiazepines
B. Barbiturates
C. Opiates

Question 64B-2:
Which of the following are likely to produce seizures during acute exposure?

A. Diazepam
B. Pentobarbital
C. Heroin
D. Cocaine

Question 64B-3:
Which of the following may develop following overdose with phencyclidine?

1. Stupor progressing to coma
2. Agitation and psychosis
3. Nystagmus
4. Rhabdomyolysis

Select: A = 1, 2, 3. B = 1, 3. C = 2, 4. D = 4 only. E = All

Question 64B-4:
Stroke rate is increased markedly in young individuals who abuse drugs. Which of the following agents is most closely correlated with stroke?

A. Heroin
B. Cocaine
C. Hydrocarbon inhalants
D. Diazepam

Question 64B-5:
How long can cocaine metabolites be detected in the urine of patients suspected of abuse?

A. 12 hours
B. 48 hours
C. 5 days
D. 15 days

Answer 64B-1: A.
Respiratory suppression may develop with any of these, but benzodiazepines are less likely to produce respiratry suppression than barbiturates or opiates. (p1523)

Answer 64B-2: D.
Cocaine is the most likely to produce seizures during acute intoxication, although opiates can rarely cause seizures. Seizures are typically a withdrawal symptom with benzodiazepines and barbiturates. (p1523)

Answer 64B-3: E.
All of these may develop in patients subjected to an overdose of phencyclidine. Rhabdomyolysis with myoglobinuria is common. Disturbance of the level of consciousness, from agitation to coma, depends on the dose. (p1525)

Answer 64B-4: B.
Cocaine is the most important cause of drug abuse–associated stroke, being implicated in approximately 50% of cases. The other agents can produce anoxia, and heroin injection has been implicated in some vascular damage, including myelopathy, which resembles anterior spinal artery syndrome. (p1526)

Answer 64B-5: B.
Cocaine and amphetamine metabolites are cleared rapidly, such that they are not reliably detectable more than 48 hours following last exposure. Benzodiazepines, barbiturates, and heroin are detectable for a longer time, and this is enhanced with chronic use. (p1522)

Chapter 64C: Effects of Toxins and Physical Agents on the Nervous System: Neurotoxins of Animals and Plants

Question 64C-1:
Which is the most common clinical presentation of a bite from the black widow spider?

A. Disseminated rash and bronchospasm
B. Respiratory arrest
C. Pain and local muscle spasm
D. No systemic symptoms

Question 64C-2:
A 24-year-old male presents with ataxia which progresses to hypotonia and weakness without sensory loss. Reflexes are absent. The clinical diagnosis is Guillain-Barré syndrome. Which would be an important differential diagnosis?

A. Tick paralysis
B. Scorpion bite
C. Black widow spider bite
D. Jimson weed poisoning

Question 64C-3:
Which are the most likely adverse effects of mushroom poisoning?

A. GI distress
B. Renal failure
C. Hepatic failure
D. Seizures and coma

Question 64C-4:
Which of the following clinical features are typical of patients with lathyrism?

1. Spastic paraparesis
2. Ascending sensory loss
3. Ataxia
4. Encephalopathy

Select: A = 1, 2, 3. B = 1, 3. C = 2, 4. D = 4 only. E = All

Question 64C-5:
A 24-year-old man reports that he was bitten by an unidentified snake. There is little local reaction. Three hours later, he develops ptosis, dysphagia, and diffuse weakness and becomes areflexic. Which type of snake is most likely responsible for the bite?

A. Rattlesnake
B. Copperhead
C. Water moccasin
D. Coral snake

Answer 64C-1: D.
Most bites of the black widow spider produce no reaction or only a local skin reaction because of the small amount of venom injected, despite the high overall potency of the venom. The other symptoms may develop but are uncommon. (p1530)

Answer 64C-2: A.
Tick paralysis may be impossible to clinically differentiate from GBS. Scorpion bite typically produces paresthesias and muscle spasms when symptoms develop, although most bites do not result in these findings. Black widow bites also produce muscle spasms and other symptoms prior to weakness. Jimson weed poisoning produces symptoms of anticholinergic toxicity. (p1531)

Answer 64C-3: A.
GI distress is common in patients with poisoning with most mushrooms. Renal and hepatic failure can develop, but luckily this is not typical. The organ dysfunction can develop with large doses. Seizures and coma may develop with severe organ dysfunction. (p1533)

Answer 64C-4: B.
Spastic paraparesis and ataxia are typical of lathyrism. Patients may complain of paresthesias, but sensory function and cognition are typically spared. (p1532)

Answer 64C-5: D.
The clinical presentation is typical of a bite from a coral snake. The three other snakes are pit vipers, which typically produce prominent local reactions before systemic symptoms develop, and when they do develop, do so with fasciculations and weakness over 12-24 hours. (p1530)

Chapter 64D: Effects of Toxins and Physical Agents on the Nervous System: Marine Toxins

Question 64D-1:
The pufferfish is potentially highly toxic, producing the powerful tetrodotoxin (TTX). Which one of the following statements regarding this toxin and the pufferfish is *not* true?

A. TTX blocks sodium channels, preventing the inward sodium current during action potentials
B. The pufferfish has a worldwide distribution in fresh and salt water.
C. TTX is unique to the pufferfish.
D. TTX poisoning resembles saxitoxin poisoning.

Question 64D-2:
Paralytic shellfish poisoning is due to a family of toxins including saxitoxin. Which one of the following statements regarding saxitoxin poisoning is *not* true?

A. Typical symptoms include paresthesias and weakness.
B. Saxitoxin is less potent then tetrodotoxin.
C. Symptoms may begin 5 minutes after ingestion of the shellfish.
D. There is no antidote.

Question 64D-3:
Ciguatera is a marine food poisoning which is occasionally seen in the US. Which of the following statements regarding ciguatera is *not* true?

A. Ciguatera toxin is formed by bacteria in the intestines of fish.
B. Reef fish are predominantly implicated in human intoxication.
C. The toxin is nontoxic to the fish.
D. The toxin acts on sodium channels of excitable membranes.

Answer 64D-1: C.
TTX is manufactured by bacteria which are not unique to pufferfish; they also produce toxin in some octopi, ocean sunfish, and some newts and salamanders. The remainder of the statements are true. (p1537)

Answer 64D-2: B.
Saxitoxin shares many features with tetrodotoxin, but it is more potent. The death rate for tetrodotoxin ingestion is approximately 50%. Nevertheless, it is a powerful agent which has a tendency to produce paresthesias and weakness, although weakness does not develop in all patients. (p1537)

Answer 64D-3: A.
Ciguatera toxin is initially formed in dinoflaggelates, then ascends the food chain. It is apparently nontoxic to the fish. The other statements are true. The toxicity is thought to be due to effects on voltage-gated sodium channels of excitable membranes of neurons, skeletal muscle, and cardiac muscle. (p1536)

Chapter 64E: Effects of Toxins and Physical Agents on the Nervous System: Effect of Physical Agents on the Nervous System

Question 64E-1:
Which of the following mechanisms has been implicated in radiation-induced encephalopathy?

A. Demyelination
B. Vascular change and necrosis
C. Breakdown of the blood-brain barrier with cerebral edema
D. All of the above

Question 64E-2:
A 27-year-old man presents with an on-the-job electrical injury to the right hand. The contact sites were the right hand and right leg. One week later, he presents with progressive myelopathy. Which is the most likely clinical formulation?

A. He has delayed transverse myelopathy following the electrical injury
B. He has developed transverse myelitis which is not directly related to the electrical injury.
C. He most likely has functional weakness due to the psychosocial issues surrounding the on-the-job injury.

Question 64E-3:
A 75-year-old male presents with coma. He is a known alcoholic and it is a cold winter night. His core temperature is 30°C. Neurologic examination does not show any cerebral or brainstem function. EEG is isoelectric. Which is the most appropriate clinical formulation?

A. The patient meets clinical and EEG criteria for brain death, and life spports should be terminated.
B. The core temperature may create the appearance of brain death, so warming and supportive measures should be continued.
C. The patient should be examined after 6 hours, and if the examination still shows no responsiveness, the life supports should be discontinued.

Answer 64E-1: D.
All of these are thought to contribute to radiation-induced encephalopathy. Early encephalopathy is probably due to opening of the blood-brain barrier with increased intracranial pressure. Early delayed encephalopathy is probably due to demyelination. Delayed radiation encephalopathy is associated with necrosis, which is likely a combination of neural and vascular effects. (p1541)

Answer 64E-2: A.
Delayed transverse myelopathy following serious electrical injury typically develops 7 days or so after the injury if the path of the current involved the cord, as in this patient. (p1542)

Answer 64E-3: B.
Profound hypothermia may produce the clinical and EEG appearance of brain death, yet the patient may recover with supportive care. Therefore, discontinuation on these grounds would not be indicated. Also, the temperature is too low for the initial examination and EEG to be used for determination of brain death as an initial assessment. (p1543)

Chapter 65: Brain Edema and Disorders of Cerebrospinal Fluid Circulation

Question 65-1:
Which of the following statements is true regarding use of corticosteroids in children with bacterial meningitis?

A. Corticosteroids improve CSF penetrance of antibiotics, thereby improving outcome of patients with meningitis.
B. Corticosteroids reduce the secondary inflammatory response and thereby reduce the risk of hearing loss and other complications of meningitis.
C. Corticosteroids impair the immune response and thereby impair treatment of meningitis.

Question 65-2:
Which of the following findings would be least likely in idiopathic intracranial hypertension (pseudotumor cerebri)?

A. Exacerbation of headache by coughing
B. Elevated protein in CSF
C. CN-6 palsy
D. Visual fields show an enlarged blind spot

Questions 65-3 through 65-5:
The following questions pertain to some important disorders of intracranial pressure. For the mini-vignettes, select the best answer from the following list.

A. Obstructive hydrocephalus
B. Mass lesion with increased intracranial pressure
C. Normal pressure hydrocephalus
D. Idiopathic intracranial hypertension
E. Low intracerebral pressure
F. Normal patient

Question 65-3:
A 26-year-old female presents with morning headache which abates through the day. Examination shows bilateral papilledema. Visual fields show incomplete left hemianopia.

Question 65-4:
A 67-year-old man presents with dementia, thought to be Alzheimer's disease by the referring physician. Examination shows markedly impaired memory plus gait ataxia. No other findings.

Question 65-5:
A 2-year-old is brought for evaluation because of increased head size. Head circumference is much larger proportionately than body size. In other respects, physical and neurologic exams are normal.

Questions 65-6 through 65-10:
The following questions regarding edema and CSF circulation are true/false. Select the best answer for each statement.

Question 65-6:
Tamoxifen may produce intracranial hypertension.

Question 65-7:
Patients with DKA are at greatest risk for cerebral edema during the phase of glucose increase.

Question 65-8:
Cerebral edema is a greater problem for acute liver failure than chronic liver failure.

Question 65-9:
Acetazolamide (Diamox) reduces CSF production.

Question 65-10:
Tight junctions are characteristic of brain capillaries but not peripheral vessels.

Answer 65-1: B.
Corticosteroids have been shown to be helpful for children but have not been proven to be of benefit for adults. The benefit is by reduction of the secondary inflammation. Meningeal inflammation aids CSF penetrance of some antibiotics, and reduction of this inflammation would not be helpful; luckily, this is not a deleterious factor for patients. In the presence of effective antibiotics, corticosteroids do not impair improvement. (p1551)

Answer 65-2: B.
CSF protein is typically reduced rather than elevated. The other findings are typical. The CN-6 lesion is a false localizing sign. (p1553)

Answer 65-3: B.
The morning headache is typical of increased intracranial pressure and, by itself, is not a very helpful localizing sign. However, the hemianopia strongly suggests a parenchymal brain lesion rather than the optic nerve visual field disturbance which can occur in some patients with idiopathic intracranial hypertension. (p1552)

Answer 65-4: C.
NPH is the most likely of the listed diagnoses, although there are other possible diagnoses which could explain ataxia and dementia, such as vitamin B12 deficiency, frontal lobe lesions and degenerations, and syndromes of parkinsonism and dementia. (p1556)

Answer 65-5: A.
Obstructive hydrocephalus, such as with congenital aqueductal stenosis, produces increased ventricular size which in the very young produces expansion of the skull before neurologic symptoms. At this young age, there may be no symptoms, but if the condition is not identified and treated, it may result in abnormal eye movements, optic atrophy, spasticity, and other symptoms. (p1554)

Answer 65-6: True.
Tamoxifen has been a powerful agent in the fight against breast cancer but has real adverse effects which can be dose limiting. Among the neurologic complications is intracranial hypertension which is unassociated with neoplastic meningitis. (p1553)

Answer 65-7: False.
The greatest risk for cerebral edema is as the glucose and sodium are being lowered. This is the time when there is the greatest driving force for fluid into the brain. (p1552)

Answer 65-8: True.
Acute liver failure from almost any reason is associated with risk for cerebral edema and secondary damage from the increased intracranial pressure. Although neurologic dysfunction is common in patients with chronic liver failure, cerebral edema is usually not the cause. (p1551)

Answer 65-9: True.
Acetazolamide reduces CSF production, but often not to a degree or for a duration which is clinically helpful. Mannitol and other osmotic agents may temporarily lower CSF production, but again the reduction is not sustained. (p1548)

Answer 65-10: True.
Tight junctions are one of a host of differences between brain vasculature and peripheral vasculature which make for complicated substrate and drug movement across the blood-brain barrier. (p1547)

Chapter 66: Developmental Disorders of the Nervous System

Question 66-1:
Which of the following statements are true regarding lissencephaly?

1. Lissencephaly may be associated with muscular dystrophy.
2. All cerebral hemispheres are devoid of sulci early in gestation.
3. Cortical lamination is disrupted in most types of lissencephaly.
4. Lissencephaly is always due to genetic defects.

Select: A = 1, 2, 3. B = 1, 3. C = 2, 4. D = 4 only. E = All

Question 66-2:
Children with mental retardation not due to anoxia or destructive processes often have pathological changes which correlate with the intellectual deficit. Which of the following is true regarding the pathological changes?

A. Most of the dendritic arborization should occur near the end of the first trimester.
B. Neuronal drop-out is prominent in most brains of patients with these causes of mental retardation.
C. Sparse dendritic arborizations and sparseness of synapses is a common pathological finding.
D. None of these are true.

Question 66-3:
Which of the following statements is not true regarding myelination of brain pathways?

A. The corpus callosum does not complete myelination until mid-adolescence.
B. Most cranial nerves are myelinated before the third trimester.
C. Axons which will be myelinated do not function electrically until the myelination is complete.
D. Hypothyroidism causes slowed myelination.

Questions 66-4 through 66-7:
The following questions concern genetic defects and timing of the insult. For each of the questions, select the best answer from the following list.

A. 1-4 weeks' gestation
B. 4-8 weeks' gestation
C. 8-20 weeks' gestation
D. > 20 weeks' gestation

Question 66-4:
Lissencephaly.

Question 66-5:
Anencephaly.

Question 66-6:
Myelomeningocele.

Question 66-7:
Agenesis of the corpus callosum.

Question 66-8:
Cerebellar degeneration may occur because of a variety of neurologic lesions. Which of the following conditions may be associated with cerebellar degeneration?

1. Tay-Sachs disease
2. Menkes' kinky-hair disease
3. Spinal muscular atrophy
4. Chromosomal abnormalities

Select: A = 1, 2, 3. B = 1, 3. C = 2, 4. D = 4 only. E = All

Answer 66-1: A.
Lissencephaly may be due to intrauterine insults other than genetic errors, such as infections, although genetic causes are important. Lissencephaly may occur in conjunction with other defects, such as Fukuyama-type muscular dystrophy. (p1566)

Answer 66-2: C.
Defective dendritic arborizations and decreased synapse formation correlate with many causes of mental retardation which are not due to anoxia or structural defects. The arborization develops predominantly during the third trimester and first few postnatal months. Neuronal dropout is common in anoxia, but the genetic and unclassified deficits have the lack of dendritic arborization as a better correlate of the mental retardation. (p1568)

Answer 66-3: C.
Axons destined for myelination will still function before myelination is complete, but they will be susceptible to conduction block and will have impaired timing of discharges because of the flow conduction velocity. (p1571)

Answer 66-4: C.
Lissencephaly is due to defective formation of sulci and gyri and is related to failure of formation of folds during this period of neuronal migration, 8-20 weeks. (p1580)

Answer 66-5: A.
Anencephaly is due to failure of closure of the anterior neuropore at about 24 days' gestation. (p1575)

Answer 66-6: A.
Myelomeningocele is due to failure of closure of the posterior neuropore at about 26 days' gestation. (p1576)

Answer 66-7: B.
Agenesis of the corpus callosum is due to either failure of formation of the commissural plate or failure of degeneration of the part of the plate which would form a barrier to axonal crossing. (p1578)

Answer 66-8: E.
All of these are potentially associated with global cerebellar degeneration. Other cases may not be associated with systemic or other neurologic disorders. (p1581)

Chapter 67: Developmental Disabilities

Question 67-1:
Which of the following is not characteristic of patients with autism?

A. Egocentric focus
B. Some patients may be intellectually gifted.
C. Most patients do not progress to have normal jobs.
D. No patients with autism will progress to near-normal behavior.

Question 67-2:
A fetus is found to have bradycardia and then delivers with Apgar scores of 4 and 7. The child requires suctioning but is otherwise apparently normal with intact respirations and good feeding. Which is the most likely outcome?

A. Normal child
B. Intellectual delay and seizures
C. Late deterioration with subsequent loss of the acquired forces

Question 67-3:
What is the expected prevalence of persistence of attention-deficit hyperactivity disorder into adult life?

A. <5%
B. 10%
C. 40%
D. 70%

Question 67-4:
Which of the following features would not be expected in a patients with ADHD?

A. Normal physical examination
B. Focal neurologic signs
C. Normal IQ
D. Motor tics

Question 67-5:
Pathologic abnormalities are most likely in which of the following disorders?

A. Dyslexia
B. ADHD
C. Autism
D. None are associated with pathological changes

Question 67-6:
Which of the following medications is not used in patients with ADHD?

A. Pemoline (Cylert)
B. Clonidine (Catapres)
C. Fluoxetine (Prozac)
D. Propranolol (Inderal)
E. All are used in selected patients with ADHD

Answer 67-1: D.

A few patients with clearly autistic features will improve substantially such that they are almost normal. Unfortunately, this is a small minority. A larger proportion will have some improvement, although most will not enter the mainstream of society with normal jobs and families. (p1587)

Answer 67-2: A.

Fetal heart rate abnormalities and the Apgar scores are of concern, and neurologic deterioration or delay could occur, but the most likely result is a normal child. (p1585)

Answer 67-3: D.

Approximately 60-70% of children diagnosed with ADHD have persistence of symptoms into adult life. Improvement in self-motivation and maturity may improve compensation abilities, although social, emotional, and performance problems persisting into adult life are common. (p1592)

Answer 67-4: B.

Focal neurologic signs would not be expected in patients with ADHD, although there are some soft signs which can be identified in some patients. Motor tics may be seen in patients with ADHD in the setting of having inherited the Tourette gene. (p1593)

Answer 67-5: C.

Autism can be associated with a variety of pathological changes including decreased axons, hypoplastic cerebellum, reduced neuronal size, hypoplastic parietal lobes, and some other findings. In addition, autism is of increased incidence in some other disorders such as tuberous sclerosis and fragile X syndrome which have their own pathological findings. (p1589)

Answer 67-6: E.

All of these agents are used in selected patients with ADHD. Stimulants are still the first line of therapy and include pemoline, methylphenidate, and dextroamphetamine. (p1594)

Chapter 68: Inborn Errors of Metabolism of the Nervous System

Question 68-1:
Which of the following are characteristic of phenylketonuria?

1. Increased phenylalanine levels
2. Prenatal diagnosis is possible
3. Musty smell to the urine
4. Increased tyrosine levels

Select: A = 1, 2, 3. B = 1, 3. C = 2, 4. D = 4 only. E = All

Question 68-2:
Which of the following statements are true regarding dietary management of PKU?

1. The diet should ideally eliminate all phenylalanine.
2. Dietary protein is reduced.
3. Treatment should be initiated within the first 6 months of life to prevent neurologic deterioration.
4. Aspartame should be avoided.

Select: A = 1, 2, 3. B = 1, 3. C = 2, 4. D = 4 only. E = All

Question 68-3:
Which of the following statements are true for Tyrosinemia I?

1. Prenatal diagnosis is possible.
2. Blood alpha-fetoprotein is markedly increased.
3. Patients may present with early metabolic encephalopathy and liver failure.
4. Restriction of phenylalanine and tyrosine stops progression.

Select: A = 1, 2, 3. B = 1, 3. C = 2, 4. D = 4 only. E = All

Question 68-4:
Which of the following are true regarding Homocystinuria I?

1. Deficiency of cystathionine synthetase
2. Autosomal dominant
3. Increased risk of thrombotic events
4. Can cause neonatal seizures and apnea

Select: A = 1, 2, 3. B = 1, 3. C = 2, 4. D = 4 only. E = All

Question 68-5:
A term neonate presents with severe encephalopathy. She was normal at birth and then over several days developed lethargy, seizures, myoclonus, hypotonia, and hiccups. EEG shows a burst suppression pattern. Which of the following is most likely?

A. PKU
B. Hartnup disease
C. Non-ketotic hyperglycinemia
D. Homocystinuria

Question 68-6:
Which of the following disorders have symptoms precipitated by protein feedings?

1. Maple syrup urine disease
2. Non-ketotic hyperglycinemia
3. Methylmalonic acidemia
4. Glutaric acidemia

Select: A = 1, 2, 3. B = 1, 3. C = 2, 4. D = 4 only. E = All

Question 68-7:
Which of the following are helpful treatments for neonatal hyperammonemia of unknown cause?

1. Hemodialysis
2. Sodium benzoate
3. Biotin
4. Lactulose

Select: A = 1, 2, 3. B = 1, 3. C = 2, 4. D = 4 only. E = All

Answer 68-1: A.
Tyrosine levels are decreased rather than increased. The remainder of the features are true. (p1597)

Answer 68-2: C.
Aspartame is metabolized, in part, to phenylalanine, and should be avoided. Protein is reduced in the diet, but some phenylalanine is needed, and levels should be kept in the normal range, not at zero. Treatment should be instituted within the first three weeks in order for normal neurologic development to occur. (p1598).

Answer 68-3: A.
The restriction of phenylalanine and tyrosine is helpful but cannot stop the progression of the hepatic and renal disease. The other statements are true. (p1600)

Answer 68-4: B.
Homocystinuria is transmitted as an autosomal recessive trait. Children are normal at birth and develop symptoms later in childhood and young adult life. (p1601)

Answer 68-5: C.
This is a typical presentation for non-ketotic hyperglycinemia, but the clinical findings are not specific. None of the other listed disorders would present in this way. Hartnup disease presents with photosensitive dermatitis and neurologic deterioration that would not be expected shortly after birth. PKU presents with neurologic deterioration later in childhood and would not be expected to have the acute encephalopathic symptoms. Homocystinuria presents with symptoms which are usually related to the thrombotic events rather than an acute neonatal encephalopathy. (p1605)

Answer 68-6: A.
Glutaric acidemia is exacerbated by diets high in lysine and tryptophan, but the other disorders are particularly exacerbated by protein administration. (p1612)

Answer 68-7: A.
Lactulose is typically not used for neonates but is used in selected adult patients with hyperammonemia. The other treatments are typical for this disorder. In addition, there are other treatments which are used for specific causes of hyperammonemia. (p1618)

Question 68-8:
Which of the following features are shared by xeroderma pigmentosum and Cockayne's syndrome?

1. Sensitivity to sunlight
2. Deafness
3. Spasticity
4. Intellectual decline

Select: A = 1, 2, 3. B = 1, 3. C = 2, 4. D = 4 only. E = All

Question 68-9:
Which of the following antiepileptic drugs is least likely to exacerbate acute intermittent porphyria?

A. Valproate
B. Phenobarbital
C. Gabapentin
D. Phenytoin

Question 68-10:
Which of the following are characterized by pigmentary degeneration of the retina?

1. Abetalipoproteinemia
2. Xeroderma pigmentosum
3. Kearns-Sayre syndrome
4. Wilson's disease

Select: A = 1, 2, 3. B = 1, 3. C = 2, 4. D = 4 only. E = All

Question 68-11:
Which of the following may present in children with hypotonia and lactic acidosis?

1. Leigh disease
2. Pyruvate dehydrogenase deficiency
3. Pyruvate decarboxylase deficiency
4. Fumarase deficiency

Select: A = 1, 2, 3. B = 1, 3. C = 2, 4. D = 4 only. E = All

Question 68-12:
Which of the following are features of MELAS?

1. Recurrent strokes
2. Seizures
3. Retinopathy
4. Severe headache in childhood

Select: A = 1, 2, 3. B = 1, 3. C = 2, 4. D = 4 only. E = All

Question 68-13:
Which is the biochemical defect in patients with Refsum's disease?

A. Catalase
B. Phytanic acid oxidase
C. Peroxisome membrane protein
D. Acyl-CoA oxidase

Questions 68-14 through 68-17:
The following questions concern enzyme defects in glycogen storage diseases. For each of the following enzymes, select the disorder from the following list.

A. Pompe's
B. Wolman's
C. Farber's lipogranulomatosis
D. None of the above

Question 68-14:
Acid alpha-glycosidase (acid maltase).

Question 68-15:
Ceramidase.

Question 68-16:
Acid lipase.

Question 68-17:
Which of the following are typical of the Hurler phenotype?

1. Normal at birth
2. Hepatosplenomegaly
3. Early cardiac disease
4. Deafness

Select: A = 1, 2, 3. B = 1, 3. C = 2, 4. D = 4 only. E = All

Answer 68-8: E.
All of these features are common between XP and Cockayne's syndrome. Both have defective DNA repair which makes them sensitive to sunlight. (p1620)

Answer 68-9: C.
Gabapentin is not metabolized by the liver and is the least likely to precipitate or exacerbate an attack of acute intermittent porphyria. (p1621)

Answer 68-10: A.
Wilson's disease is characterized by corneal abnormalities but does not have the retinal degeneration of the other disorders. (p1622)

Answer 68-11: E.
All of these present with lactic acidosis and hypotonia, although the degree of lactic acidosis in fumarase deficiency is modest. (p1630)

Answer 68-12: E.
All of these are typical features of MELAS: mitochondrial encephalopathy, lactic acid, and stroke. Infarcts have an occipital predominance. (p1634)

Answer 68-13: B.
Refsum's disease is due to a deficiency of phytanic acid oxidase. Catalase deficiency is usually asymptomatic. Peroxisomal membrane protein defect causes Zellweger's syndrome. Acyl-CoA oxidase deficiency is also called pseudoneonatal adrenoleukodystrophy. (p1637-1641)

Answer 68-14: A.
Pompe's disease is due to a deficiency of acid maltase. (p1643)

Answer 68-15: C.
Farber's lipogranulomatosis is due to a defect in ceramidase. (p1646)

Answer 68-16: B.
Wolman's disease is due to a defect in acid lipase. (p1649)

Answer 68-17: E.
All of these are typical features of the Hurler phenotype, along with short stature, multiple skeletal abnormalities, thick coarse hair, and small, widely-spaced teeth. (p1648)

Questions 68-18 through 68-20:
The following questions concern the enzyme defects in mucopolysaccharidosis. For the enzymes, select the associated disorder from the following list.

A. Hurler's
B. Hunter's
C. Sanfilippo's
D. None of these

Question 68-18:
Heparan-*N*-sulfatase.

Question 68:-19:
L-Iduronidase.

Question 68-20:
Iduronate-2-sulfatase.

Question 68-21:
A 26-year-old man presents with progressive intellectual decline and ataxia. MRI shows extensive white matter changes. NCV shows marked slowing and dispersion of the waveforms. Which is the most likely diagnosis?

A. Adrenoleukodystrophy
B. Metachromatic leukodystrophy
C. Neuronal ceroid lipofuscinosis
D. Gaucher's disease

Answer 68-18: C.
Sanfilippo's syndrome type A is due to a deficiency of heparan-*N*-sulfatase. (p1649)

Answer 68-19: A.
Hurler's syndrome is due to deficiency of L-iduronidase. (p1649)

Answer 68-20: B.
Hunter's syndrome is due to deficiency of iduronate-2-sulfatase. (p1649)

Answer 68-21: B.
Although the clinical presentation is certainly not specific, MLD is the most likely of the disorders listed here. The combination of central and peripheral demyelination suggests the disorder. Although ALD in adults may have some mild neuropathy, marked slowing with central involvement would be unusual. (p1661)

Chapter 69: Neurocutaneous Syndromes

Question 69-1:
Which clinical finding is least likely in a child with tuberous sclerosis complex?

A. Shagreen patch
B. Seizures
C. Hypomelanotic macules
D. Cognitive abnormalities

Question 69-2:
Which of the following would have the least cutaneous lesions?

A. Tuberous sclerosis complex
B. Neurofibromatosis type 1
C. Neurofibromatosis type 2
D. Osler-Weber-Rendu syndrome

Questions 69-3 through 69-6:
The following questions pertain to some important neurocutaneous disorders. For each of the questions, select the best answer from the following list of disorders.

A. NF1
B. NF2
C. Tuberous sclerosis complex
D. Ehlers-Danlos syndrome
E. Osler-Weber-Rendu syndrome
F. Sturge-Weber syndrome
G. Ataxia telangiectasia

Question 69-3:
Progressive ataxia with hypersensitivity to ionizing radiation.

Question 69-4:
Child with hemiparesis, focal and generalized seizures, and an erythematous skin lesion.

Question 69-5:
Café-au-lait lesions in a patient with optic glioma.

Question 69-6:
Cutaneous hyperelasticity.

Question 69-7:
Which of the following clinical features is least likely in a patient with Fabry's disease?

A. Painful dysesthesias of the limbs
B. Stroke in childhood as the presenting symptom
C. X-linked inheritance
D. Corneal opacity

Questions 69-8 through 69-10:
The following statements all concern neurocutaneous syndromes. For each statement, select whether the statement is true or false.

Question 69-8:
Von Hippel-Lindau syndrome causes retinal and cerebral hemangioblastomas.

Question 69-9:
Neurologic complications of xeroderma pigmentosum consist of progressive dementia, hearing loss, and motor system abnormalities.

Question 69-10:
Epidermal nevus syndrome produces most of its neurologic complications by a markedly increased frequency of primary CNS tumors.

Answer 69-1: A.
The shagreen patch is found on only 20-30% of adult patients with TSC and is found on an even smaller number of children with the disorder. Cognitive abnormalities are common in TSC, although not as prevalent as previously thought. (p1667)

Answer 69-2: C.
Patients with NF2 will have fewer skin lesions than patients with the other listed disorders. These patients present with intracranial lesions. The typical lesions of NF1, including café-au-lait spots, Lisch nodules, and subcutaneous neurofibromas, are not commonly seen. (p1674)

Answer 69-3: G.
Ataxia telangiectasia results in progressive ataxia along with typical skin lesions on the sclerae, earlobes, and bridge of the nose. Patients have immunodeficiency and heightened sensitivity to ionizing radiation. (p1685)

Answer 69-4: F.
This is a classic presentation of Sturge-Weber syndrome. Not all patients with the cutaneous lesions have intracranial lesions, but when focal findings are present, intracranial complications are suspected. Focal deficit is more likely with this disorder than the other disorders. (p1683)

Answer 69-5: A.
NF1 is the most likely diagnosis in a patient with café au lait spots and optic glioma. Diagnostic criteria would be met with just these two findings. (p1675)

Answer 69-6: D.
Ehlers-Danlos syndrome is associated with cutaneous hyperelasticity and may be associated with arterial dissection or aneurysm formation. Occasionally patients may develop peripheral neuropathy. (p1675)

Answer 69-7: B.
Fabry's disease is due to an X-linked deficiency of alpha-galactosidase A. Patients often present with symptoms of peripheral neuropathic involvement but later develop a propensity to cerebral arterial thrombosis and hemorrhage. Stroke may occur in youth but is rare. (p1680)

Answer 69-8: True.
VHL causes these vascular abnormalities plus visceral cysts and tumors. While hemangioblastomas may occur sporadically, the multiple occurrence suggests VHL. (p1694)

Answer 69-9: True.
XP and associated disorders typically produce dementia, ataxia, and tremor as well as hearing loss. The most clinically obvious features are non-neurologic, e.g., the skin changes which are due to UV exposure. (p1698)

Answer 69-10: False.
Epidermal nevus syndrome produces skin lesions; a majority of patients have some neurologic manifestations. Common deficits are cognitive changes and seizures, among others. An increased frequency of some gliomas is possible, but this is not a prominent part of the neurologic manifestations of the disease. (p1691)

Chapter 70: The Dementias

Questions 70-1 through 70-5:
The following questions concern the differentiation between cortical and subcortical dementias. For the questions, select the clinical association from the following list.

A. Cortical dementia
B. Subcortical dementia
C. Both
D. Neither

Question 70-1:
Progressive supranuclear palsy.

Question 70-2:
Vascular dementia.

Question 70-3:
Alzheimer's disease.

Question 70-4:
Apraxia is a common feature.

Question 70-5:
Psychomotor slowing.

Question 70-6:
EEG findings are occasionally helpful in the diagnosis of dementia. Which of the following statements regarding EEG in dementia are true?

1. EEG in Creutzfeldt-Jakob disease shows periodic complexes which suggest but do not make the diagnosis.
2. A normal EEG indicates pseudodementia rather than organic dementia.
3. The most common EEG finding in Alzheimer's disease is background slowing.
4. The most common EEG finding in vascular dementia is frontal intermittent rhythmic delta activity (FIRDA).

Select: A = 1, 2, 3. B = 1, 3. C = 2, 4. D = 4 only. E = All

Answer 70-1: B.
PSP is a prototypic subcortical dementia. (p1701)

Answer 70-2: C.
Vascular dementia can produce both cortical and subcortical findings. Sustained hypertension and diabetes typically result in multiple small-vessel infarcts which give a predominance of subcortical lesions. In contrast, atrial fibrillation may produce numerous small-cortical infarcts from showers of microemboli. (p1701)

Answer 70-3: A.
Alzheimer's disease is a prototypic cortical dementia. There can be some subcortical damage as well, but this is very small compared to the magnitude of cortical damage with Alzheimer's disease. (p1701)

Answer 70-4: A.
Cortical dementias are expected to produce apraxia and other cortical signs rather than subcortical dementias. (p1701)

Answer 70-5: B.
Psychomotor slowing is typical with subcortical dementias rather than cortical dementias, especially early in the course. (p1701)

Answer 70-6: B.
EEG is helpful if abnormal but is not as helpful if normal, since some patients with early degenerative dementias will have normal examinations. The most common finding in dementia is slowing of the background. While vascular dementia may produce subcortical damage to a degree sufficient to produce FIRDA, this is not expected. (p1701)

Chapter 70A: The Dementias: Primary Degenerative Dementia

Question 70A-1:
Which of the following statements are true regarding familial Alzheimer's disease?

1. Mutation on chromosome 14 is the most common defect causing early-onset AD.
2. Familial AD and sporadic AD cannot be differentiated on the basis of clinical features.
3. The defect is in the presenilin I gene.
4. Late-onset AD is often associated with inheritance of the apolipoprotein E4 alleles.

Select: A = 1, 2, 3. B = 1, 3. C = 2, 4. D = 4 only. E = All

Question 70A-2:
Which of the following statements are true regarding imaging in patients with Alzheimer's disease?

1. Virtually all patients with dementia should have some sort of imaging procedure performed.
2. Atrophy of the medial temporal lobe and adjacent structures is the most characteristic finding on MRI.
3. PET shows temporoparietal hypometabolism in the absence of MRI abnormalities in the area.
4. A normal PET indicates that AD or vascular dementia is not present.

Select: A = 1, 2, 3. B = 1, 3. C = 2, 4. D = 4 only. E = All

Question 70A-3:
Clinical findings in AD typically include memory and other cognitive deficits with a paucity of focal signs. Which one of the following features would strongly suggest an alternative diagnosis?

A. Seizures
B. Rigidity with passive limb movement
C. Hallucinations
D. Personality change
E. None of these would indicate an alternative diagnosis

Question 70A-4:
Which of the following statements regarding pathological changes in Alzheimer's disease are true?

1. Neurofibrillary tangles are found in other dementing illnesses.
2. The number of neuritic plaques and neurofibrillary tangles correlates with severity of disease.
3. Loss of synapses is a better correlate to severity of disease than other pathological findings.
4. Spongiform changes may develop in some patients with AD.

Select: A = 1, 2, 3. B = 1, 3. C = 2, 4. D = 4 only. E = All

Question 70A-5:
Which of the following are major risk factors for developing Alzheimer's disease?

1. Family history
2. Lack of education
3. Age
4. Not smoking

Select: A = 1, 2, 3. B = 1, 3. C = 2, 4. D = 4 only. E = All

Question 70A-6:
Which of the following agents is not a symptomatic treatment for patients with Alzheimer's disease?

A. Tacrine
B. Selegiline
C. Rivastigmine
D. Donepezil

Answer 70A-1: E.
All of these statements are thought to be true. Inheritance of the E4 allele increases the odds of developing AD, but not all patients with E4 alleles will develop AD and not all patients with AD have one or both E4 alleles. (p1706)

Answer 70A-2: A.
PET is a sensitive functional imaging tool, but even it is not 100% sensitive. There are well-documented cases of AD with normal PET scans. The other statements are true. (p1707)

Answer 70A-3: E.
All of these are findings which can be encountered in otherwise typical AD. Seizures occur in approximately 10-20% of patients. Rigidity suggestive of parkinsonism or frontal lobe dysfunction may develop in half. Hallucinations and delusions may develop in 30%, and personality change develops in the majority of patients. (p1705)

Answer 70A-4: E.
All of these are correct. Neurofibrillary tangles can be seen in other dementing conditions including prion diseases and dementia pugilistica. Spongiform changes may suggest prion diseases but can be seen in some patients with AD, although the appearance is different than that seen in Creutzfeldt-Jakob disease. (p1709)

Answer 70A-5: B.
Family history confers significant risk of AD with APO-E4 typing and other genetic predispositions. Age is also a major risk factor, with the risk continuing to increase with age. Education has only a minor protective effect. Smoking was initially thought to be protective, but this relationship is in doubt. (p1711)

Answer 70A-6: B.
Selegiline is a MAO-inhibitor which was developed for treatment of Parkinson's disease but which is felt to have a small protectant effect for both Parkinson's disease and Alzheimer's disease. The other agents are acetylcholinesterase inhibitors. Tacrine was the first released in the US. Donepezil and rivastigmine are newer agents which have a lower frequency of adverse effects. (p1712)

Question 70A-7:
Down syndrome is associated with an increased frequency of developing progressive dementia in adult life. Which of the following statements regarding the association between Down syndrome and Alzheimer's-like dementia are true?

1. Neuritic plaques and neurofibrillary tangles are seen in patients with dementia with Down syndrome.
2. Patients have altered expression of the APP gene.
3. Patients with Down syndrome have dementia rates of up to 75% at age 60.
4. The neurotransmitter deficit differs from AD in that there is a serotonin deficit rather than a cholinergic deficit.

Select: A = 1, 2, 3. B = 1, 3. C = 2, 4. D = 4 only. E = All

Question 70A-8:
A 72-year-old man with memory loss is found on examination to have stooped posture, increased tone of appendicular muscles, postural instability, and positive glabellar reflex. He has had some occasionally visual hallucinations. All of the following would be true except which statement?

A. He exhibits hypersensitivity to the extrapyramidal effects of some neuroleptics.
B. Response of the cognitive deficit to donepezil would not be expected.
C. Delusions are likely even with a mild cognitive deficit.
D. He shows prominent fluctuations in functional status.

Question 70A-9:
Pick's disease is characterized by dementia which can resemble AD. Which one of the following statements regarding Pick's disease is not true?

A. EEG changes are more prominent than in AD.
B. A serotonin receptor deficit is prominent.
C. Personality changes are prominent early in the course of the disease.
D. There is loss of muscarinic cholinergic receptors.

Answer 70A-7: A.
There is a substantial cholinergic deficit with dementia associated with AD and Down syndrome. Serotonin receptor dysfunction is more associated with Pick's disease than AD or Down syndrome. (p1713)

Answer 70A-8: B.
This patient has typical features of dementia with Lewy bodies. All of the statements are true except the poor expectation of response to donepezil, an acetylcholinesterase inhibitor. The magnitude of cholinergic deficit in dementia with Lewy bodies is even greater than in AD. The early onset of hallucinations and delusions is a helpful feature for diagnosis of this disorder. (p1713)

Answer 70A-9: A.
EEG changes are usually less prominent than in AD, although this discrepancy is not sufficient to be a diagnostic test. The other statements are true. The personality changes may appear to be premorbid with disorders of impulse control and loss of some social inhibitions before cognitive changes develop. (p1715)

Chapter 70B: The Dementias: Dementia as Part of Other Degenerative Diseases

Question 70B-1:
Which of the statements regarding cognitive changes in ALS is true?

A. Family history of ALS makes cognitive changes more likely.
B. Patients develop a frontal dementia.
C. 2-3% of patients with ALS have a dementia.
D. All of these are true.

Question 70B-2:
Which of the following statements about dementia in Huntington's disease are true?

1. Huntington's disease produces a cortical dementia.
2. Language is affected early in the disease.
3. Memory deficit is more severe than in Alzheimer's disease
4. Behavioral disturbance and affective disturbance are prominent early in the course of the disease.

Select: A = 1, 2, 3. B = 1, 3. C = 2, 4. D = 4 only. E = All

Question 70B-3:
What is the approximate frequency of dementia in patients with Parkinson's disease?

A. 5-10%
B. 15-20%
C. 50%
D. 70%

Question 70B-4:
Which of the following statements are true regarding dementia in progressive supranuclear palsy?

1. Dementia may precede the parkinsonian features.
2. The dementia is subcortical.
3. There are commonly frontal lobe signs.
4. PET typically shows biparietal hypometabolism.

Select: A = 1, 2, 3. B = 1, 3. C = 2, 4. D = 4 only. E = All

Answer 70B-1: D.
All of these statements are true. The correlation between ALS and dementia is not great. Some patients with ALS will have subtle cognitive changes, even in the absence of dementia. (p1720)

Answer 70B-2: D.
Huntington's disease is a subcortical dementia, although some cortical changes can be seen. Language content is not often affected early in patients with cortical dementia. Memory deficit is not affected as early in the course as in Alzheimer's disease. However, behavioral and affective changes are common early in Huntington's disease. (p1720)

Answer 70B-3: B.
Approximately 15-20% of patients with Parkinson's disease have dementia; however, a greater proportion exhibit at least some mild cognitive difficulty. (p1719)

Answer 70B-4: A.
Dementia may precede the parkinsonian features of PSP, which makes the diagnosis of PSP initially elusive. PSP is a typical subcortical dementia with common frontal lobe findings including frontal release signs. PET shows hypometabolism frontally rather than in the parietal region. (p1719)

Chapter 70C: The Dementias: Vascular Dementia

Questions 70C-1 through 70C-5:
The following questions relate to vascular dementia. For each of the vignettes, select the most likely disorder from the following list.

A. Multi-infarct dementia
B. Subcortical arteriosclerotic encephalopathy
C. Cognitive changes after a single stroke
D. Any of these
E. None of these

Question 70C-1:
A 78-year-old man presents with mental status changes with apathy and psychomotor slowing. Examination shows clumsiness and slurred speech. MRI shows extensive white matter changes.

Question 70C-2:
A 46-year-old female presents with confusion, bilateral leg weakness, and diplopia. She has a remote history of transient loss of vision in one eye which resolved after several days. No other medical problems or risk factors for atherosclerotic disease.

Question 70C-3:
A 78-year-old man presents with stroke resulting in left hemiparesis and neglect along with short-term memory loss. Six months later, he is found to have no more neglect but continues to have memory loss associated with some depression.

Question 70C-4:
A 70-year-old female presents with progressive dementia. Previously, she had known small cerebral infarctions and TIAs.

Question 70C-5:
A 56-year-old man presents with sudden onset of leg weakness and impaired bladder control associated with apathy and short-term memory loss. Past history is remarkable for hypertension and diabetes mellitus.

Question 70C-6:
Dementia is common in patients with stroke, but not universal. Which of the following statements are true regarding the differentiation between patients with dementia and those without?

1. Patients with dementia are more likely to have dominant hemisphere lesions than patients without dementia.
2. Patients with dementia are more likely to have bihemispheric damage than patients without dementia.
3. Increased ventricular size is a risk factor for dementia in patients with a history of stroke.
4. MCA infarcts are more likely than other large cerebral vessels to be associated with memory loss.

Select: A = 1, 2, 3. B = 1, 3. C = 2, 4. D = 4 only. E = All

Question 70C-7:
Which of the following statements regarding imaging in vascular dementia are true?

1. MRI cannot distinguish between demyelinating disease and leukoaraiosis.
2. Virtually all patients with white matter changes suggestive of leukoaraiosis have memory loss.
3. PCA infarcts are more likely to be associated with memory change than are MCA infarcts.
4. Extensive white matter changes are suggestive of atrial fibrillation and proximal emboli.

Select: A = 1, 2, 3. B = 1, 3. C = 2, 4. D = 4 only. E = All

Answer 70C-1: B.

SAE (Binswanger's disease) presents with multiple mental status changes often with motor abnormalities. MRI findings are suggestive but not diagnostic. (p1723)

Answer 70C-2: E.

This history suggests MS rather than vascular disease. The remote history of monocular visual loss despite youth and absence of vascular risk factors and the duration of previous visual loss would be unusual for vascular causes. (p1723)

Answer 70C-3: C.

Cognitive changes after a single stroke differ depending on the location of the lesion. Right hemisphere lesions due to MCA infarctions commonly produce left hemiparesis and neglect, of course, but can also produce deficit in short-term memory and depression. These latter findings do not always improve along with the motor symptoms and may require antidepressant medication. (p1723)

Answer 70C-4: A.

The progression of dementia in a patient with known CVAs and TIAs is strongly suggestive of multi-infarct dementia; however, this clinical diagnosis cannot be so secure that other potential causes can be ignored. Also, vascular disease may predispose to a degenerative dementia, which may be difficult to diagnose in the setting of extensive cerebrovascular disease. (p1723)

Answer 70C-5: C.

The presentation of leg weakness and urinary dyscontrol suggests a myelopathy, but a medial frontal lesion can produce these symptoms along with the memory loss and apathy. Anterior cerebral artery infarction can produce all of these findings. (p1723)

Answer 70C-6: A.

MCA infarcts may produce memory loss, but they are less likely to do so than PCA and ACA infarcts. The rest of the statements are true. (p1725)

Answer 70C-7: B.

MRI is sensitive but cannot distinguish between demyelinating and vascular disease. Patients with memory loss and stroke are more likely to have anterior and posterior cerebral artery damage than patients with middle cerebral artery infarcts, although at least some mild memory loss can develop in any of these. Not all patients with the imaging findings of leukoaraiosis have dementia. Atrial fibrillation is more likely to produce multiple cortical infarctions than subcortical infarctions. (p1726)

Question 70C-8:
Which of the following statements are true regarding leukoaraiosis?

1. The pathophysiological changes involve the arterioles.
2. The most important risk factors for dementia in stroke are hypertension and stroke.
3. Most patients with dementia and stroke have a history of previous CVA and/or TIA.
4. Some patients with dementia following strokes have pathological changes which suggest Alzheimer's disease.

Select: A = 1, 2, 3. B = 1, 3. C = 2, 4. D = 4 only. E = All

Question 70C-9:
A 72-year-old man with dementia and ataxia has an evaluation which shows ventricular dilatation out of proportion to cortical atrophy, suggestive of normal pressure hydrocephalus. Radionucleotide cisternography shows reflux of tracer into the lateral ventricles. MRI not only shows the ventricular dilatation but also shows some white matter changes. The patient also has hypertension and hyperlipidemia. Which would be the most appropriate clinical formulation?

A. Ventriculoperitoneal shunt should be placed for NPH and the vascular disease will have to be treated with management of hypertension and hypercholesterolemia and use of antiplatelet agents.
B. Treat the vascular disease as in choice A, but shunt should be avoided since, in the presence of vascular disease, it is unlikely to be of long-term benefit.
C. Treat the vascular disease as in choice A, and if there is no improvement within 2-3 months, proceed to shunt placement.

Answer 70C-8: E.
All of these statements are true. The overlap between vascular dementia and degenerative dementias is controversial, but general thought is that vascular disease may induce the degenerative cascade. (p1725)

Answer 70C-9: B.
The diagnosis of NPH is made by ventricular dilatation out of proportion to cortical atrophy plus the reflux of tracer into the lateral ventricles on radionucleotide cisternography. Some white matter disease is present in most patients at this age, but its presence should not preclude offering shunt. However, in the presence of extensive white matter change, the response to shunt is typically disappointing. (p1728)

Chapter 70D: The Dementias: Progressive Focal Cortical Syndromes

Question 70D-1:
Which of the following behavioral disturbances are prominent in fronto-temporal dementia?

1. Disinhibited
2. Apathetic
3. Premorbid personality change
4. Increased affection for sweets

Select: A = 1, 2, 3. B = 1, 3. C = 2, 4. D = 4 only. E = All

Question 70D-2:
Progressive non-fluent aphasia is associated with which of the following clinical features?

1. Memory is relatively preserved
2. Absence of focal motor signs
3. Spongiform changes most prominent in the left anterior temporal, frontal, and frontoparietal regions
4. Poor reception and expression but preserved repetition

Select: A = 1, 2, 3. B = 1, 3. C = 2, 4. D = 4 only. E = All

Question 70D-3:
Which statement best describes the relationship between Alzheimer's disease and the focal cortical degeneration syndromes?

A. AD is a diffuse process, although with a predilection for certain regions, while the focal syndromes are isolated degenerations with eventual extension of involvement. They are pathophysiologically distinct.
B. AD and focal syndromes are on a continuum of degenerative processes with focal predilection but with extensive spread of degeneration.
C. Focal cortical degenerations are clinically distinct from AD.

Answer 70D-1: E.
All of these are behavioral changes which can occur in patients with FTD. The premorbid personality change with inappropriate comments and gestures may precede the dementia for years. (p1732)

Answer 70D-2: B.
Memory is preserved, although testing can be difficult because of the impaired language function. Focal motor signs can develop including rigidity, tremor, and akinesia affecting predominantly the right arm and leg. Language reception and expression are certainly affected, but repetition is severely affected. Spongiform changes are seen in the mentioned areas. (p1733)

Answer 70D-3: B.
There are pathophysiological similarities between the neurodegenerative diseases, especially the degenerative dementias and focal cortical degenerative syndromes. All of these begin with seemingly selective destruction of a certain group of neurons but then develop extension of the degeneration with more symptoms. (p1734)

Chapter 70E: The Dementias: Other Causes of Dementias

Question 70E-1:
Which of the following features would be unexpected in a patient with suspected HIV dementia?

A. There are no other clinical features of HIV infection.
B. CSF shows oligoclonal bands.
C. MRI shows prominent white matter changes.
D. Pathological changes include prominent degeneration of cortical gray and subcortical white matter.

Questions 70E-2 and 70E-3:
The following two questions are linked. Consider them together, but answer them in order.

Question 70E-2:
A 56-year-old man with dementia has no focal findings on examination. Head CT shows mild atrophy but no other findings. Laboratory studies are normal except for positive serum RPR at a low titer. Which of the following is the most likely diagnosis?

A. Neurosyphilis
B. Alzheimer's disease
C. Parkinson's-dementia complex
D. HIV dementia

Question 70E-3:
The same patient was lost to follow-up for 6 months, at which time he returned, now with advancing dementia, hypertonia, tremor, and dysarthria. MRI shows atrophy plus areas of increased signal intensity on T2-weighted images in the white matter. RPR is positive. CSF shows increased protein and mononuclear pleocytosis with a positive VDRL. Which is the most likely diagnosis?

A. Neurosyphilis
B. Alzheimer's disease
C. Parkinson's-dementia complex
D. HIV dementia

Question 70E-4:
Which of the following can produce dementia in adults?

A. Neuronal ceroid lipofuscinosis
B. Adrenoleukodystrophy
C. Mitochondrial encephalopathy
D. Wilson's disease
E. All of these

Question 70E-5:
A 36-year-old man with malignant glioma infiltrating the white matter of the left occipital region is treated with radiation chemotherapy and radiation therapy. He had a good initial response, but 18 months later he returns for evaluation of progressive cognitive decline. Which of the following should be considered in the differential diagnosis?

1. Infiltrating tumor of the white matter
2. Hydrocephalus
3. Radiation necrosis
4. Paraneoplastic encephalopathy

Select: A = 1, 2, 3. B = 1, 3. C = 2, 4. D = 4 only. E = All

Answer 70E-1: D.
Pathological changes in HIV dementia include degeneration of subcortical gray and white matter, but the cerebral cortex is relatively preserved. The remainder of the statements are true. (p1739)

Answer 70E-2: B.
With the information presented, the most likely diagnosis is AD. The positive RPR deserves further evaluation, but neurosyphilis as a cause of uncomplicated dementia is uncommon. (p1740)

Answer 70E-3: A.
This latter information suggests neurosyphilis, even though the initial presentation of dementia is not the most common finding. The extrapyramidal findings might have suggested a Parkinson's-dementia complex, although the CSF findings would be inconsistent with this. (p1740)

Answer 70E-4: E.
All of these can produce dementia in adults, although most will usually have other neurologic signs. In all, early cognitive changes may precede obvious neurologic deficit. Neuronal ceroid lipofuscinosis, Wilson's disease, and adrenoleukodystrophy are associated with prominent motor findings, while mitochondrial encephalopathies may be associated with stroke-like episodes or neuromuscular abnormalities. (p1741)

Answer 70E-5: A.
Paraneoplastic encephalopathy is not expected with primary gliomas but rather mainly with lung and breast cancer. (p1741)

Question 70E-6:
A 49-year-old man develops prominent dementia over a 6-month period. MRI shows prominent atrophy. There is a history of heavy ethanol consumption. LFTs are mildly elevated. Which is the most likely diagnosis?

A. Wernicke's encephalopathy
B. Korsakoff's syndrome
C. Alcoholic dementia
D. Lead intoxication

Question 70E-7:
A 64-year-old woman presents for evaluation of memory loss. She has an MMSE of 20. Examination reveals poor concentration and flat affect. Upon further questioning, she admits to hypersomnia and crying spells and loss of interest in her previous hobbies. Which is the most appropriate clinical formulation?

A. The patient shows signs of depression and dementia. Neuropsychological testing should be performed to determine whether the patient has pseudodementia or an organic dementia complicated by depression.
B. The patient's apparent cognitive difficulties are due to depression, so antidepressant medication and counseling are required.
C. The patient has dementia plus depression. The patient should be treated with donepezil or other symptomatic agent to determine whether both cognitive difficulty and affective disturbance will improve.

Answer 70E-6: C.
Alcoholic dementia is the most likely diagnosis. Korsakoff's syndrome is characterized by memory difficulty out of proportion to other cognitive deficits. Wernicke's encephalopathy is a more acute syndrome usually with other neurologic findings such as oculomotor defect. Lead intoxication has to be considered in alcoholic patients with dementia; however, this is now rare and would be also associated with other findings in most individuals. (p1742)

Answer 70E-7: A.
Depression is part of many dementing disorders, and in most instances is not a reaction to the diagnosis, but rather part of the chemical abnormality. In patients with AD, behavioral and affective symptoms may improve with administration of donepezil or other related symptomatic agent, but since this is rarely a completely effective treatment, management of the depression with an antidepressant is often necessary. (p1743)

Chapter 71: The Epilepsies

Question 71-1:
The incidence of epilepsy is greatest in which of the following age groups?

A. 0-15 years
B. 15-30 years
C. 30-50 years
D. over 50 years

Question 71-2:
Which of the following seizure types has the best prognosis?

A. Juvenile myoclonic epilepsy (JME)
B. Rolandic epilepsy
C. Complex partial seizures
D. Infantile spasms

Questions 71-3 through 71-5:
The following questions concern identification of seizure types which can be easily confused; prominent convulsive activity is not seen in these entities. For each of the following questions, select the most likely diagnosis from the following list.

A. Complex partial seizures of frontal origin
B. Complex partial seizures of temporal origin
C. Absence seizures
D. Non-epileptic episodes

Question 71-3:
A 50-year-old man has episodes of unresponsiveness which are preceded by olfactory hallucinations. He has prominent lip smacking during the episode. After the episode, he has lost the thread of the previous conversation.

Question 71-4:
An 18-year-old woman has episodes of unresponsiveness along with lip smacking. She otherwise has a blank stare during the episodes. She returns to normal conversation after the episodes.

Question 71-5:
A 51-year-old woman presents with very brief episodes of unresponsiveness with complex motor automatisms. The patients is confused after the episode, but quickly recovers.

Question 71-6:
Which statements regarding routine EEG in epilepsy are true?

1. EEG is more likely to show a defined focus in complex partial seizures of frontal origin than of temporal origin.
2. EEG during aura of a partial seizure may show attenuation.
3. Normal EEG during an apparent partial seizure indicates non-epileptic event (pseudoseizure).
4. Interictal EEG may be normal in up to 50% of patients with seizures.

Select: A = 1, 2, 3. B = 1, 3. C = 2, 4. D = 4 only. E = All

Question 71-7:
An 8-year-old female develops seizures characterized by left focal clonic activity. They initially respond to anticonvulsants, but the response wanes over 6-7 months. She subsequently develops progressively decreased use of the left arm. Which of the following should be considered in the differential diagnosis?

1. Rolandic epilepsy
2. Rasmussen's encephalitis
3. Herpes encephalitis
4. Brain tumor

Select: A = 1, 2, 3. B = 1, 3. C = 2, 4. D = 4 only. E = All

Answer 71-1: A.
The greatest incidence of epilepsy is in children less than 15 years of age, and many of those develop seizures at less than 1 year of age. The incidence of epilepsy declines through adult life then increases again in older patients greater than 60 years of age. (p1746)

Answer 71-2: B.
Rolandic epilepsy is one of the benign focal epilepsies of childhood and has a very favorable outcome. Many patients do not have to be treated with anticonvulsants since the seizures are limited in clinical features, frequency, and nocturnal pattern. (p1749)

Answer 71-3: B.
Complex partial seizures of temporal origin can produce this presentation. The olfactory hallucinations can also occur with a frontal focus. (p1750)

Answer 71-4: C.
This is a typical history of absence epilepsy. Some patients will have lip smacking, but the complex motor automatisms seen in some partial seizures are not seen. (p1750)

Answer 71-5: A.
This is a typical history of complex partial seizures of frontal origin The onset is abrupt, the duration short, and the post-ictal period is brief. (p1750)

Answer 71-6: C.
A defined focus is more likely to be identified on routine EEG monitoring with temporal than frontal seizure origins. Some patients with especially complex partial epilepsy may have no discharges evident on routine surface EEG. The other statements are true. (p1751)

Answer 71-7: C.
Rasmussen's encephalitis is characterized by focal seizures followed by loss of extremity use. With time, the seizures and neurologic deficit extend and become bilateral. Infiltrating neoplasm would be the main differential diagnosis. Herpes encephalitis would be expected to develop acutely. Rolandic epilepsy would not produce neurologic deficit. (p1752)

Question 71-8:
Which of the following characteristics of atypical absence seizures differentiates this condition from absence epilepsy?

1. Abnormal EEG background
2. Cognitive deficit
3. Loss of postural tone
4. Occurrence of generalized tonic-clonic seizures in the same patient

Select: A = 1, 2, 3. B = 1, 3. C = 2, 4. D = 4 only. E = All

Question 71-9:
Which one of the following features would make the diagnosis of febrile seizure in doubt?

A. Focal onset of the seizure
B. Duration of 20 minutes
C. No family history of febrile seizures
D. Patient age of 13 years

Question 71-10:
A 13-year-old female presents with generalized tonic-clonic seizures. Additional history reveals that she has had irregular jerks of the arms upon awakening. Her father has epilepsy. Examination is normal. EEG shows bilateral poly-spike and wave complexes at a frequency of 3-4 Hz with a frontal predominance. Which is the most likely diagnosis?

A. Rolandic epilepsy
B. West syndrome
C. Juvenile myoclonic epilepsy
D. Batten's disease
E. None of these

Question 71-11:
An 8-year-old boy presents with acquired aphasia and seizures and is diagnosed with the Landau-Kleffner syndrome. Which of the following features would be expected with this diagnosis?

A. Partial and generalized seizures
B. Myoclonus
C. Word deafness
D. EEG shows multifocal spike-and-wave discharges.
E. All of the above may occur.

Question 71-12:
Which of the following statements are true regarding post-traumatic epilepsy?

1. Post-traumatic epilepsy is more common with depressed skull fractures than closed head injuries.
2. Prophylactic phenytoin decreases the chance of late-onset post-traumatic seizures.
3. Subdural hematoma predisposes to development of post-traumatic seizures.
4. Children are less likely to develop early post-traumatic epilepsy than adults.

Select: A = 1, 2, 3. B = 1, 3. C = 2, 4. D = 4 only. E = All

Question 71-13:
Which of the following statements are true regarding psychogenic seizures?

1. No specific motor activity is expressly diagnostic of psychogenic seizures.
2. Normal prolactin level after a generalized tonic-clonic seizure excludes the diagnosis of epilepsy.
3. Generalized tonic-clonic activity without change in electrocerebral activity on EEG makes the diagnosis of psychogenic seizure.
4. Documentation of a psychogenic seizure on monitoring should cause anticonvulsants to be withdrawn.

Select: A = 1, 2, 3. B = 1, 3. C = 2, 4. D = 4 only. E = All

Question 71-14:
Which of the following statements are true regarding anticonvulsants in pregnancy?

1. Total levels of phenytoin are decreased.
2. Free levels of valproate increase.
3. Free levels of phenobarbital decrease.
4. Free fraction of phenytoin is decreased.

Select: A = 1, 2, 3. B = 1, 3. C = 2, 4. D = 4 only. E = All

Answer 71-8: A.

Atypical absence seizures are associated with other types of seizures including generalized tonic-clonic, myoclonic, and atonic seizures. However, the co-occurrence of generalized tonic-clonic seizures is not a differentiating feature alone, since these can occur in otherwise typical absence epilepsy. (p1754)

Answer 71-9: D.

Febrile seizures are usually brief and generalized, although they can be focal and can occasionally have a duration in excess of 15 minutes. The occurrence of two or more atypical features in the same patient would make the diagnosis of febrile seizures unlikely. Many patients with febrile seizures have no relevant family history. However, most patients with febrile seizures are under 5 years of age, and onset after age 10 is not expected and warrants careful search for other cause. (p1755)

Answer 71-10: C.

This is a typical presentation of JME. Rolandic epilepsy would not have the myoclonus or the EEG findings. West syndrome presents in younger children with infantile spasms plus other findings. Batten's disease, neuronal ceroid lipofuscinosis, would be expected to have other neurologic and ophthalmological findings. (p1757)

Answer 71-11: E.

These are all features of the Landau-Kleffner syndrome. The EEG may alternatively show bilateral centrotemporal spikes. (p1758)

Answer 71-12: B.

Prophylactic phenytoin decreases the chance of early post-traumatic seizures but not late seizures, so long term prophylaxis is seldom indicated. Children are more likely than adults to have early post-traumatic seizures. (p1761)

Answer 71-13: B.

Not all seizures are followed by an elevation in prolactin level, even when the seizure was generalized tonic-clonic. Many patients with psychogenic seizures also have epileptic seizures, so anticonvulsants should only be withdrawn if there is good evidence that all of the patient's episodes are non-epileptic. (p1763)

Answer 71-14: A.

The free fraction of phenytoin is increased, which is why the total level is decreased; there is a greater fraction available for metabolism. The other statements are true. Free levels of valproate increase because of the decrease in protein binding. Phenobarbital is the only one of the first generation anticonvulsants to show a reduction in free drug during pregnancy. (p1764)

Question 71-15:
Fetal complications of epilepsy are a matter of grave concern to women with epilepsy and their physicians. Which one of the following statements is not true regarding fetal malformations and complications in epileptic women?

A. The risk of congenital malformations is increased in children of women with epilepsy even in the absence of exposure to anticonvulsant drugs.
B. Polytherapy and high levels of anticonvulsants are thought to play a role in increasing the risk for congenital malformations.
C. Folate supplementation reduces the risk of neural tube defects in mothers with epilepsy on anticonvulsants.
D. Fetal exposure to anticonvulsants is an independent risk factor for later development of mental retardation.

Question 71-16:
Which of the following statements is true regarding positron emission tomography (PET) findings in patients with partial epilepsies?

A. Interictal imaging is most likely to show areas of hypometabolism.
B. Interictal imaging is most likely to show no abnormality.
C. PET shows essentially the same data as SPECT, although with lower spatial resolution.
D. Regions of hypometabolism indicate areas of structural damage and neuronal loss.
E. None of these are true.

Questions 71-17 through 71-20:
A 34-year-old woman with intractable complex partial seizures is being treated with phenytoin. The seizures are characterized by lip smacking and unresponsiveness with a brief post-ictal period. She has the seizures approximately twice per month. The seizures started when she was 22 years old, without a precipitating event. She has never had a generalized tonic-clonic seizure. For each of the following 4 questions, select the best answer.

Question 71-17:
What is the most likely finding on MRI?

A. Normal
B. Temporal lobe abnormality
C. Frontal lobe abnormality

Question 71-18:
Valproate is added and she has perfect control of the seizures for more than two years. Phenytoin is withdrawn with no recurrence of seizures. She decides she wants to get pregnant. EEG is normal. Which would be the most appropriate clinical formulation?

A. Continue the valproate.
B. Change back to phenytoin.
C. Withdraw all anticonvulsants.
D. Change to gabapentin.

Question 71-19:
The patient in Question 71-18 never does get pregnant and decides to remain on valproate since she is seizure free. At a routine follow-up visit, her laboratory studies are normal except for a valproate level of 46 ug/ml. Which is the most appropriate next step?

A. Increase the valproate dose and recheck to maintain in the therapeutic range.
B. Keep the valproate dose the same, advising her regarding compliance with the medication.
C. Give an extra dose of valproate that day and recheck the level again two weeks later without changing daily dose.

Answer 71-15: D.
Fetal exposure to anticonvulsants was once thought to be an independent risk factor for later development of mental retardation, but when other factors were considered, the risk increase evaporated. The remainder of the statements are true. (p1764)

Answer 71-16: A.
The best correlate of PET with EEG is the observation of regions of hypometabolism on the PET with seizure focus on EEG. This is best seen in patients with temporal lobe foci. (p1768)

Answer 71-17: B.
The seizures are most likely to be of temporal origin. High-resolution MRI shows abnormalities in most patients with intractable seizures of temporal lobe origin. (p1768)

Answer 71-18: C.
The patient has never had a generalized tonic-clonic seizure, has been seizure free for more than two years, and has a normal EEG, so withdrawal of the anticonvulsant is warranted. There is the possibility of returning to having complex partial seizures, at which point reintroduction of phenytoin or another anticonvulsant could be performed. If possible, the patient should be off anticonvulsants for several months before getting pregnant to determine whether complex partial or secondary generalized seizures will occur. All women contemplating pregnancy, especially those on anticonvulsants, should be advised to have folate supplementation. (p1765)

Answer 71-19: B
Therapeutic ranges are guidelines. There is nothing magic about a level of 50 ug/ml. After a patient has been seizure free for so long, she may become a little lax about taking the medication regularly, especially with valproate, which is multidosed. (p1770)

Question 71-20:
Two more years go by and the patient in the previous 3 questions has now been seizure free for 4 years. She asks about discontinuation of the valproate. EEG is still normal. How would you advise her?

A. The risk of having a seizure when she had them for 14 years makes recurrence a virtual certainty. Valproate should be continued.
B. She has a very high risk of having recurrent seizures when off the valproate, but since she has done well recently, change to a second generation anticonvulsant should be considered, which may allow her to get off the valproate with its required monitoring and risk of adverse effects.
C. The risk of recurrent seizure is high because of the long duration of focal epilepsy, but the risk is not certain. Considering that she had partial seizures without secondary generalization, discontinuation of the valproate would be warranted.

Question 71-21:
What is the drug of choice for a 16-year-old male with absence epilepsy complicated by generalized tonic-clonic seizures?

A. Ethosuximide
B. Valproate
C. Felbamate
D. Lamotrigine

Answer 71-20: C.
If she is ever to get off anticonvulsants, this is the time. It is true that the chance of staying off anticonvulsants is not certain, but it is not zero. Most of the second generation agents are approved for adjunctive therapy (in combination with another agent) rather than monotherapy, although there is reason to believe that effectiveness in monotherapy would be reasonable. (p1775)

Answer 71-21: B.
Mixed absence and generalized tonic-clonic seizures are more likely to be responsive to valproate than ethosuximide. Opinion differs on this point; in a new patient with predominantly absence epilepsy with an occasional tonic-clonic seizure, ethosuximide may be of benefit, but most of these patients will have had their absence seizures already treated with ethosuximide at the time when they then manifest the tonic-clonic seizures. (p1771)

Chapter 72: Sleep Disorders

Question 72-1:
Melatonin has been implicated in maintenance of the normal circadian rhythm. Which of the following statements are true regarding melatonin and its role in sleep?

1. Melatonin is secreted mainly at night.
2. Melatonin is synthesized from L-tryptophan.
3. Melatonin production is suppressed by exposure to bright light.
4. Melatonin is synthesized in the suprachiasmatic nucleus.

Select: A = 1, 2, 3. B = 1, 3. C = 2, 4. D = 4 only. E = All

Question 72-2:
Penile tumescence is most prominent during which phase of the sleep-wake cycle?

A. Stage II sleep
B. Slow wave (stage III and IV) sleep
C. REM sleep
D. There is no consistent prominence.

Question 72-3:
Sleep disturbance has been implicated in generation of which of the following problems?

A. Motor vehicle accidents
B. On-the-job judgment errors
C. Airplane accidents
D. Peptic ulcer disease

Select: A = 1, 2, 3. B = 1, 3. C = 2, 4. D = 4 only. E = All

Question 72-4:
A 30-year-old man presents because of excessive daytime sleepiness. He reports that he sleeps well at night, needing a loud alarm clock to awaken. During the day he has difficulty staying awake. If he is not stimulated, he will fall asleep easily, such as in seminars, as a passenger in a car, or at his desk. He has had a couple of episodes of sleep paralysis in the past. Which is the most appropriate clinical formulation?

A. He most likely has narcolepsy, with sleep attacks during the day plus episodes of sleep paralysis. The normal nocturnal sleep indicates that he is not sleep deprived.
B. He most likely has excessive daytime sleepiness without narcolepsy. The episodes of sleep paralysis are commonly seen in patients with narcolepsy but are not diagnostic. He needs evaluation for nocturnal sleep disorder and medical causes of EDS.
C. He has no sleep disorder, and most likely has an affective disorder as the cause for his change in sleep pattern.

Question 72-5:
Which of the following would be considered in the differential diagnosis of cataplectic attacks?

1. Complex partial seizures
2. Vertebrobasilar insufficiency
3. Arrhythmia
4. Periodic paralysis

Select: A = 1, 2, 3. B = 1, 3. C = 2, 4. D = 4 only. E = All

Question 72-6:
Which of the following are significant risk factors for obstructive sleep apnea syndrome?

1. Obesity
2. Large neck circumference
3. Males
4. Menopause

Select: A = 1, 2, 3. B = 1, 3. C = 2, 4. D = 4 only. E = All

Answer 72-1: A.
Melatonin is synthesized in the pineal gland. Control over melatonin synthesis is by the suprachiasmatic nucleus. The remainder of the statements are true. (p1784)

Answer 72-2: C.
Penile and clitoral tumescence is much more prominent during REM sleep than in other sleep states. (p1784)

Answer 72-3: E.
Sleep disturbance from shift work or other causes of sleep deprivation has been implicated in all of these and many more. In addition, chronic sleep deprivation may contribute to personality changes and chronic pain syndromes. (p1789)

Answer 72-4: B.
It is impossible to be certain about the diagnosis, but the clinical presentation is most typical of excessive sleepiness rather than sleep attacks. The sleep attacks of narcolepsy usually occur in inappropriate settings, such as when walking, talking, eating, sexual activity, etc. (p1792)

Answer 72-5: A.
Periodic paralysis may produce weakness to the point that the patient is immobile, but does not have the abrupt onset which would characterize cataplexy. The differential diagnosis includes seizures, particularly atonic and complex partial seizures. (p1794)

Answer 72-6: E.
All of these are significant risk factors for production of OSAS. While males are more likely than females to develop OSAS, there is an increased incidence in females who are postmenopausal. (p1797)

Question 72-7:
The most common cause of restless legs syndrome is thought to be which of the following?

A. Peripheral neuropathy
B. Parkinson's disease
C. Neuroleptic use
D. Idiopathic

Question 72-8:
Which of the following statements concerning sleep disturbance and stroke is not true?

A. Patients with obstructive sleep apnea syndrome (OSAS) have an increased incidence of stroke.
B. Patients with stroke have an increased incidence of OSAS.
C. Brainstem infarction may produce primary automatic respiration during sleep.
D. Stroke may reduce total and REM sleep.
E. All of these are true.

Questions 72-9 through 72-12:
The following questions concern sleep disturbance in medical conditions. For each, select whether the statement is true or false.

Question 72-9:
Sleep disturbance is no more common in Parkinson's disease than in normal age-matched controls.

Question 72-10:
Cluster headaches are most closely related to REM sleep.

Question 72-11:
Benign rolandic epilepsy produces discharges and clinical seizures which are most prominent in REM sleep.

Question 72-12:
Sleep deprivation increases the chance of identifying epileptiform discharges during the transition from wakefulness to light sleep.

Answer 72-7: D.
Most cases of RLS are idiopathic. Peripheral neuropathy is the most important specific disorder in the differential diagnosis, since clinical symptoms of RLS may occur superimposed on typical signs and symptoms of peripheral neuropathy. Neuroleptic use may give akathisia, or a type of motor restlessness, but this is not the most common cause of the presentation of RLS. Other important causes of RLS include Parkinson's disease, hypothyroidism, motor neuron diseases, iron deficiency anemia, and uremia. (p1799)

Answer 72-8: E.
All of these are true. There is a reciprocal relationship between OSAS and stroke, although at least part of this may be that they share some common risk factors, such as weight, age, and hypertension. Brainstem infarction may produce variable effects on sleep including reduced REM and total sleep in the case of some patients with locked-in syndrome. Loss of automatic respiration during sleep (Ondine's curse) develops classically with bilateral brainstem lesions below the mid-pons but can also develop in patients with unilateral infarction. (p1807)

Answer 72-9: False.
Approximately 70-90% of patients with PD have sleep disturbance, which can be due to primary effects of the disease, such as difficulty initiating sleep or sleep fragmentation, or due to secondary factors, such as depression and dementia. (p1808)

Answer 72-10: True.
Cluster headaches in sleep usually develop out of REM sleep, although they can develop out of NREM sleep. (p1805)

Answer 72-11: False.
Benign rolandic epilepsy is characterized by EEG discharges and clinical seizures which are most prominent in drowsiness and NREM sleep. (p1803)

Answer 72-12: True.
Sleep deprivation serves two functions, causing a patient to sleep who did not during routine daytime EEG testing and probably also increasing cerebral cortical excitability. This is an excellent activation method for patients with normal interictal EEGs yet with the serious clinical concern for seizures. (p1803)

Chapter 73: Headache and Other Craniofacial Pain

Question 73-1:
What is the most likely MRI finding in a patient with occipital headache which is produced and exacerbated by cough?

A. Normal
B. Chiari malformation
C. Posterior fossa mass lesion
D. Hydrocephalus

Question 73-2:
A 50-year-old man presents with onset of headache after a motor vehicle accident which is positional, much better when recumbent and exacerbated when sitting or standing. Examination is otherwise normal. MRI shows enhancement of the meninges. CSF shows 20 WBCs, all mononuclear cells, with mild increase in protein. Which is the most likely diagnosis?

A. Post-traumatic meningitis
B. Low CSF pressure
C. Subarachnoid hemorrhage

Question 73-3:
Migraine headache may be confused with more serious causes of headache involving vascular structures. Which of the following statements is not true regarding this differential diagnosis?

A. Consistent one-sided headaches strongly suggest a vascular abnormality rather than migraine headache.
B. Most aneurysms which would produce headache will be visible on MRA.
C. Acute development of headache warrants evaluation for possible subarachnoid hemorrhage.
D. LP should be preceded by CT for evaluation of possible intracranial hemorrhage.

Question 73-4:
A 42-year-old man presents with the hyperacute onset of the worst headache of his life. He describes it as a feeling of a grenade going off in his head. Emergent CT is normal. LP is also normal. Angiography shows segmental vasoconstriction. What is the most likely diagnosis?

A. Subarachnoid hemorrhage
B. Thunderclap headache
C. Migraine headache
D. Vasculitis

Question 73-5:
Which of the following statements are true regarding headache in stroke?

1. New onset of headache in an older patient may suggest an impending stroke.
2. Visual prodromes make the diagnosis of stroke unlikely, favoring migraine.
3. Visual changes in ischemia are more likely to be negative (visual loss), while visual changes in migraine are more likely to be positive.
4. Ischemic stroke is rarely associated with headache.

Select: A = 1, 2, 3. B = 1, 3. C = 2, 4. D = 4 only. E = All

Answer 73-1: A.
Although cough headache is worrisome for posterior fossa lesion or Chiari malformation, normal MRI is the most likely finding. (p1831)

Answer 73-2: B.
The patient almost certainly has a dural tear which has resulted in CSF leak. This can occur in the intracranial or intraspinal dura. The mononuclear pleocytosis in the CSF and the enhancement on MRI may suggest secondary CSF inflammation from infection or blood, but this is unlikely. (p1833)

Answer 73-3: A.
Physicians evaluating patients with consistently one-sided headache often worry about a structural abnormality or vascular anomaly, but this is rarely the case. Other features are more important in this suspicion, such as sudden onset or associated meningeal signs. Modern high-resolution MRA seldom misses clinically significant aneurysms, but if there is continued suspicion, then angiography may be warranted. LP is often needed to rule out SAH, but some patients will have intracerebral hematoma which may make LP dangerous; therefore, CT should precede LP for the vast majority of patients. (p1837)

Answer 73-4: B.
This is a typical presentation of thunderclap headache. This is certainly worrisome for SAH, but the latter would be expected to produce abnormal CSF unless the LP is done very soon after the event. Also, the segmental vasoconstriction would not be expected in SAH this early, since vasospasm does not develop this soon. (p1837)

Answer 73-5: B.
Approximately 40% of patients with ischemic stroke have headache, and the headache may precede the stroke. Visual prodromes may be present in retinal or occipital ischemia as well as with migraine. (p1839)

Questions 73-6 through 73-10:
For each of the mini-vignettes which follow, select the most likely diagnosis from the following list.

A. Cerebral infarction
B. Intraparenchymal hemorrhage
C. Subarachnoid hemorrhage
D. Carotid dissection
E. Giant cell arteritis
F. Migraine

Question 73-6:
A 40-year-old man presents with new left-sided headache without a previous history of headache. Examination is normal except for left miosis and ptosis.

Question 73-7:
A 55-year-old man presents with sudden onset of headache followed by neck pain. No focal findings. No prior events.

Question 73-8:
A 65-year-old female with severe headache in the left temporal region, but the temporal artery appears normal. She also complains of aching in the shoulders and upper arms.

Question 73-9:
A 58-year-old man develops a frontal headache with left-sided predominance associated with progressive left hemiparesis. The symptoms develop over the course of two hours.

Question 73-10:
A 50-year-old woman presents with left hemianopia associated with occipital headache and nausea. No history of previous migraines.

Question 73-11:
Which of the following clinical features would be expected in basilar migraine?

1. Loss of consciousness
2. Ataxia
3. Numbness of face, hands, and feet
4. Onset at the age of 35

Select: A = 1, 2, 3. B = 1, 3. C = 2, 4. D = 4 only. E = All

Question 73-12:
A 13-year-old female presents with severe retro-orbital headache, nausea, and vomiting. She then develops partial CN-3 headache with ptosis and external ophthalmoplegia. Which is the most likely diagnosis?

A. Intracavernous aneurysm
B. Cavernous sinus thrombosis
C. Ophthalmoplegia migraine
D. None of these

Question 73-13:
Which of the following statements most accurately represents current theories on generation of migraine aura?

A. Platelet aggregation produces a phase of vasoconstriction leading to neuronal depression followed by reactive vasodilatation producing the headache phase.
B. A wave of cortical neuronal activation is followed by a wave of neuronal depression which is related to a change in energy metabolism.
C. Synchronous cortical neuronal discharge produces a wave of neuronal inhibition which produces the aura.

Question 73-14:
Which of the following dietary components have been implicated in exacerbating migraine?

1. Monosodium glutamate
2. Nitrites
3. Tyramine
4. Caffeine

Select: A = 1, 2, 3. B = 1, 3. C = 2, 4. D = 4 only. E = All

Answer 73-6: D.
The unilateral headache with ipsilateral Horner's syndrome suggests carotid dissection. (p1839)

Answer 73-7: C.
The prototypic presentation of SAH is sudden onset of headache with meningeal signs. The onset at the age of 55 years would argue against this being simple migraine. (p1837)

Answer 73-8: E.
Giant cell arteritis typically presents with temporal headache, and the vast majority have elevated sedimentation rate. Not all patients have temporal artery tenderness, however. Systemic symptoms such as proximal muscle pain, joint pain, and morning stiffness comprise the syndrome of polymyalgia rheumatica. (p1841)

Answer 73-9: B.
The progressive hemiparesis at the time of the progressive headache is most suggestive of intraparenchymal hemorrhage. One would expect that the headache should localize over the side of the affected hemisphere, but poor anatomic localization is common; the side of the headache does not always predict the side of pathology. (p1839)

Answer 73-10: A.
She is most likely to have had an occipital infarction. The development of vascular migraine at 50 years of age is unlikely. Also, the visual changes with migraine are more likely to be positive phenomena rather than negative phenomena, although the scintillating scotomata may progress to hemianopia. (p1839)

Answer 73-11: A.
Most patients with basilar migraine will develop symptoms at youth; onset at an older age would not be expected, and a search for other causes would be undertaken. (p1849)

Answer 73-12: C.
This is a typical history of ophthalmoplegia migraine. The other diagnoses are unlikely at this age but would be considered, especially in older patients. MRI with MRA would usually be ordered in a patient with this presentation upon the first occurrence of the symptoms. (p1849)

Answer 73-13: B.
The vasoconstrictive theory of migraine aura generation was popular for years, but recent evidence indicates that the reduction in local cerebral blood flow is reactive rather than causative. A spreading depression of neuronal excitability is currently thought to be responsible for the negative component of the aura, while the preceding wave of excitation may be responsible for positive symptoms as the wave marches across the cortex. (p1851)

Answer 73-14: E.
All of these have been implicated in producing migraine. While caffeine is a component of several migraine medications and caffeine withdrawal is well known to produce migraine, caffeine may produce migraine in selected individuals and at high doses. (p1853)

Question 73-15:
The triptans have been a major advance in the treatment of migraine. What is thought to be the chemical mechanism of action of this class of agents?

A. 5-HT1B receptor block produces vasoconstriction and 5-HT1D receptor block produces inhibition of neuropeptide release.
B. 5-HT1B receptor activation produces vasoconstriction and 5-HT1D receptor activation produces inhibition of neuropeptide release.
C. 5-HT1B receptor activation produces inhibition of neuropeptide release and 5-HT1D receptor activation produces vasoconstriction.

Question 73-16:
Which of the following symptoms respond well to triptans?

1. Photophobia
2. Nausea
3. Phonophobia
4. Headache

Select: A = 1, 2, 3. B = 1, 3. C = 2, 4. D = 4 only. E = All

Question 73-17:
Which of the following classes of substances have been found to be helpful for migraine prophylaxis?

1. Calcium channel blockers
2. Serotonin antagonists
3. Beta-adrenergic blockers
4. Magnesium supplementation

Select: A = 1, 2, 3. B = 1, 3. C = 2, 4. D = 4 only. E = All

Question 73-18:
All of the following features help to differentiate cluster headache from migraine except which?

A. Duration
B. Age of onset
C. Distribution
D. Nocturnal occurrence
E. Periodicity

Question 73-19:
Which of the following medications would be least likely to help in abortive therapy of cluster headache?

A. Sumatriptan
B. Inhaled oxygen
C. Hydrocodone
D. Ergotamine

Question 73-20:
Which of the following medications would be least likely to prevent subsequent cluster headaches?

A. Ergotamine
B. Corticosteroids
C. Histamine desensitization
D. Valproate
E. Lithium

Question 73-21:
A 27-year-old female presents with intractable headache affecting the left side of the head. The headache started 3 weeks ago and has been unrelenting. Neurologic examination is normal except for ipsilateral miosis. MRI of the brain is normal. What is the most likely diagnosis?

A. Status migrainosis
B. Hemicrania continua
C. Temporal arteritis
D. Cluster status
E. None of these

Answer 73-15: B.
The triptans are agonists for both the 5-HT1B and 5-HT1D receptors, the former mediating vasoconstriction and the latter mediating inhibition of neuropeptide release from trigeminal afferents. (p1855)

Answer 73-16: E.
All of these fundamental symptoms of migraine respond to triptans, although the proportion of responders differs between symptoms, individual triptans, and individual patients. (p1856)

Answer 73-17: E.
All of these classes of agents have been found to be helpful in migraine prophylaxis. Calcium channel blockers may be more helpful for migraine with aura than common migraine. Serotonin antagonists include cyproheptadine and methysergide, which are peripheral serotonin antagonists but also have central effects which may be more complex; e.g., methysergide is a central serotonin agonist. The exact mechanism of action of these agents is uncertain. Magnesium supplementation has the least supporting evidence of the classes listed. (p1859)

Answer 73-18: C.
The periorbital distribution of cluster headache is not unique. Distribution is only helpful if the pain extends to a whole side of the head or bilaterally, in which case cluster is not the diagnosis. Duration of cluster headaches is shorter and age of onset is generally older than in patients with migraine. Migraines may occur at night, but frequent awakening from sleep is much more typical of cluster. Migraines may have waxing and waning frequency, but the brief frequent clusters interspersed by paucity or absence of headache is suggestive of cluster. (p1863)

Answer 73-19: C.
There is little or no place for hydrocodone for treatment of cluster or, for that matter, migraine. Pure analgesics seldom help because of the short duration of the headaches, and dependence and rebound headache can develop. The other agents are viable alternatives for abortive therapy. (p1866)

Answer 73-20: C.
Histamine desensitization was used years ago to prevent subsequent cluster headaches, but its use been abandoned by most specialists. There is no convincing evidence of benefit. The other agents are all helpful for some patients with cluster, but the most important omission from this list is methysergide. (p1866)

Answer 73-21: B.
Hemicrania continua is an uncommon condition which presents with continuous unilateral headache which may have few interspersed periods of relief. Because of the distribution of the headache, imaging is necessary to rule out structural abnormality. Temporal arteritis would not be expected in this age, but if suspected, ESR should be checked. Note that not all patients with giant cell arteritis have temporal artery swelling and tenderness. (p1868)

Question 73-22:

A 28-year-old man is seen in the ER for the acute onset of headache at the cranio-cervical junction and occipital region while having intercourse. The onset of the headache was quick but not explosive, but peaked at orgasm. He admits to some occasional similar headaches with and without exertion, but not of this magnitude. CT head without contrast is normal. What is the most appropriate clinical formulation?

A. He has coital headache, which is usually benign. The presence of some similar events and the normal CT are reassuring and further evaluation is not needed. He is treated with a symptomatic agent.
B. He probably has coital headache, as above, but subarachnoid hemorrhage cannot be ruled out on the basis of history and CT. LP should be performed.
C. He most likely has subarachnoid hemorrhage, and since neurological status is so good, angiography should be performed.

Question 73-23:

Which of the following statements are true regarding zoster?

1. Acyclovir prevents postherpetic neuralgia if given at the onset of the eruption.
2. Corticosteroids may reduce the frequency of postherpetic neuralgia.
3. Zoster of the geniculate ganglion has a high risk of stroke from carotid involvement.
4. Postherpetic neuralgia develops in about 10% of patients with herpes zoster ophthalmicus.

Select: A = 1, 2, 3. B = 1, 3. C = 2, 4. D = 4 only. E = All

Answer 73-22: B.
Coital headache is usually benign, but because of the possibility of subarachnoid hemorrhage, CT should be done. If the CT is normal, LP should usually be performed since not all SAH shows on CT. (p1874)

Answer 73-23: C.
Acyclovir does not prevent the development of postherpetic neuralgia but it does reduce acute pain and speeds healing of the lesions. Zoster of the geniculate ganglion does not increase the risk for stroke from carotid involvement. (p1875)

Chapter 74: Cranial Neuropathies

Question 74-1:
A 74-year-old male with a history of hypertension and diabetes presents with inability to abduct the right eye without other ocular motor deficit. Which is the most likely etiology?

A. Small-vessel ischemia
B. Aneurysm formation
C. Brainstem infarction
D. Increased intracranial pressure

Question 74-2:
"Crocodile tears" is typically a manifestation of repair of which of the following cranial nerves?

A. Oculomotor
B. Trigeminal
C. Facial
D. Glossopharyngeal

Question 74-3:
Facial palsy following trauma raises the suspicion of which of the following structural abnormalities?

A. Basilar skull fracture
B. Mandibular fracture
C. Epidural hematoma
D. Subdural hematoma

Question 74-4:
Which of the following cranial neuropathies may develop as a result of lesion in the cavernous sinus?

1. Oculomotor
2. Trochlear
3. Abducens
4. Optic

Select: A = 1, 2, 3. B = 1, 3. C = 2, 4. D = 4 only. E = All

Question 74-5:
Which of the following statements is not true regarding damage to the lingual nerve?

1. May occur during extraction of the lower third molar
2. Can result from dental anesthesia
3. Patients complain of paresthesias on the ipsilateral tongue.
4. Patients have loss of taste on the ipsilateral tongue.

Select: A = 1, 2, 3. B = 1, 3. C = 2, 4. D = 4 only. E = All

Answer 74-1: A.
The patient has an abducens nerve paresis. Small vessel ischemia is the most likely cause, although the other listed entities can produce this lesion. Other clinical findings would normally be expected. (p1883)

Answer 74-2: C.
Abberant regeneration with recovery of facial palsy may result in involuntary tearing on the affected side. (p1885)

Answer 74-3: A.
Facial palsy following trauma raises concern over basilar skull fracture. Both longitudinal and transverse fractures of the temporal bone may produce facial palsy. (p1884)

Answer 74-4: A.
The optic nerve does not course through the cavernous sinus, so damage would not occur from lesions within the cavernous sinus. The three listed ocular motor nerves pass through the cavernous sinus en route to the orbit. (p1880)

Answer 74-5: A.
Taste is not carried in the lingual nerve, so lesion results in paresthesias but no alteration in taste.

Chapter 75: Movement Disorders

Questions 75-1 through 75-8:
The following questions present mini-vignettes of some important movement disorders. While each patient profile is not a classic case of the disease, the clinical findings do not depart from those expected in evaluation of patients. Select the best diagnosis from the list.

A. Parkinson's disease
B. Dementia with Lewy bodies
C. Essential tremor
D. Progressive supranuclear palsy
E. Multiple system atrophy
F. Cortical-basal ganglionic degeneration
G. Idiopathic dystonia
H. Rheumatic chorea
I. Huntington's disease
J. Tourette's syndrome
K. None of these

Question 75-1:
A 70-year-old man with rigidity and bradykinesia and frequent backwards falls.

Question 75-2:
A 30-year-old man with arrhythmic jerking of the extremities. He has a recent history of psychiatric problems with paranoia and personality change.

Question 75-3:
A 67-year-old female presents with stiffness, stooped posture, severe orthostatic hypotension, and constipation.

Question 75-4:
A 76-year-old female with rigidity and resting tremor, decreased postural reflexes, frequent forward falls.

Question 75-5:
A 8-year-old male with jerking of the shoulders associated with snorting and grunting. Goes away in sleep. Has problems with attention.

Question 75-6:
A 76-year-old man with action and intention tremor. Poor writing. Examination is otherwise normal.

Question 75-7:
A 56-year-old man with akinesia and rigidity associated with limb dystonia. Has some spontaneous movements of an arm, the alien hand syndrome.

Question 75-8:
A 58-year-old man with rigidity and stooped posture. Has prominent hallucinations and memory loss.

Question 75-9:
Which neuroleptic is lease likely to exacerbate Parkinson's disease?

A. Risperidone
B. Thioridazine
C. Haloperidol
D. Clozapine

Question 75-10:
Which of the following medications require routine blood monitoring?

1. Clozapine
2. Amantadine
3. Tolcapone
4. Ropinerole

Select: A = 1, 2, 3. B = 1, 3. C = 2, 4. D = 4 only. E = All

Answer 75-1: D.
The clinical presentation would have been suggestive of Parkinson's disease except for the backward falling. PD typically presents with forward falling. The backward falling is common with PSP and is associated with the neck being extended with difficulty looking upwards. (p1900)

Answer 75-2: I.
Huntington's disease is characterized by progressive psychological and cognitive changes associated with a movement disorder. In adults, the chorea is prominent, while in children, rigidity may be more evident. (p1914)

Answer 75-3: E.
MSA presents with a parkinsonism flavor or a cerebellar flavor. Some autonomic difficulty is expected with PD, but the severe orthostatic hypotension and other autonomic findings suggest MSA rather than garden-variety PD. (p1900)

Answer 75-4: A.
This is a common presentation of Parkinson's disease. There are no atypical features which would suggest another parkinsonian syndrome. The presence of tremor is important; its absence would raise concern over another disease. (p1894)

Answer 75-5: J.
This is a typical presentation of Tourette's syndrome. The attentional deficit may prompt treatment with stimulants which may then exacerbate the tics. (p1917)

Answer 75-6: C.
Essential tremor presents with action and intention tremor without other findings. Some patients with PD may have a similar tremor, separate from the resting tremor, but this would be associated with other obvious stigmata of PD. (p1905-1906)

Answer 75-7: F.
CBGD is the only one of these conditions which commonly is associated with the alien hand syndrome. There are parkinsonian features and commonly also signs of cortical dysfunction with apraxia plus dementia, corticospinal signs, and cortical and subcortical language deficits. (p1904)

Answer 75-8: B.
DLB is associated with cognitive changes and parkinsonism and is suspected when there are hallucinations early in the course of the disease. (p1895)

Answer 75-9: D.
Clozapine is the least likely to exacerbate extrapyramidal symptoms, although it requires frequent blood monitoring. In addition, clozapine has fairly significant anticholinergic effects which may exacerbate cognitive deficits. (p1898)

Answer 75-10: B.
Clozapine and tolcapone require routine blood monitoring while the other agents do not. For any of these agents, the practitioner should well document that the monitoring and risks were explained to the patient and consider alternatives. (p1898)

Question 75-11:
Which of the following statements are true regarding post-anoxic action myoclonus?

1. The pathophysiology likely involves serotonin deficiency.
2. The myoclonus usually responds to 5-hydroxytryptophan.
3. Most patients also have a seizure disorder.
4. The myoclonus usually responds to valproate.

Select: A = 1, 2, 3. B = 1, 3. C = 2, 4. D = 4 only. E = All

Question 75-12:
Which of the following statements are true regarding drug-induced parkinsonism?

1. 15% of patients on neuroleptics develop parkinsonian features.
2. Careful examination can distinguish drug-induced from idiopathic parkinsonism in most patents.
3. Tremor is less prominent in drug-induced parkinsonism than in idiopathic parkinsonism.
4. Parkinsonism typically persists for months or years following discontinuation of the neuroleptic.

Select: A = 1, 2, 3. B = 1, 3. C = 2, 4. D = 4 only. E = All

Questions 75-13 through 75-15:
The following questions pertain to differentiation between tardive dyskinesia and tardive dystonia. For the three questions, select the best answer from the following associations:

A. Tardive dyskinesia
B. Tardive dystonia
C. Both
D. Neither

Question 75-13:
More prominent in older patients.

Question 75-14:
May typically persist following discontinuation of the neuroleptic.

Question 75-15:
May respond to reserpine.

Question 75-16:
Which of the following features are typical of Wilson's disease?

1. Elevated serum ceruloplasmin
2. Copper deposition in the cornea
3. Seizures are common
4. Fine action tremor is common

Select: A = 1, 2, 3. B = 1, 3. C = 2, 4. D = 4 only. E = All

Question 75-17:
Hemifacial spasm is a focal movement disorder which may be difficult to treat. Which of the following statements is true?

A. May be treated by botulinum toxin injection
B. May be treated by microvascular decompression
C. May follow Bell's palsy
D. There may be bilateral involvement
E. All are true

Answer 75-11: E.
All of these are correct. 5-HTP is usually not available, so valproate and clonazepam are usually the drugs of choice. (p1920)

Answer 75-12: B.
Drug-induced parkinsonism cannot be reproducibly differentiated from idiopathic parkinsonism on the basis of neurologic examination. Tremor is less prominent with drug-induced parkinsonism than with idiopathic parkinsonism, but this difference is not diagnostic. Parkinsonism that persists for many months or even years following discontinuation of the neuroleptic probably is a manifestation of early or subclinical Parkinson's disease that was exacerbated by the medication. Note that there are other agents besides neuroleptics that may produce parkinsonian features, but this is less likely. (p1922)

Answer 75-13: A.
Tardive dystonia does not have an age predilection. (p1923)

Answer 75-14: C.
Unfortunately, both tardive dyskinesia and tardive dystonia may persist following discontinuation of the neuroleptic. (p1923)

Answer 75-15: C.
Both tardive dyskinesia and tardive dystonia can respond to reserpine, which depletes presynaptic catecholamines. (p1923)

Answer 75-16: C.
Serum ceruloplasmin is low rather than high. Seizures may occur but are uncommon. The copper deposition in the cornea produces the Kayser-Fleischer ring. A fine action tremor is common, whereas the prototypic wing-beating tremor is less common. (p1924)

Answer 75-17: E.
All of these statements are true. Bilateral involvement may rarely occur, although the development of the second side involvement is independent. (p1929)

Chapter 76: Cerebellar and Spinocerebellar Disorders

Question 76-1:
Which is the most common antibody seen in paraneoplastic cerebellar degeneration?

A. Anti-Hu
B. Anti-Yo
C. Anti-Ri
D. None of these

Question 76-2:
Paraneoplastic cerebellar degeneration is seen in which of the following malignancies?

A. Ovarian cancer
B. Breast cancer
C. Hodgkin's disease
D. Small-cell lung cancer
E. All of these

Question 76-3:
Which of the following features would not be expected with ataxia telangiectasia?

A. X-linked inheritance
B. Reduction in serum IgG
C. Elevation in serum alpha-fetoprotein
D. Predisposition to malignancies
E. All are characteristic

Question 76-4:
Which of the following conditions is associated with vitamin E deficiency?

A. Cystic fibrosis
B. Biliary atresia
C. Abetalipoproteinemia
D. All of the above

Questions 76-5 through 76-10:
The following questions are True/False. For each statement, select the best answer on the basis of current practice and information.

Question 76-5:
Chronic cerebellar ataxia in alcoholics is due to thiamine deficiency rather than being a direct effect of the ethanol.

Question 76-6:
Wernicke-Korsakoff syndrome is a specific abnormality of alcoholics.

Question 76-7:
Friedreich's ataxia is the most common hereditary ataxia.

Question 76-8:
Autosomal dominant cerebellar ataxias may be caused by expansion of trinucleotide repeats.

Question 76-9:
Ornithine transcarbamylase (OTC) deficiency is the only X-linked hyperammonemia.

Question 76-10:
Females are unaffected in adrenoleukomyeloneuropathy.

Answer 76-1: B.
Anti-Yo antibody is the most common antibody seen in paraneoplastic cerebellar degeneration. About half of patients with PCD have a demonstrable antibody against neurons. Occasional patients with anti-Hu antibody may present with a clinical picture of PCD, although the neurological involvement is typically more extensive. (p1933)

Answer 76-2: E.
All of these have been implicated in producing paraneoplastic cerebellar degeneration, although the antibodies may be different. (p1933)

Answer 76-3: A.
Inheritance of ataxia telangiectasia is autosomal recessive, with patients being homozygous for the gene on chromosome 11, or compound heterozygotes for null allele. (p1937)

Answer 76-4: D.
All of these can cause vitamin E deficiency. Almost any cause of malabsorption may produce vitamin E deficiency. Of the listed disorders, the neurologic complications of the deficiency are most prominent with abetalipoproteinemia. (p1939)

Answer 76-5: True.
Ethanol is the acute intoxicant, but thiamine deficiency is felt to be responsible for the chronic cerebellar ataxia. (p1940)

Answer 76-6: False.
Wernicke-Korsakoff syndrome has been well documented in patients with malnutrition in the absence of ethanol intake, e.g., cancer patients. (p1940)

Answer 76-7: True.
Friedreich's ataxia is the most common of the inherited ataxias, and has autosomal recessive inheritance. (p1941)

Answer 76-8: True.
Expansion of trinucleotide repeats has been associated with several disorders including some of the dominantly inherited cerebellar ataxias. (p1948)

Answer 76-9: True.
All of the other inherited hyperammonemias are autosomal recessive. (p1935)

Answer 76-10: False.
Although ALMN is X-linked, about 8% of carrier females have neurologic abnormalities. (p1935)

Chapter 77: Disorders of Bones, Joints, Ligaments, and Meninges

Question 77-1:
Basilar impression may be associated with which of the following anomalies?

A. Chiari I
B. Chiari II
C. Down syndrome
D. Syringomyelia
E. All of the above

Question 77-2:
The most common neurologic finding in the Klippel-Feil anomaly is which of the following?

A. Hydrocephalus
B. Cervical radiculopathy
C. Myelopathy
D. Normal neurologic function

Questions 77-3 through 77-5:
The following 3 questions concern the Chiari malformation. For each question, select the best answer from the following choices.

A. Chiari I
B. Chiari II
C. Chiari III
D. Chiari IV
E. All of the above

Question 77-3:
Resembles the Dandy-Walker malformation.

Question 77-4:
Occipital meningoencephalocele.

Question 77-5:
Syringomyelia.

Question 77-6:
A 16-year-old female presents with left leg weakness and has a combination of upper and lower motor neuron findings. There is a tuft of hair overlying the spinous processes at the L3-4 levels. Examination is otherwise normal. Which is the most likely diagnosis?

A. Transverse myelitis
B. Myelomeningocele
C. Familial spastic paraparesis
D. Diastematomyelia

Question 77-7:
Which of the following complications of achondroplasia is not expected to produce signs and symptoms in childhood?

A. Hydrocephalus
B. Spinal stenosis
C. Sleep apnea
D. Neural compression at the foramen magnum
E. All may occur in childhood

Question 77-8:
Myelomeningocele may be associated with which of the following malformations?

A. Polymicrogyria
B. Hydrocephalus
C. Chiari malformation
D. Syringomyelia
E. All may be associated

Answer 77-1: E.
All of these may be associated with basilar impression of the skull. Other associations include Hurler's syndrome, Klippel-Feil anomaly, and achondroplasia. Familial cases may occur without other abnormalities. (p1953)

Answer 77-2: D.
Although the spectrum of neurologic signs is wide, the most common findings are none at all. All of the other listed complications can occur. (p1954)

Answer 77-3: D.
Chiari IV is probably a variant of the Dandy-Walker malformation. (p1956)

Answer 77-4: C.
Chiari III is displacement of the cerebellar and brainstem tissue associated with an infratentorial encephalocele. (p1956)

Answer 77-5: E.
All of the Chiari types may have associated syringomyelia or hydrocephalus. (p1956)

Answer 77-6: D.
Diastematomyelia is one important cause of the tethered cord syndrome. The tuft of hair is common but not invariable. Tethered cord from diastematomyelia can produce both upper and lower motor neuron signs. Myelomeningocele would have other neurologic signs. (p1961-1962)

Answer 77-7: B.
Spinal stenosis is not expected to produce complications in childhood, but it is a common cause of neurologic deficit in later life in patients with achondroplasia. (p1959)

Answer 77-8: E.
All of these may develop in patients with myelomeningocele. Chiari malformation and hydrocephalus are prominent associated neurologic associations. (p1961)

Question 77-9:
A 54-year-old man presents with left arm pain and weakness. The weakness is most prominent in the biceps and brachioradialis. He has altered sensory perception on the thumb and radial aspect of the index finger. Biceps tendon reflex is reduced. Which of the following statements is most likely true?

A. He has a C6 radiculopathy due to acutely herniated disk.
B. He has a C6 radiculopathy due to foraminal stenosis.
C. He has an upper brachial plexus lesion due to infiltrating tumor.
D. None of these are likely.

Questions 77-10 through 77-12:
The following 3 questions pertain to neurogenic and vascular claudication. For each clinical feature, select the best association from the following:

A. Lumbar spinal stenosis
B. Peripheral vascular disease
C. Both
D. Neither

Question 77-10:
Pain with walking which abates with sitting.

Question 77-11:
Relief of pain within seconds of cessation of walking.

Question 77-12:
Commonly have sphincter control deficit.

Answer 77-9: B.
Foraminal stenosis is the most common cause of radiculopathy in a man of this age; disc herniation is more common in younger patients, usually under 45 years of age. Tumor infiltration of the upper brachial plexus is rare compared with the other listed entities. (p1969)

Answer 77-10: C.
Both neurogenic and vascular claudication commonly produce pain with walking, although the pattern differs between patients. (p1975)

Answer 77-11: B.
The relief of pain within seconds is characteristic of vascular claudication rather than neurogenic claudication. With spinal stenosis, the improvement typically takes minutes. (p1975)

Answer 77-12: D.
Neither vascular nor neurogenic claudication are commonly associated with sphincter disturbance, although spinal stenosis can progress to the point of cauda equina damage, and can occasionally present with urinary incontinence. (p1975)

Chapter 78: Disorders of Upper and Lower Motor Neurons

Question 78-1:
Which of the following findings would be expected in spinal muscular atrophy (SMA) type 1?

A. Reduced compound muscle action potential amplitude.
B. Normal sensory conduction velocity.
C. Active denervation on electromyography.
D. All of the above.

Question 78-2:
Which of the following differentiates adult-onset SMA from PMA?

A. Autosomal dominant inheritance of some patients with SMA.
B. More rapid progression of SMA than PMA.
C. Active denervation without signs of reinnervation in SMA but with signs of reinnervation in PMA.
D. Biopsy signs of fiber-type grouping more prominent in PMA than SMA.

Question 78-3:
Which of the following statements is *not* true regarding hereditary spastic paraplegia?

A. Urinary urgency may develop.
B. The most common inheritance pattern is autosomal recessive.
C. There are no disease-modifying treatments for HSP.
D. Patients may have loss of vibratory sensation in the legs.
E. Upper extremities may become involved.

Question 78-4:
A 56-year-old man is diagnosed with multifocal motor neuropathy. He has progressive weakness affecting the arms more than the legs. Self-care is beginning to be affected. Which would be the most appropriate treatment?

A. Prednisone orally
B. Solumedrol at high-dose intravenously for 3-5 days
C. Intravenous immunoglobulin
D. Azathioprine

Question 78-5:
Which of the following statements is *not* true regarding the role of the immune system in patients with ALS?

A. Patients with ALS may have monoclonal gammopathy.
B. Immune suppression slows the progression of ALS.
C. Patients with ALS may have antibodies to L-type voltage-gated calcium channels.
D. Patients with lymphoproliferative disorders are more likely than the general population to develop ALS.

Question 78-6:
Which of the following clinical features would not be expected in patients with ALS?

A. Head droop
B. Muscle fasciculations
C. Muscle cramps
D. Unsteady gait
E. Sphincter dysfunction

Answer 78-1: D.
All of these findings can be seen in patients with SMA type 1. These findings are more likely to be identified in patients who are several months of age rather than in newborns. (p1999)

Answer 78-2: A.
Approximately 30% of patients with adult-onset SMA have autosomal dominant inheritance, the remainder have autosomal recessive inheritance. PMA typically progresses more rapidly than SMA. SMA is associated with more prominent signs of reinnervation on EMG and biopsy than PMA, which is characterized by signs on active denervation. (p2001)

Answer 78-3: B.
The most common inheritance pattern is autosomal dominant, responsible for 70-85% of cases. The remaining cases are autosomal recessive or X-linked. Urinary urgency and upper extremity involvement can occur, especially with a prolonged course. The degeneration can involve the posterior columns, so loss of vibratory sensation can develop. (p1989)

Answer 78-4: C.
IVIG is an accepted treatment for patients with MMN, and is given at a total dose of 2 g.kg divided into 2-5 days. Corticosteroids are ineffective and may actually worsen the condition. Another effective treatment is cyclophosphamide, which is helpful in gaining long-term benefit, although at a cost of significant long-term side effects. (p1995)

Answer 78-5: B.
The autoimmune theory of ALS is not popular. Immunosuppressant therapy does not appear to alter the clinical course of ALS. However, patients with monoclonal gammopathy and some patients with lymphoproliferative disorders are more likely to develop ALS. Also, patients with ALS may have antibodies to the L-type voltage-gated calcium channel, although this antibody is seen in other autoimmune diseases as well. (p2007)

Answer 78-6: E.
Sphincter dysfunction is not expected in ALS. The other findings are typical. Head droop can develop in ALS, although it can also develop in myasthenia gravia and polymyositis. Unsteady gait may be an initial sign of upper motor neuron dysfunction, even before lower motor neuron dysfunction affects gait. (p2007-2009)

Question 78-7:
A 66-year-old man is evaluated for weakness and diagnosed as having ALS on the basis of upper and lower motor neuron degeneration. Examination is notable for personality change and mild dementia, with impairments in memory as well as other spheres of cognitive function. Which is the most likely clinical formulation?

A. The patient has the chance association of Alzheimer's disease with ALS. The two degenerative diseases are not associated.
B. The patient has ALS with a fronto-temporal dementia, a separate pathological entity from Alzheimer's disease.
C. Approximately 15% of patients with ALS develop dementia as part of the disease process.

Question 78-8:
Which are the expected EMG findings in patients with ALS?

A. Active denervation
B. Chronic reinnervation
C. Fasciculations
D. Early recruitment of motor units

Answer 78-7: B.
About 5% of patients with ALS will develop dementia and this usually has the appearance of fronto-temporal dementia clinically and pathologically. The CNS pathology is distinct from that expected in uncomplicated ALS. (p2014)

Answer 78-8: D.
Reduced number of motor units is expected in patients with ALS. Early recruitment would be expected in myopathic disorders. Fasciculations are not specific for ALS, but are usually identified in patients with ALS. Active denervation and polyphasic motor units indicative of chronic reinnervation are typical. (p2009)

Chapter 79: Disorders of Nerve Roots and Plexuses

Question 79-1:
Diabetic polyradiculoneuropathy may produce which of the following findings?

1. Low back pain
2. Abdominal pain
3. Proximal leg weakness
4. Arm and leg weakness

Select: A = 1, 2, 3. B = 1, 3. C = 2, 4. D = 4 only. E = All

Question 79-2:
A 38-year-old female with breast cancer has neoplastic meningitis. Which of the following clinical findings may be caused by the meningeal tumor?

1. Radicular pain
2. Confusion
3. Cranial neuropathies
4. Cerebellar ataxia

Select: A = 1, 2, 3. B = 1, 3. C = 2, 4. D = 4 only. E = All

Question 79-3:
AIDS patients may develop a CMV polyradiculoneuropathy. Which of the following features would not be expected in this condition.

A. Coexisting signs of CMV gastroenteritis
B. Urinary retention
C. Areflexia
D. A presenting sign of HIV infection
E. All would be typical

Question 79-4:
Which of the following statements regarding metastatic brachial plexopathy is not true?

A. The lower plexus is usually affected.
B. The plexopathy is usually painless, although there may be some dysesthesias.
C. Lung cancer is a common cause.
D. All are true

Question 79-5:
Which of the following statements are true regarding neurologic complications of herpes zoster?

1. Late development of contralateral hemiparesis develops commonly after zoster of the geniculate ganglion.
2. Prednisone is contraindicated in patients with zoster.
3. Early administration of acyclovir prevents development of postherpetic neuralgia.
4. Segmental motor weakness may develop as a complication of zoster.

Select: A = 1, 2, 3. B = 1, 3. C = 2, 4. D = 4 only. E = All

Question 79-6:
Patients have an increased tendency to develop a brachial plexopathy in which of the following medical conditions?

1. Hereditary neuropathy with liability to pressure palsies
2. After influenza infection
3. Post-immunization
4. Postpartum

Select: A = 1, 2, 3. B = 1, 3. C = 2, 4. D = 4 only. E = All

Question 79-7
A 32-year-old man presents with pain and weakness in the right shoulder region. The weakness is most prominent in the biceps and deltoid and there is a reduced biceps tendon reflex. Which of the following would be serious considerations in the differential diagnosis?

1. Cervical radiculopathy
2. Idiopathic brachial plexopathy
3. Neoplastic plexus infiltration
4. Monomelic amyotrophy

Select: A = 1, 2, 3. B = 1, 3. C = 2, 4. D = 4 only. E = All

Answer 79-1: E.
All of these are potential manifestations of diabetic radiculoneuropathy. Diffuse arm and leg weakness is a rare complication but can occur with extension of the radiculopathy to the upper dermatomes. Symptoms other than the classic diabetic amyotrophy findings usually trigger a search for structural abnormalities. (p2026)

Answer 79-2: A.
Cerebellar ataxia in a patient with breast cancer may be due to a direct effect of posterior fossa tumor or a remote effect of tumor as a paraneoplastic cerebellar degeneration. However, carcinomatous meningitis would not be expected to produce cerebellar ataxia on its own. (p2027)

Answer 79-3: D.
CMV polyradiculoneuropathy typically occurs late in the course of the illness, when CD4 counts are low. Patients present with extremity and perineal pain progressing to ascending sensory and motor loss with areflexia and urinary incontinence. (p2028)

Answer 79-4: B.
Neoplastic plexopathy is usually very painful, which aids in differentiation from radiation plexopathy which may be characterized by dysesthesias but with much less pain. (p2035)

Answer 79-5: D.
Segmental motor weakness may develop up to 5 weeks after an eruption of zoster. Luckily, this develops in 5% or less of patients. Prednisone may be given to healthy patients with zoster but should not be given to immunosuppressed patients because of the possibility of disseminated zoster infection. Early administration of acyclovir improves the speed of healing of the vesicles and helps initial symptoms to abate but probably does not alter the frequency of postherpetic neuralgia. Zoster of the geniculate ganglion produces the Ramsay-Hunt syndrome, but it is ophthalmic zoster that may be associated with late development of hemiparesis due to angiitis, although this is not a common complication. (p2030)

Answer 79-6: E.
All of these conditions increase the susceptibility to brachial plexopathy, although perhaps half of patients have none of these conditions. (p2037)

Answer 79-7: A.
The most likely diagnosis would be cervical radiculopathy, but the next two diagnoses should be considered. Neoplastic plexus infiltration would be unusual for a patient with no known cancer. Monomelic amyotrophy, a focal motor neuron disease, could produce focal weakness but would not be expected to be painful. (p2037)

Questions 79-8 and 79-9:
These two questions concern the same patient. A 56-year-old man presents with a 3-month history of progressive weakness of the extremities without sensory loss, weight loss, dysarthria, and dysphagia. Examination shows prominent atrophy plus fasciculations in the extremities. Reflexes are present but not pathologic, and there are no definite corticospinal tract signs.

Question 79-8:
Which is the most appropriate clinical formulation?

A. The patient probably has amyotrophic lateral sclerosis despite the absence of upper motor neuron signs. EMG and laboratory testing are ordered.
B. The patient probably has a late-onset spinal muscular atrophy.
C. The patient probably has an autoimmune neuromuscular disorder.

Question 79-9:
EMG shows denervation in distal muscles plus slow nerve motor conduction velocities which are out of proportion to the axonal changes. CSF protein is increased. SIEP shows a monoclonal gammopathy. Which is the most appropriate clinical formulation?

A. The patient has ALS.
B. The patient has SMA.
C. The patient has an autoimmune motor polyradiculoneuropathy.

Question 79-10:
A 55-year-old female develops left leg weakness within one day following coronary angiography. She has pain which extends from the groin down the medial aspect of the leg. She has paresthesias which extend medially and laterally on the upper and lower leg. Weakness is most prominent in the iliopsoas and quadriceps, but tibialis anterior and gastrocnemius are both affected. Which is the most likely diagnosis?

A. Direct needle-stick damage to the femoral nerve
B. Retroperitoneal hematoma from arterial blood
C. Compression of the femoral nerve and lumbosacral plexus by the sandbag

Answer 79-8: A.
Despite the absence of long-track signs, progressive motor neuronopathy is most likely to be ALS. When the patient is followed over time, the long-track signs are likely to develop. Late onset SMA would be very unlikely at this age. An autoimmune neuromuscular disorder could be responsible for this but need not be implicated with these data. (p2031)

Answer 79-9: C.
This would be a typical presentation of a motor polyradiculoneuropathy, but this will be a minority of patients with apparent motor neuron disease. (p2031)

Answer 79-10: B.
The most likely diagnosis is bleeding from the puncture site resulting in a retroperitoneal hematoma. The blood produces a depolarizing block of nerve conduction, producing paresthesias followed by numbness and weakness. Direct needle stick of the femoral nerve is unlikely with angiography, but the occurrence would be obvious at the time of initial stick, and the symptoms would not develop over subsequent hours. Moreover, the weakness and sensory loss extend beyond the distribution of the femoral nerve. Compression by sandbag can affect the femoral nerve but would not be expected to produce compression of the plexus. (p2040)

Chapter 80: Disorders of Peripheral Nerves

Question 80-1:
Onion bulb formation refers to which of the following pathophysiologic processes?

A. Attempts to reinnervate missing tissues resulting in neuroma formation
B. Repeated episodes of demyelination and remyelination
C. Aberrant reinnervation of skeletal muscle giving ineffectual muscle fiber contraction
D. Segmental regions of demyelination interspersed by relatively normal tissue

Question 80-2:
Which of the following causes of neuropathy is least likely to have autonomic involvement?

A. Amyloid
B. Guillain-Barré syndrome
C. CIDP
D. Diabetes

Questions 80-3 through 80-6:
The following questions pertain to the type of neuromuscular condition and relevant clinical findings. For each of the questions, select the most likely associated disorder from the following list.

A. Axonal neuropathy
B. Demyelinating neuropathy
C. Neuromuscular junction disorder
D. Myopathy
E. Both A and B

Question 80-3:
Mild weakness with total areflexia.

Question 80-4:
Proximal weakness with preservation of distal muscle strength.

Question 80-5:
Dysproteinemia.

Question 80-6:
Most toxins.

Questions 80-7 through 80-11:
The following questions pertain to symptoms manifest in patients with neuropathy. For each of the definitions listed in the questions, select the best choice from the following terms.

A. Paresthesias
B. Dysesthesia
C. Fasciculation
D. Hyperalgesia
E. Allodynia
F. None of these

Question 80-7:
Diagnostic of motor neuron disease.

Question 80-8:
Abnormal unpleasant sensation in response to an ordinary non-noxious sensory stimulus.

Question 80-9:
Abnormal unpleasant spontaneous sensation with a tingling or prickling character.

Question 80-10:
Painful sensation in response to a non-noxious stimulus.

Question 80-11:
Exaggerated pain from a noxious stimulus.

Answer 80-1: B.
An onion bulb is a structure with a central axon, usually thinly myelinated, surrounded by multiple redundant thin Schwann cell processes, resulting from repeated demyelination and remyelination. (p2047)

Answer 80-2: C.
CIDP is the least likely to have prominent autonomic dysfunction, although the autonomic nerves may be affected. All of the others commonly have autonomic neuropathy as a prominent feature. (p2050)

Answer 80-3: B.
Demyelinating disorders such as Guillain-Barré syndrome are characterized by loss of reflexes at a time when weakness is quite mild. The other disorders will have suppression of reflexes which is roughly proportional to the weakness. (p2049)

Answer 80-4: D.
Proximal weakness is the prototypic presentation of a myopathy, though it can also be seen in CIDP. (p2049)

Answer 80-5: E.
Dysproteinemias have produced both axonal and demyelinating neuropathies. (p2052)

Answer 80-6: A
Most toxins produce an axonal neuropathy, although there are a few exceptions. (p2052)

Answer 80-7: F.
Fasciculations are a typical feature of motor neuron disease. Patients may or may not be aware of them. They are seen especially on EMG, but can often be seen on examination in many patients. However, fasciculations can be seen in other neuropathies, some metabolic states, and in some otherwise normal patients. (p2048)

Answer 80-8: B.
Dysesthesia is due to misperception of a sensory stimulus such that an unpleasant tingling or prickling sensation is produced by touching an object that normally lacks that sensory characteristic. (p2048)

Answer 80-9: A.
Paresthesia resembles dysesthesia, except that the sensations are not in response to a stimulus but develop spontaneously. (p2048)

Answer 80-10: E.
Allodynia is a painful perception when the sensory stimulation is non-noxious. (p2054)

Answer 80-11: D.
Hyperalgesia is exaggeration of the painful perception of a normally noxious stimulus. (p2054)

Question 80-12:
Which is the most common entrapment neuropathy?

A. Ulnar nerve compression at the elbow
B. Median nerve compression at the wrist
C. Radial nerve compression at the spiral groove
D. Peroneal nerve compression at the fibular neck

Question 80-13:
Which is the most sensitive electrodiagnostic test for carpal tunnel syndrome?

A. Motor distal latency
B. Sensory latency
C. Electromyography of the abductor pollicis brevis
D. Palmar autonomic testing

Question 80-14:
Which of the following conditions have been shown to predispose to carpal tunnel syndrome?

1. Pregnancy
2. AV shunt for hemodialysis
3. Repetitive overuse syndromes
4. Obesity

Select: A = 1, 2, 3. B = 1, 3. C = 2, 4. D = 4 only. E = All

Question 80-15:
Which of the following muscles would be denervated in a patient with lesion of the posterior interosseus nerve?

1. Brachioradialis
2. Extensor carpi radialis longus and brevis
3. Supinator
4. Extensor carpi ulnaris

Select: A = 1, 2, 3. B = 1, 3. C = 2, 4. D = 4 only. E = All

Question 80-16:
Which of the following is the most common entrapment neuropathy in the leg?

A. Tibial nerve
B. Fibular (peroneal) nerve
C. Sciatic nerve
D. Femoral nerve
E. None of these

Question 80-17:
A 30-year-old female presents with pain on the lateral aspect of the left thigh. She has burning pain with dysesthesias. No known acute trauma. Sensory threshold is increased on the lateral thigh, and does not extend below the knee. Which of the following is least likely to be a potential contributor to this abnormality?

A. Pregnancy
B. Weight gain
C. Tight-fitting clothes or belt
D. Renal tumor

Questions 80-18 through 80-21:
The following questions pertain to hereditary neuropathies. For each of the questions, select the best answer from the following list.

A. CMT1
B. CMT2
C. CMT3
D. CMT4
E. None of these

Question 80-18:
Dejerine-Sottas disease.

Question 80-19:
Usually autosomal recessive.

Question 80-20:
Dominantly inherited axonal neuropathy.

Question 80-21:
Latest onset of this group.

Answer 80-12: B.
Median nerve compression at the wrist, as in carpal tunnel syndrome (CTS), is the most common entrapment neuropathy. All of the others are relatively common in clinical practice, but are less common than CTS. (p2056)

Answer 80-13: B.
Sensory conduction through the wrist is the most sensitive study for CTS. Motor conduction is often abnormal, as well, although with less sensitivity. EMG is only abnormal if there has been loss of axonal integrity, implicating a much more severe neural entrapment. (p2058)

Answer 80-14: E.
All of these conditions may predispose to CTS. Others include rheumatoid arthritis, amyloid, some mucopolysaccharidoses, gout, hypothyroidism, and diabetes. (p2058)

Answer 80-15: D.
All of these muscles are innervated by the radial nerve, but only the extensor carpi ulnaris is innervated by the deep pure-motor branch of the radial nerve, the posterior interosseus nerve. (p2060)

Answer 80-16: B.
The fibular (peroneal) nerve is the nerve most likely to be damaged by entrapment neuropathy. (p2061)

Answer 80-17: D.
This is a typical case of meralgia paresthetica. Retroperitoneal tumors can rarely produce damage to the lateral femoral cutaneous nerve, but the other potential contributors would be far more likely. (p2062)

Answer 80-18: C.
Dejerine-Sottas disease is CMT3, a childhood-onset hypertrophic neuropathy which is usually apparently sporadic. (p2066)

Answer 80-19: D.
CMT4 is autosomal recessive while the others tend to be dominantly-inherited or sporadic. There are some reports of recessive inheritance with CMT1 and CMT2; however, this is not expected, and many of these patients may be the products of new mutations. (p2064)

Answer 80-20: B.
CMT2 is the axonal form of CMT, with NCVs which are near normal and prominent axonal changes on EMG. (p2064)

Answer 80-21: B.
CMT2 has onset even later than CMT1 with onset in the second decade. The others begin even younger, with CMT 3 and CMT4 having symptoms beginning in early childhood. (p2065)

Question 80-22:
Genetic testing may be helpful in which of the following conditions?

1. Chronic demyelinating neuropathy with a family history of neuropathy
2. Chronic demyelinating neuropathy without a family history of neuropathy
3. Multiple mononeuropathies in the absence of diabetes or a family history of neuropathy
4. Pre-symptomatic screening of children of patients with CMT2

Select: A = 1, 2, 3. B = 1, 3. C = 2, 4. D = 4 only. E = All

Question 80-23:
Which of the following features are characteristic of hereditary sensory and autonomic neuropathy type III (familial dysautonomia, Riley-Day syndrome)?

1. Autosomal dominant inheritance
2. Hyporeflexia
3. Anhydrosis
4. Insensitivity to pain

Select: A = 1, 2, 3. B = 1, 3. C = 2, 4. D = 4 only. E = All

Question 80-24:
Which of the following disorders are X-linked?

1. Adrenomyeloneuropathy
2. Metachromatic leukodystrophy
3. Pelizaeus-Merzbacher disease
4. Globoid cell leukodystrophy (Krabbe's disease)

Select: A = 1, 2, 3. B = 1, 3. C = 2, 4. D = 4 only. E = All

Question 80-25:
A 23-year-old man presents with rapidly-progressive ascending weakness and areflexia. NCVs show slowed motor and sensory NCVs, and F-waves, where elicitable, are markedly prolonged. Which of the following findings would be expected in this patient at the time of admission?

1. Fibrillation potentials and positive sharp waves confined to distal muscles
2. Increased CSF protein
3. Moderate CSF pleocytosis
4. Report of a recent infection

Select: A = 1, 2, 3. B = 1, 3. C = 2, 4. D = 4 only. E = All

Question 80-26:
Which of the following conditions should be specifically considered in the differential diagnosis of a patient with Guillain-Barré syndrome?

1. Tick paralysis
2. Botulism
3. Acute porphyria
4. Lyme disease

Select: A = 1, 2, 3. B = 1, 3. C = 2, 4. D = 4 only. E = All

Question 80-27:
Which of the following interventions for Guillain-Barré syndrome are felt to have documented beneficial effects?

1. Corticosteroids
2. Intravenous immunoglobulin
3. Azathioprine
4. Plasma exchange

Select: A = 1, 2, 3. B = 1, 3. C = 2, 4. D = 4 only. E = All

Question 80-28:
Chronic inflammatory demyelinating polyradiculoneuropathy is usually idiopathic, but may develop in association with which of the following medical conditions?

1. Monoclonal gammopathy
2. SLE
3. HIV infection
4. Hodgkin's lymphoma

Select: A = 1, 2, 3. B = 1, 3. C = 2, 4. D = 4 only. E = All

Answer 80-22: A.
Genetic testing can be helpful to guide counseling in all of these conditions except CMT2, for which there is no specific associated gene which can be tested. There may be disagreement on testing of pre-symptomatic children, but this should still be considered. (p2068)

Answer 80-23: C.
Hyporeflexia and insensitivity to pain are late features of HSAN-III. Inheritance is autosomal recessive. Episodes of profuse sweating, vasomotor changes, and hypertension are signs of the autonomic instability. (p2070)

Answer 80-24: B.
ADMN and Pelizaeus-Merzbacher disease are both X-linked disorders, although the latter does not have PNS manifestations as do the other entities on this list. (p2076)

Answer 80-25: C.
This patient has typical Guillain-Barré syndrome. Increased CSF protein is typical, although about 10% of patients have normal proteins, and more at the time of presentation. A mononuclear pleocytosis would not be expected, and when present suggests GBS as a complication of HIV infection. A majority of patients report recent infection, although many of these are inconsequential. (p2081)

Answer 80-26: E.
All of these should be considered in the differential diagnosis of patients with presumed GBS. The first two would be expected to produce only motor symptoms and signs, but early in the presentation, the sensory findings can be subtle and are certainly subjective. (p2082)

Answer 80-27: C.
IVIG and plasma exchange have been shown to be effective in impacting the course of GBS. (p2086)

Answer 80-28: E.
All of these conditions predispose to development of a neuropathy which meets criteria for CIDP. The pathogenic role of the immunoglobulin is debatable in many patients with monoclonal gammopathy. (p2087)

Question 80-29:
Which of the following are accepted treatments for CIDP?

1. Corticosteroids
2. Plasmapheresis
3. IVIG
4. Azathioprine

Select: A = 1, 2, 3. B = 1, 3. C = 2, 4. D = 4 only. E = All

Question 80-30:
Which of the following features help to differentiate multifocal motor neuropathy from ALS?

1. ALS has weakness most prominent in the arms while MMN has weakness most prominent distally in the legs.
2. Muscle cramps and fasciculations are common in ALS but uncommon in MMN.
3. Weakness may be profound in muscles of normal bulk in ALS while patients with MMN have weakness proportional to atrophy.
4. Depressed tendon reflexes are common in MMN while hyperreflexia is expected in ALS.

Select: A = 1, 2, 3. B = 1, 3. C = 2, 4. D = 4 only. E = All

Question 80-31:
Which of the following statements regarding neuropathy in diabetes are true?

1. Mononeuropathy of CN-3 usually spares pupillary fibers.
2. Mononeuropathy may develop from peripheral nerve infarction.
3. Unilateral pain and weakness in the hip and thigh is often due to diabetic lumbar radiculoplexopathy.
4. Pure autonomic neuropathy is common.

Select: A = 1, 2, 3. B = 1, 3. C = 2, 4. D = 4 only. E = All

Question 80-32:
A 30-year-old female presents with left-sided peri-orbital pain, associated with malaise and fever. Swelling in the periorbital region develops, followed by numbness of the skin above the eye plus an ocular motor deficit which spans several single nerves. The patient is a brittle diabetic and is markedly acidotic. What is the most likely clinical formulation?

A. Orbital abscess, possibly staphylococcal, with destruction of the posterior orbital structures.
B. Diabetic ketoacidosis, mucormycosis, with ocular motor nerve and trigeminal nerve involvement.
C. Cavernous sinus thrombosis due to bacterial thrombophlebitis.

Question 80-33:
Which of the following features are characteristic of critical illness polyneuropathy?

1. Flaccid weakness and hyporeflexia
2. Setting of sepsis and/or multi-organ failure
3. Gradual recovery over 3-6 months
4. Prominent distal pain and paresthesias

Select: A = 1, 2, 3. B = 1, 3. C = 2, 4. D = 4 only. E = All

Answer 80-29: E.
All of these treatments are used for CIDP, although azathioprine would certainly be the last choice in this group; there are no studies which definitively show efficacy of this agent. Therefore, you would be on solid ground if you selected A, eliminating azathioprine from this group of treatments. (p2088)

Answer 80-30: D.
Both ALS and MMN have weakness which is most prominent in the arms. Muscle cramps and fasciculations are prominent in both conditions. MMN quite typically has muscles which may be profoundly weak despite normal bulk. However, differences in reflexes can be a helpful differentiating tool. (p2090).

Answer 80-31: A.
Autonomic component to diabetic neuropathy is common; pure autonomic neuropathy is rare, but may occur. Mononeuropathy of CN-3 usually spares pupillary fibers because the vascular supply to the segments of the nerve which serve the extraocular muscles differs from that of the nerves destined for the pupil. (p2100-2101)

Answer 80-32: B.
Mucormycosis is the most likely diagnosis in this patient. There is extension to involve not only the sinus cavities but also the trigeminal and ocular motor nerves; any of CN-3, 4, or 6 can be affected. (p2101)

Answer 80-33: A.
Pain and other sensory symptoms are uncommon in patients with critical illness polyneuropathy. The remainder of the statements are true. (p2116)

Chapter 81: Disorders of the Autonomic Nervous System

Question 81-1:
Which one of the following statements is true regarding multiple system atrophy?

A. MSA has a familial predisposition.
B. Pathological signs of degeneration are confined to the nigro-striatal, cerebellar, and brainstem pathways.
C. Patients with MSA are unlikely to have their parkinsonian symptoms respond to dopaminergic agents.
D. In MSA, Lewy bodies are not confined to the basal ganglia but rather extend to cortical tissue.

Question 81-2:
Sweating changes are common in patients with traumatic myelopathy. Which of the following indicates the most common sweating disorder with myelopathy?

A. Hyperhydrosis above the lesion and anhydrosis below the lesion
B. Anyhdrosis above the lesion and hyperhydrosis below the lesion
C. Normal sweating above the lesion and anhydrosis below the lesion
D. Normal sweating above the lesion and hyperhydrosis below the lesion

Question 81-3:
Which of the following statements regarding the sympathetic skin response is not true?

A. The SSR is usually absent in axonal neuropathies.
B. The SSR is usually preserved in demyelinating neuropathies.
C. The SSR is usually absent in autonomic neuropathies
D. Prolonged SSR latency or reduced amplitude indicates incipient autonomic failure, regardless of cause.

Question 81-4:
Suggestions to patients with nocturnal micturition syncope would include all of the following except which?

A. Sit on the toilet at night, rather than stand.
B. Avoid Valsalva maneuver when attempting to initiate urination.
C. Administer amitriptyline before bed.
D. Elevate the head of the bed.

Question 81-5:
Which of the following statements are true regarding fatal familial insomnia?

1. It is a prion disease.
2. Autonomic function is impaired.
3. Circadian rhythm is altered.
4. The ventral pons and medulla are predominantly involved.

Select: A = 1, 2, 3. B = 1, 3. C = 2, 4. D = 4 only. E = All

Question 81-6:
Which of the following agents may be helpful for treating postural hypotension?

1. Midodrine
2. Fludrocortisone
3. Desmopressin
4. Selegiline

Select: A = 1, 2, 3. B = 1, 3. C = 2, 4. D = 4 only. E = All

Answer 81-1: C.
MSA patients usually fail to respond to dopaminergic agents, although some patients may respond initially. There is no familial predisposition to MSA. Pathologic signs of degeneration are widespread in MSA, but diffuse Lewy bodies are not seen; this would be expected with Lewy body dementia. The parkinsonian symptoms are due to striatonigral degeneration. (p2136-2138)

Answer 81-2: A.
Hyperhydrosis above the lesion may be so prominent that medications are needed to control the bothersome sweating on the upper body and face. Anhydrosis below the lesion is typical. (p2145)

Answer 81-3: D.
SSR is either present or absent. While every laboratory has normative values for latency and amplitude, the variability is so great that these parametric data are not used for analysis. (p2154)

Answer 81-4: C.
The anticholinergic effects of amitriptyline would make vasomotor compensatory mechanisms even more impaired and would make initiating urination even more difficult. This is one of the medications to generally avoid in the elderly, especially if orthostasis, dementia, or ataxia is already present. Elevation of the head of the bed reduces recumbency-induced diuresis and therefore is less of an exacerbation of hypotension. (p2160)

Answer 81-5: A.
Fatal familial insomnia is a prion disease which affects predominantly the thalamus. There are multiple changes in autonomic function including increases in blood pressure, heart rate, lacrimation, salivation, sweating, and temperature. (p2138)

Answer 81-6: A.
Midodrine acts by constriction of resistance vessels. Fludrocortisone results in reduced salt loss and fluid expansion. Desmopressin reduces nocturnal polyuria. Selegiline is commonly used for symptomatic treatment of patients with parkinsonism, but can exacerbate the postural hypotension. (p2162)

Chapter 82: Disorders of Neuromuscular Transmission

Question 82-1:
Which of the following statements is true regarding acetylcholine receptor antibodies in myasthenia gravis?

A. Patients with negative antibody titers are unlikely to respond to plasma exchange.
B. Approximately 80% of patients with ocular myasthenia have positive antibody testing.
C. Patients with thymoma without myasthenia gravis usually have detectable binding antibodies.
D. Almost all patients with thymoma and myasthenia have elevated AChR-binding antibodies.

Question 82-2:
Which of the following findings is least likely in patients with generalized myasthenia gravis?

A. Normal CMAP amplitude
B. Decremental response to repetitive stimulation more prominent in proximal muscles than distal muscles
C. Increased jitter on single-fiber EMG
D. Fibrillation potentials and positive sharp waves in affected muscles

Question 82-3:
Which of the following statements regarding thymectomy for myasthenia gravis is true?

A. Thymectomy usually produces maximum improvement 1-2 months after operation.
B. Thymectomy can only be performed once.
C. The best response to thymectomy is in young patients early in their disease.
D. The procedure of choice for most patients is endoscopic thymectomy.
E. Thymectomy is of no value in seronegative patients.

Question 82-4:
Which of the following treatments is least likely to be helpful for myasthenic crisis?

A. Corticosteroids
B. Plasma exchange
C. Azathioprine
D. IVIG

Question 82-5:
Which of the following is not a legitimate concern with administration of IVIG for myasthenia gravis?

A. Anaphylactic reaction in patients with IgA deficiency
B. Transmission of HIV
C. Transmission of hepatitis
D. Vascular headache
E. All are real concerns

Question 82-6:
Which is the treatment of choice for initial treatment of patients with pure ocular myasthenia?

A. Corticosteroids
B. Immunosuppressant drugs
C. Thymectomy
D. IVIG
E. Cholinesterase inhibitors

Answer 82-1: D.
Patients with myasthenia gravis without elevated antibodies may still respond to plasma exchange. Approximately 55% of patients with ocular myasthenia have binding antibodies, and approximately 80% of patients with generalized myasthenia have binding antibodies. (p2172)

Answer 82-2: D.
Fibrillation potentials and positive sharp waves are a hallmark of muscle fiber excitability and can be seen in myopathies and neuropathies. The other findings would be expected in generalized myasthenia. (p2173)

Answer 82-3: C.
Thymectomy usually produces maximal improvement 2-5 years after surgery. Repeat thymectomy can be performed, especially if the patient initially responded to thymectomy then relapsed. Transthoracic thymectomy is generally the preferred surgical approach since endoscopic and other limited procedures may not allow for complete exploration and resection. Thymectomy may be helpful not only for seropositive patients but also seronegative patients. (p2174)

Answer 82-4: C.
Azathioprine is the agent least likely to be helpful for a patient in myasthenic crisis, since it takes weeks to months for improvement to occur. Of the others, plasma exchange and IVIG are used most frequently, with often an increase in corticosteroid dose. (p2174)

Answer 82-5: B.
HIV transmission has not been documented in patients receiving IVIG. Hepatitis transmission has been described although is uncommon. Vascular headache may be sufficient to limit the administration of IVIG. Patients with IgA deficiency may have an anaphylactic reaction to IVIG which contains IgA; therefore, all patients scheduled to receive IVIG should have IgA levels measured before the first infusion. (p2178)

Answer 82-6: E.
Cholinesterase inhibitors are the first agents used for ocular myasthenia. Rarely corticosteroids may be used for patients with complete debilitating ptosis or complete ophthalmoplegia. If the myasthenia spreads, further treatment options have to be considered. (p2178)

Questions 82-7 through 82-9:
The following questions concern individual neuromuscular conditions which may produce weakness in children and adults. For the following questions, select the best diagnosis from the following list.

A. Myasthenia gravis
B. Ocular myasthenia
C. Lambert-Eaton myasthenic syndrome
D. Botulism
E. None of these

Question 82-7:
Antibodies to voltage-gated calcium channels.

Question 82-8:
Decremental response to repetitive nerve stimulation at 3/sec.

Question 82-9:
Response to cholinesterase inhibitors is not expected.

Question 82-10:
A 56-year-old man is sent to you for NCV and EMG. Nerve conductions are normal, although CMAP amplitude is low for some nerves. Sensory conductions are normal. EMG shows normal insertional activity, widespread fibrillation potentials and positive sharp waves, and rare fasciculations. Motor unit potentials are large-amplitude, long-duration, polyphasic in appearance. Repetitive nerve stimulation produces a pronounced decremental response at 3/sec. Single fiber EMG shows increased jitter and blocking. Which is the most likely diagnosis?

A. Myasthenia gravis with superimposed peripheral neuropathy
B. ALS
C. Slow channel syndrome
D. Cannot narrow differential diagnosis with these data

Answer 82-7: C.
LEMS is associated with antibodies against the voltage-gated calcium channels in most patients. (p2182)

Answer 82-8: A.
The decremental response to low-frequency stimulation is expected in patients with myasthenia gravis. (p2172)

Answer 82-9: D.
Cholinesterase inhibitors may be helpful in all of the listed conditions except botulism. (p2184)

Answer 82-10: B.
ALS is the most likely diagnosis with the pure motor findings, signs of active and chronic denervation. Patients with denervation often have a decremental response to repetitive stimulation and abnormal SFEMG, indicative of abnormal neuromuscular transmission, but this is because of poor neuronal health rather than a primary neuromuscular defect. (p2185)

Chapter 83: Disorders of Skeletal Muscle

Questions 83-1 through 83-4:
The following questions concern muscle biopsy and diagnosis of neuromuscular conditions. For each of the biopsy findings listed in the questions, select the most likely associated pathophysiological cause from the following list:

A. Denervation
B. Myopathy
C. Both
D. Neither

Question 83-1:
Fiber-type grouping.

Question 83-2:
Increased central nuclei.

Question 83-3:
Perifascicular atrophy.

Question 83-4:
Atrophy of an entire fascicle.

Question 83-5:
Which of the following conditions have a defect in the dystrophin gene?

1. Duchenne's muscular dystrophy
2. MDX mouse
3. Becker's muscular dystrophy
4. Myotonic dystrophy

Select: A = 1, 2, 3. B = 1, 3. C = 2, 4. D = 4 only. E = All

Question 83-6:
Which test should be used for confirmation of the diagnosis of Duchenne muscular dystrophy?

A. Muscle biopsy
B. EMG
C. Serum CK and aldolase assay
D. Dystrophin gene assay

Question 83-7:
When performing genetic counseling of a mother of a patient with DMD, which of the following statements would be correct?

A. 30% of cases may be sporadic.
B. Genetic analysis of the carrier is recommended.
C. Prenatal diagnosis is possible.
D. Carrier state may not be definitively determined in all carriers.
E. All are correct.

Question 83-8:
Which of the following disorders are autosomal dominant?

1. Duchenne's muscular dystrophy
2. Emery-Dreifuss dystrophy
3. Limb girdle muscular dystrophy type 2
4. Facioscapulohumeral dystrophy

Select: A = 1, 2, 3. B = 1, 3. C = 2, 4. D = 4 only. E = All

Question 83-9:
A child presents with progressive external ophthalmoplegia, pigmentary degeneration of the retina, and diffuse weakness. Which is the most likely diagnosis?

A. Neuronal ceroid lipofuscinosis
B. Kearns-Sayre syndrome
C. Oculopharyngeal dystrophy
D. Juvenile myasthenia gravis

Question 83-10:
Which of the following clinical features of myotonic dystrophy is least likely?

A. Cataracts
B. Somnolence
C. Cardiac involvement
D. Diabetes mellitus

Answer 83-1: A.
Denervation characteristically produces fiber-type grouping, best seen on oxidative stains. The grouping is due to reinnervation of denervated muscle fibers by adjacent motor nerves. (p2189)

Answer 83-2: C.
Increased central nuclei are typically thought of as being caused by myopathy, although some increase may be seen in neuropathic disorders, especially long-term denervation, such as juvenile SMA. (p1290)

Answer 83-3: B.
Perifascicular atrophy is typically seen in patients with dermatomyositis, a myopathy, but is not typically seen with other myopathies. (p2191)

Answer 83-4: A.
Atrophy of an entire fascicle is typically seen in chronic progressive denervation. Fiber-type grouping has progressed to the point that the patient has innervation of some entire fascicles by single motoneurons. The subsequent loss of this neuron will result in atrophy of the entire fascicle with little hope of attracting new neuronal sprouts. (p2189)

Answer 83-5: A.
A defect in the dystrophin gene may be seen in all of these conditions except myotonic dystrophy. (p2193, 2208)

Answer 83-6: D.
Examination of the dystrophin gene can establish the diagnosis in the majority of patients. Muscle biopsy, EMG, and enzyme levels are usually done, although they are not specific for DMD but are supportive of the diagnosis in the appropriate clinical situation. (p2194)

Answer 83-7: E.
All of these statements are correct. Unfortunately, genetic analysis may not be able to detect carrier status if the defect is small. Prenatal diagnosis can be accomplished by amniocentesis or chorionic villus sampling. (p2197)

Answer 83-8: D.
Only FSH is autosomal dominant, of these disorders. DMD and Emery-Dreifuss dystrophy are X-linked, and LGMD2 is autosomal recessive while LGMD1 is dominant. (p2198-2199)

Answer 83-9: B.
The combination of pigmentary degeneration of the retina plus external ophthalmoplegia suggests KSS. Juvenile myasthenia would not produce the retinal changes. Neuronal ceroid lipofuscinosis would produce the retinal changes but has more central findings than peripheral and ocular motor findings. (p2207)

Answer 83-10: D.
DM is probably not more likely in patients with myotonic dystrophy than in the general population. The remainder of the listed findings are much more prominent. (p2209)

Question 83-11:
Which of the following would be the best confirmatory test for myotonic dystrophy?

A. Myotonia on EMG
B. DNA analysis
C. Muscle biopsy
D. CK and aldolase assays

Question 83-12:
A 19-year-old man presents with attacks of weakness which affect mainly the quadriceps and biceps muscles. Examination during an episode reveals affected muscles to be tight and areflexic. Potassium was 2.3 during one episode. Which of the following would be expected to exacerbate the condition?

1. Catecholamines
2. Rest after exercise
3. Corticosteroids
4. Heavy carbohydrate meal

Select: A = 1, 2, 3. B = 1, 3. C = 2, 4. D = 4 only. E = All

Question 83-13:
A 23-year-old female presents with complaints of weakness and muscle cramps. Examination shows increased tone at rest. Walking is initially stiff but she improves with time, having near-normal gait after several minutes of walking. EMG shows myotonia. Muscle biopsy shows absent type 2B fibers and increased internal nuclei. Which is the most likely diagnosis?

A. Myotonic dystrophy
B. Myotonic fluctuans
C. Myotonic congenita
D. Paramyotonia congenita

Question 83-14:
A 13-year-old male presents with easy fatigue, poor athletic performance, and has pain and tightness of muscles with contractures on exercise. During the contractures, the muscles are tender to stretch. Which of the following are likely?

1. EMG shows repetitive muscle fiber action potentials during the contracture.
2. He exhibits the second-wind phenomenon; i.e., if he slows his activity at the onset of the contractures, he can largely overcome the symptoms.
3. Forearm ischemic exercise testing shows marked increase in lactate.
4. He has phosphorylase deficiency.

Select: A = 1, 2, 3. B = 1, 3. C = 2, 4. D = 4 only. E = All

Question 83-15:
A 50-year-old male presents with proximal weakness and is diagnosed with polymyositis without known connective tissue disorder or malignancy. There are no skin changes. Which of the following would *not* be expected?

A. Increased CK
B. Perifascicular atrophy on muscle biopsy
C. Cardiomyopathy
D. Small-amplitude polyphasic potentials on EMG

Question 83-16:
Which of the following are viable options for treatment of polymyositis?

1. Corticosteroids
2. Cyclophosphamide
3. Azathioprine
4. Methotrexate

Select: A = 1, 2, 3. B = 1, 3. C = 2, 4. D = 4 only. E = All

Answer 83-11: B.
DNA analysis is a noninvasive assay for myotonic dystrophy. Myotonia on EMG is seen in other disorders, so this is not a specific finding. Muscle biopsy findings are suggestive but more invasive than DNA analysis. CK and aldolase are frequently measured but certainly are not diagnostic. (p2210)

Answer 83-12: E.
This patient has typical hypokalemic periodic paralysis. All of these are recognized exacerbating factors in this condition. (p2213)

Answer 83-13: C.
This is a typical presentation for myotonic congenita. The biopsy findings are not invariable, and biopsy is not needed for most patients. Myotonia fluctuans is characterized by muscle stiffness which is made worse by exercise. Paramyotonia involves the face, eyes, tongue, and hands, and is exacerbated by forced contracture. In contrast, myotonia congenita involves predominantly the limbs. (p2215-2216)

Answer 83-14: C.
This is a typical presentation of muscle phosphorylase deficiency, McArdle's disease. EMG during a cramp would be electrically silent rather than show muscle fiber activity. The forearm ischemic exercise test would show absence of increase in lactate rather than an increase. (p2217)

Answer 83-15: B.
Perifascicular atrophy is a typical feature of dermatomyositis and is typically not seen in uncomplicated polymyositis. (p2226)

Answer 83-16: E.
All of these are viable options for treatment of patients with polymyositis, although corticosteroids are typically the first agents used. The information supporting efficacy of the other treatments is far less strong. (p2227)

Question 83-17:
A 55-year-old man presents with weakness which is most prominent in distal muscles of the arms and legs plus involvement of the quadriceps. There is no pain. Laboratory studies show mild elevation in CK. EMG shows myopathic features. He declines biopsy and is subsequently treated with high-dose corticosteroids, without any improvement. He finally agrees to biopsy. Which is the most likely result?

A. Polymyositis refractory to corticosteroid therapy
B. Inclusion body myositis
C. Motor neuron disease
D. Corticosteroid myopathy in the setting of resolving inflammatory myopathy

Questions 83-18 through 83-21:
The following questions pertain to biopsy of patients with congenital myopathies. For each of the questions, select the best answer from the following disorders.

A. Central core disease
B. Nemaline myopathy
C. Centronuclear (myotubular) myopathy
D. Congenital fiber-type disproportion
E. Any of these

Question 83-18:
Floppy infant.

Question 83-19:
It is typically X-linked.

Question 83-20:
Oxidative stains show unstained central zones.

Question 83-21:
Oxidative stains show many fibers with a dark central spot.

Answer 83-17: B.
This is a typical presentation for inclusion body myositis, although the findings are not specific, short of biopsy. The vast majority of patients with polymyositis improve with corticosteroids, so failure of this regimen would suggest alternatives to the diagnosis of polymyositis. (p2228)

Answer 83-18: E.
All of these conditions can present as a floppy infant. (p2230-2231)

Answer 83-19: C.
Centronuclear myopathy is typically X-linked, but there is also an autosomal dominant form. (p2232)

Answer 83-20: A.
This is a typical appearance of central core disease. (p2230)

Answer 83-21: C.
Centronuclear myopathy may resemble central core in that there is a pale center on oxidative stains, but the presence of the additional dark-staining bodies and central nuclei on H&E stain makes the diagnosis. (p2231)

Chapter 84: Neurological Problems of the Newborn

Question 84-1:
Which of the following are potential causes of neonatal seizures?

1. Hypoxic encephalopathy
2. Meningitis
3. Drug withdrawal
4. Inherited epilepsy

Select: A = 1, 2, 3. B = 1, 3. C = 2, 4. D = 4 only. E = All

Question 84-2:
Which is usually the first-line anticonvulsant for neonatal seizures?

A. Phenytoin
B. Phenobarbital
C. Carbamazepine
D. Valproate
E. None of the above

Question 84-3:
A term child from a difficult delivery with prolonged labor is admitted to the neonatal ICU with hypotonia, lethargy, hyporeflexia, and recurrent seizures. She is ventilator independent but requires tube feedings. Which of the following are likely to be true?

1. The chance of good neurologic outcome is less than 20%.
2. Increased intracranial pressure is likely to develop.
3. Autonomic failure is likely.
4. The seizures are likely to be difficult to control.

Select: A = 1, 2, 3. B = 1, 3. C = 2, 4. D = 4 only. E = All

Question 84-4:
A term neonate with hypoxic encephalopathy initially has an improvement in neurologic status but two days later becomes less responsive, loses some brainstem functions, and has an exacerbation of the seizures. Which is the most likely clinical formulation?

A. The patient has metabolic derangements complicating the hypoxic encephalopathy.
B. The patient has had an intracranial hemorrhage.
C. The patient is suffering from delayed deterioration following hypoxia.

Question 84-5:
Which of the following statements regarding prognosis of neonates with hypoxic encephalopathy are true?

1. Patients who suffer perinatal asphyxia but do not have clinical evidence of hypoxic encephalopathy are not expected to have late neurologic sequelae.
2. The severity of the encephalopathy is the most important prognostic factor.
3. APGAR scores at 10 and 20 minutes are more predictive of outcome than at 1 and 5 minutes.
4. Occurrence of seizures is not an independent prognostic sign.

Select: A = 1, 2, 3. B = 1, 3. C = 2, 4. D = 4 only. E = All

Question 84-6:
Which is the most common pathogen in patients with neonatal meningitis?

A. *Escherichia coli*
B. *Streptococcus pneumoniae*
C. *Haemophilus influenzae*
D. *Staphylococcus aureus*
E. None of these

Answer 84-1: E.
All of these are potential causes of epilepsy in the newborn period. All of these are expected except inherited epilepsy. However, there is a benign familial neonatal epilepsy which is due to a defect on chromosome 20. (p2239)

Answer 84-2: B.
Phenobarbital is the drug of choice for most patients with neonatal seizures. Anticonvulsant therapy should not be a substitute for treatment of the underlying disorder, e.g., hypocalcemia or hypoglycemia. (p2239)

Answer 84-3: D.
The first three statements are likely to be the case with severe hypoxic encephalopathy, whereas the patient as presented suffers from moderate encephalopathy. The chance of good outcome exceeds 50%. (p2241)

Answer 84-4: C.
Delayed deterioration following hypoxia can develop in neonates just as it can develop in adults. In neonates, the deterioration may occur between 1 and 3 days following delivery. The delayed deterioration is thought to be related to reperfusion injury and free radical generation. Metabolic disturbances may aggravate hypoxic encephalopathy but they do not need to be implicated to explain the deterioration. Post-anoxic hemorrhage is more a problem of premature infants than term infants. (p2240)

Answer 84-5: A.
The occurrence of seizures is an independent prognostic sign in neonates with hypoxic encephalopathy. The other statements are true. (p2344)

Answer 84-6: A.
Escherichia coli is the most common pathogen in patients with neonatal meningitis.

Question 84-7:
Which of the following are potential outcomes of congenital cytomegalovirus infection?

1. Microcephaly
2. Hepatosplenomegaly
3. Blindness
4. Normal child

Select: A = 1, 2, 3. B = 1, 3. C = 2, 4. D = 4 only. E = All

Question 84-8:
Subarachnoid hemorrhage may develop as a complication of a difficult delivery. Which of the following statements are true regarding primary subarachnoid hemorrhage in the newborn?

1. Prognosis is good, with 90% being normal.
2. The SAH is usually venous blood.
3. Seizures are common.
4. Hydrocephalus is common.

Select: A = 1, 2, 3. B = 1, 3. C = 2, 4. D = 4 only. E = All

Question 84-9:
A term infant of a difficult delivery presents with decreased use of the right arm. The hand appears to work, although there is no visible contraction of proximal arm muscles and the biceps reflex is absent on that side. The patient also has tachypnea and mild hypoxia. Which is the most likely clinical formulation?

A. The patient has damage to the upper plexus from brachial plexus stretch. The respiratory symptoms are likely from damage to the innervation of the diaphragm.
B. The patient has damage to the lower plexus resulting in arm weakness. The respiratory compromise is probably another sequela of the difficult delivery and not directly related to the arm symptoms.
C. The child has injury to the high cervical spine with incomplete segmental damage and myelopathy.

Question 84-10:
Many medications may have a teratogenic effect on the fetus. Which of the following statements regarding drug effects on the fetus is not true?

A. Early gestation exposure to valproate carries a 5% risk of neural tube defects.
B. Folate supplementation is only helpful if given prior to or very early in pregnancy.
C. Microcephaly occurs in 40% of neonates of mothers addicted to heroin.
D. Maternal ethanol abuse causes children who are large for gestational age.

Answer 84-7: E.
All of these are potential results of congenital CMV infection. Most are asymptomatic at birth. Other findings may include jaundice, petechiae, periventricular calcifications, and chorioretinitis. (p2249)

Answer 84-8: A.
SAH in the newborn does not have the same clinical implications as in adults. Hydrocephalus may occur but is rare. The other statements are true. (p2251)

Answer 84-9: A.
This is the presentation of a patient with an upper plexus injury. In neonates, the C3 through C5 roots may be damaged sufficiently that the diaphragm is denervated on that side. The lack of leg findings would argue against myelopathy from cervical spine injury. The pattern of weakness does not suggest a lower plexus injury. (p2252)

Answer 84-10: D.
Maternal ethanol addiction typically causes growth retardation along with intellectual deficits. The other statements are correct. (p2253)

Chapter 85: Neurological Problems of Pregnancy

Question 85-1:
Which of the following statements are true regarding headache in pregnancy?

1. Most patients with migraine show worsening during pregnancy.
2. Meperidine increases the risk of fetal malformations.
3. Migraines usually are worst during the second and third trimester.
4. Ergotamine is contraindicated in pregnancy.

Select: A = 1, 2, 3. B = 1, 3. C = 2, 4. D = 4 only. E = All

Question 85-2:
Which of the following features characterize the relationship between pregnancy and myotonic dystrophy?

1. Fertility is reduced.
2. Weakness is worse during the latter half of pregnancy.
3. Delivery may be impaired by reduced fetal contractions.
4. One half of the children of mothers with myotonic dystrophy inherit the disorder.

Select: A = 1, 2, 3. B = 1, 3. C = 2, 4. D = 4 only. E = All

Question 85-3:
Which of the following statements regarding Bell's palsy is not true?

A. Facial nerve palsy is 3 to 4 times more likely during pregnancy.
B. Varicella zoster virus is the causative agent in most cases of Bell's palsy.
C. Corticosteroids improve the prognosis in non-pregnant adults.
D. Acyclovir improves the prognosis in non-pregnant adults.

Question 85-4:
A 34-year-old female with pseudotumor cerebri develops increasing headache during pregnancy. Examination shows optic disc edema but no visual loss. Which of the following clinical approaches is most appropriate?

A. Corticosteroids are administered to reduce the possibility of visual loss.
B. Optic sheath fenestration should be performed as early as possible during pregnancy.
C. Headaches should be treated with analgesics and lumbar puncture done serially if needed.

Question 85-5:
Which of the following statements regarding AEDs and pregnancy is true?

A. The rate of birth defects is increased in children of epileptic mothers, independently of anti-epileptic drugs.
B. Phenytoin produces no significant increase in risk of major congenital anomalies.
C. The fetal hydantoin syndrome does not develop with AEDs other than phenytoin.
D. Carbamazepine produces no significant increase in risk of major congenital anomalies.

Answer 85-1: D.
Ergotamine and related drugs are associated with a high rate of fetal malformations and are contraindicated during pregnancy. Meperidine is not known to increase the risk of fetal malformations. About 80% of patients with migraine have improvement during pregnancy, with substantial improvement during the second and third trimesters. (p2258)

Answer 85-2: E.
All of the statements are true. Fertility is decreased, presumable due to primary ovarian failure. (p2259)

Answer 85-3: B.
HSV-1 is the most common agent implicated in Bell's palsy with VZV a distant second. (p2259)

Answer 85-4: C.
Headache should be treated with analgesics, and serial lumbar punctures can be done. Corticosteroids and optic nerve fenestration are reserved for visual loss. (p2262)

Answer 85-5: A.
Epilepsy is an independent risk factor for birth defects. (p2263)

Chapter 86: Geriatric Neurology

Question 86-1:
Which of the following are functional changes with normal aging?

1. Decreased vibratory sensation
2. Reduction in digit span
3. Decreased olfaction
4. Decreased visual acuity

Select: A = 1, 2, 3. B = 1, 3. C = 2, 4. D = 4 only. E = All

Question 86-2:
An 80-year-old man is evaluated for memory loss. He is found on neuropsychological testing to have depression with impaired concentration but no organic dementia. MRI shows moderate diffuse atrophy with mild enlargement of the ventricular system. What would be the most likely clinical formulation?

A. The atrophy indicates a degenerative dementia and the depression is an affective component of the disease.
B. The patient has memory loss due to depression and the atrophy is not indicative of another neurologic condition.
C. The patient is normal for age in imaging and neuropsychological testing.

Question 86-3:
Which is the most common cause of dementia in the elderly?

A. Alzheimer's disease
B. Vascular dementia
C. Frontotemporal dementia
D. Medications

Question 86-4:
Which of the following statements is not true regarding syncope in the elderly?

A. About 40% of patients do not have a specific diagnosis after evaluation.
B. Rate of recurrent syncope is higher for elderly than middle-aged people.
C. Subclavian steal is a common cause of non-cardiac syncope.
D. Ventricular tachycardia is the most common cause of cardiac syncope in the elderly.

Question 86-5:
Which of the following statements characterizes changes in sleep patterns with advancing age?

A. Altered sleep patterns contributes to a higher frequency of stroke and myocardial infarction.
B. Sleep disturbance is a common cause of patients being admitted to nursing homes.
C. Sleep in the elderly contains more stage I and less stages III and IV than in younger patients.
D. Older patients spend more time in bed than younger adult patients.
E. All are true.

Answer 86-1: E.
All of these are normal changes in neurologic function with aging. (p2276-7)

Answer 86-2: B.
Patients with Alzheimer's disease and other degenerative dementias have cerebral atrophy, but there is considerable overlap in atrophy with normal aging. The diagnosis of degenerative dementia would have been made by the neuropsychological testing rather than the imaging. (p2277)

Answer 86-3: A.
AD is by far the most common cause of dementia in elderly patients. Medications and vascular dementia are two other very important causes. (p2280)

Answer 86-4: C.
Subclavian steal is only rarely a cause of syncope in the elderly, although it is a potential cause. Orthostatic hypotension, situational syncope, TIA, and medications are much more important causes. (p2286)

Answer 86-5: E.
All of these statements are true. While older patients spend more time in bed, they spend less time asleep. (p2287)

From THE Neurology publisher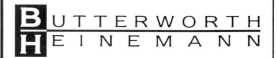

The authoritative standard for the diagnosis and management of neurological disorders.

Neurology in Clinical Practice, Third Edition

Walter G. Bradley, Robert B. Daroff, Gerald M. Fenichel, C. David Marsden

0-7506-9973-6, Hardcover, 2000, 2296 pp., $450.00

www.NICP.com

NICP is now on-line providing you with the most comprehensive neurology resource available. Receive a one-year subscription, from the time of registration, to the on-line version with the purchase of the book.

The companion handbook - Perfect for quick reference

Pocket Companion to Neurology in Clinical Practice Third Edition

0-7506-7264-1, Paperback, 2000, 768 pp., $45.00

The ideal book for exam preparation!

Review Manual for Neurology in Clinical Practice Third Edition

Karl E. Misulis, Walter G. Bradley, Robert B. Daroff, Gerald M. Fenichel

0-7506-7192-0, Paperback, March 2000, 368 pp., $45.00

Five Ways to Order!
- Order on-line at www.bh.com
- Call us at: 1-800-366-2665 or 781-904-2500
- Fax your order to: 1-800-446-6520 or 781-933-6333
- E-Mail your order to: orders@bhusa.com
- Mail your order to: Butterworth-Heinemann, Fulfillment Center, 225 Wildwood Avenue, Woburn, MA 01801

227-1832